# LATINO FAMILIES IN THERAPY

# THE GUILFORD FAMILY THERAPY SERIES
## Michael P. Nichols, Series Editor

## Recent Volumes

# LATINO FAMILIES IN THERAPY
## A Guide to Multicultural Practice

CELIA JAES FALICOV, PhD

THE GUILFORD PRESS
New York    London

*For all those who had the courage to weave new lives and embroider them with the dignity of old meanings*

© 1998 The Guilford Press
A Division of Guilford Publications, Inc.
72 Spring Street, New York, NY 10012
www.guilford.com

Printed in the United States of America

This book is printed on acid-free paper.

Last digit is print number:  9  8  7  6  5  4

**Library of Congress Cataloging-in-Publication Data**

Falicov, Celia Jaes.
    Latino families in therapy  :  a guide to multicultural practice  /
Celia Jaes Falicov.
        p.    cm. — (The Guilford family therapy series)
    Includes bibliographical references and index.
    ISBN 1-57230-364-6 (hc.) ISBN 1-57230-593-2 (pbk.)
    1. Hispanic Americans—Mental health.   2.  Family psychotherapy—
United States.  3. Minorities—United States—Family relationships.
4.  Emigration and immigration—Psychological aspects.      I.  Title.
II. Series.
RC451.5.H57F35   1998
616.89′0089′68073—dc21                                              98-2636
                                                                              CIP

# Preface

## A CASE OF CULTURAL MISUNDERSTANDING

My original interest in the crossroads between culture and psychotherapy arose from an emotional personal experience—an upsetting cross-cultural encounter I witnessed in the early 1970s. Fresh out of graduate school and interning at the Neuropsychiatric Institute in Chicago, I was asked to help out as an interpreter/translator between the staff of the University of Illinois Hospital Pediatric Cardiology Unit and a Puerto Rican great aunt with a 7-year-old grand nephew, Ricki. This is what happened:

Inside the hospital room lay a thin child who, failing to recover from open-heart surgery, was very weak, pale, and lethargic. His great aunt, a small woman in her late sixties, dressed in unadorned style—a plain, black cotton house dress and flat cotton shoes—sat beside him, clutching her rosary and fervently praying. The nurses and doctors had grown to dislike her. They secretly blamed her for slowing down the child's recovery. In their view, she was overanxious, overprotective, and even spoiled Ricki when she should have vigorously encouraged him to do more, be more self-sufficient, and eat the healthy hospital food instead of the "greasy stuff" she pushed on him. The consulting psychiatrist had a psychological explanation for the great aunt's behavior. He noticed, and had it confirmed by the nurses, that the child's mother was seldom seen at the hospital. He presumed then that the mother had abandoned her child to the care of the great aunt, who naturally would be resentful and bitter about losing her freedom and assuming such dire responsibility. He proceeded to write in the hospital chart that the great aunt's overprotectiveness was probably a "reaction formation" against her "unconscious anger and resentment" toward the child. The boy's pervasive respiratory distress after surgery was diagnosed as psychologically induced, and it remained so until he died.

In the aftermath, it seemed clear that Ricki's true condition—and especially the hospital staff's understanding of it—had fallen prey to cultural misunderstandings. Tension and alienation between the family and staff led to attributions that frankly jeopardized the boy's treatment, and an undercurrent of quietly tacit, institutional discrimination flowed against the dark-skinned, foreign family.

What was missing here? What had this group of professional caregivers failed to understand? I brooded over Ricki's case and the clear role culture played in it. I knew, for example, that reliance on a grandmother or a great aunt for caretaking when mother is absent is a common survival mechanism of female-headed, poor families. In the Latino culture, three-generational help and support throughout life is expected and valued. In this particular case, Ricki's mother had herself been raised by an aunt while her own single mother worked. As in so many Latino families, older people play enormous roles in raising children—a practice that ensures positions of authority and a sense of purpose.

I thought of Ricki's great aunt hovering over the child's bedside, a reminder that to pamper and "overprotect" children, especially sick children, is a cultural feature of many Latinos. In Ricki's case, a cultural heritage of strong kinship bonds, shared parenting, and three-generational involvement had been misinterpreted in favor of other, more mainstream ideals of leisure, autonomy, and freedom from parenting in old age.

As in most cases of cultural misunderstanding, one could think compassionately about both sides, the family and the hospital staff. A child was dying; naturally everyone was upset. Each side relied on its own cultural coping mechanisms. The nurses and doctors had been trained to trust the American or European medical values of mastery over nature and self-sufficiency as better avenues for recovery than feeding, cuddling, and praying. These were the great aunt's ways of comforting and facing destiny with the acceptance and resignation of her culture and her religion. The psychiatrist applied his interpretations with good intentions, but he had no cultural, class, or gender perspective on the use of his psychoanalytic meanings.

Social disadvantages also played a part. Ricki's family had been rendered essentially powerless to complain or confront hospital staff by virtue of their different ethnicity, class, language, and skin color. The staff, in turn, could more easily find a way out of their sense of failure by projecting their own feelings of helplessness and defeat on the great aunt, a mechanism called "blaming the victim."

To be fair, cultural misunderstanding didn't kill this child, but much grief could have been spared. Better support and even admiration for the tireless nurturing the great aunt provided the dying child could have replaced distancing and blaming. Collaboration and mutual respect might have eased at least some aspects of a very bad situation.

I left that heart-wrenching setting with a driving ambition to do something to increase cultural sensitivity in the helping professions. At first glance, I have very little in common with an elderly Puerto Rican woman caring for a sick child. But I share collective identities and cultural borderlands with both groups in that hospital encounter. A very personal interest and empathy for the predicament of the "culturally different" stems from my own history and cultural circumstances.

## A PERSONAL NARRATIVE

Since names can be windows to the culture of people, let me start with an analysis of my full name, Celia Haydée Jaes de Falicov. If you are familiar with Latin American populations, the name might clue you to the possibility that you are dealing with a Latin American Jew, or at least a Latin American married to a Russian Jew. You might have doubts about the origin of my maiden name, Jaes, which was probably shortened and distorted by immigration authorities when my father's family arrived in Argentina from Lithuania, fleeing from ethnic and religious persecution and economic hardship. My mother's family, Zisman, escaped the anti-Semitism of Rumania, after her grandfather was arbitrarily and publicly shot to death by the Cossacks.

From a young age, I was aware that history and sociopolitical events shape a family's destiny. Growing up in a country where families' lives are profoundly altered by political ideologies and economic instability, I knew that to understand family distress, one must always include events that occur outside the boundaries, control, and wishes of the family.

My parents met in Argentina. I was their firstborn and the first Argentine national on both sides of two very large families, fragmented in time and space by migration. The oldest child of immigrants, and later an immigrant myself, I shared perspectives that connected me to the encounter of languages and cultures at Ricki's hospital bed. First, I know something about the protection of closely knit extended families in difficult environments.

My uncles, aunts, and cousins all lived within half a block of my house. Most important, there was my maternal grandmother—she cooked special dishes for me, and I could always seek her love to fill yearnings left by my nuclear family. The daily life of the neighborhood reproduced the protectiveness of the extended family in many ways. Nurturance and control could come from the butcher, baker, or shoemaker, all of whom knew who I was then and still recognize me and my siblings 40 years later. Second, I know something about the ravages of internal cultural wars, such as the one that was waged both within me and inside my family throughout my developing years. I refused to speak Yiddish, but I loved the Spanish language and Argentinian culture, from the patriotic songs to the milk sweets bought at the kiosks in the streets. It was my language, my culture.

Like other young people of my generation, I immersed myself in the hard facts of life in Argentina. Incensed by terrible social and political injustices, I volunteered in a Buenos Aires slum called, with a mixture of sarcasm and romanticism, *Villa Miseria* (Misery Village). There I was deeply shaken by seeing very poor, very young women who used knitting needles to provoke abortions as a desperate way out of an impossible predicament. When their attempts to abort were unsuccessful, their newborns were often left under the care of an older relative, just as Ricki's young Puerto Rican mother had been forced to do.

My maternal grandfather worried about my lack of allegiance to Judaism and often questioned me about where my loyalties would be in the case of a war between Argentina and Israel. He warned me about the dangers of getting involved with gentiles, particularly young men. He believed they would ultimately reject me because of my ethnicity. He was sharp enough, I think, to realize that I was fascinated by Catholicism (and by Catholic young men). Both the religion (and the men) were prohibited within my family and in the public school, which segregated Jewish children from the compulsory classes in Catholicism. The exclusion and segregation, of course, made everything Roman Catholic more alluring, and Judaism more shameful, less valued.

My rebellion consisted of sneaking in the back of churches to hear Catholic mass. In the churches of Argentina, and later in Mexico, I saw many women clutching rosaries—reminiscent, today, of Ricki's great aunt—softly praying for their sick friends and relatives. I learned about Catholicism and came to feel that the resignation and magic in the wishes of its prayers resembled the prayers I heard from my Orthodox Jewish grandparents. Only later did I understand the emotional value of prayer as the wish for a turn of fate when life's suffering is pervasive and the possibility of control bleak.

Not surprisingly, my first boyfriend came from a devout Catholic family and was the proud owner of not only two Castilian last names, but three, and lived in a most distinguished upper-class neighborhood. He didn't suspect that I was Jewish, and I wasn't eager to reveal it (although I never openly lied about it). When I finally did disclose my Jewish heritage, a new appreciation for my grandfather's predictions flourished in me. My "Latin lover" didn't reject me outright; he claimed to like me, even "love" me very much, but he suddenly remembered that his mother had designs for him to marry a particular somebody of the same social class, religion, and of course with a distinguished set of last names. He gallantly offered to continue to see me on the side. Had I accepted, I may have become his first *casa chica* (little house), a woman and children existing secretly as a private family while the legally married wife and children represent the public nuclear family and its extended context in the *casa grande* (large house).

The sting of that experience taught me about the protection of sticking to my people in certain areas, but my strong connection with the Spanish language and culture continued. Like many children of immigrants, I absorbed the new culture many hours of the day and brought it home, tango and all, while living partially in the old culture of my family.

Only much later did I realize that shame was a driving force behind my powerful attraction to Catholicism. Shame at living in a Jewish ghetto in an uneducated, working-class family that lived in cramped, small quarters with adults who had heavy accents and practiced a marginalized religion. I felt my parents' shame and my own shame at trying to pass for non-Jewish, internal shame that silenced me in many settings where injustices were lurking and should have been confronted. My own sensitivity to shame allows me to resonate with the powerlessness and helplessness engendered in marginalized, discriminated minorities faced with the mainstream institutions.

Marriage propelled me into a different cultural world. My husband's parents were an Argentinian-born, middle-class, Russian, Jewish, professional couple. They taught me how families function when they value reason over emotion, and education and assimilation over tradition and religion. These excursions into the educated middle-class opened an avenue to understand the white, European values that I would find embedded in so many professions and institutions—the hospital setting and the training of the psychiatrist who diagnosed Ricki's family are later examples.

My own immigration to the United States took place in 1961. I came newly married with my husband who was a physician in residency training. So here we were, at the start of an interclass marriage, getting first-hand experience on being first-generation immigrants by learning to speak a new language and grappling with new ways of life. Later we had to learn to raise children born in a new land, who spoke a different native language and espoused some similar and other quite different values. My children are now becoming adolescents and young adults in the United States in an ideological climate that is beginning to acknowledge diversity and a societal context that encourages self-definition. Each one of them is developing selections about which Latin, with a dash of Jewish, parts of her parents' background to incorporate.

I never abandoned my intense and ambivalent love affair with the Argentinian culture and language, and was probably too old or too "Latin-looking" and sounding to assimilate fully in the United States, in spite of considerable acculturation. When my husband died 9 years ago, I gradually became aware that part of the excruciating pain wasn't only that I had lost him as a person, but that with his death I had also lost my language, my country, and my culture more than ever before. He was love and family, but he was also continuity and culture. He and I had managed over the years to co-create meanings that reflected shared history and ideology, preserved an Argentinian brand of Spanish with some Anglicized expressions, and maintained old social gestures and customs while acquiring new ones. Those continuities must have mitigated some of the losses of the uprooting and incorporated the myriad experiences of a shared migration.

If I had never reflected before on the alteration of the family life-cycle transitions suffered by immigrants, this unexpected loss made it patently clear that one person can embody and signify a country and a culture for another person. I had to face anew the issue of belongingness, the agony of whether I should return to my roots or stay close to the new life created in my adoptive country, only to conclude, at least for now, that where I belong is here *and* there, or in between, perennially sitting *con el culo entre dos sillas,* (with my ass between two chairs) (Ciola, 1996). Sitting between two mostly comfortable close chairs, of course, is a much more appealing metaphor than seeing my heart broken down the middle, one large piece in the warmth of the south, the other in the cold of the north.

Over many years a tapestry of personal and professional experiences, including those with so many Latino clients, has informed and invigorated my quest toward cultural sensitivity in family therapy. This book is the culmination of my effort to bridge the gap between the contexts and cultures of our clients and ourselves—a map for cultural inclusion in psychotherapy.

## ACKNOWLEDGMENTS

I feel deeply grateful to the many families, past and present, who continue to teach me about Latinos. Their trust and will to better their lives provided the inspiration for this book.

Special thanks go to Leita McIntosh-Koontz, whose outstanding editorial capacities and sensitivity toward the subject matter resulted in a much better finished product. Jocelyn M. Steer's skillful reading of the manuscript was also very helpful. My thanks also go to Ramona Romero, Valerie Loewe, and Lisa Reynaga for patiently typing and retyping various drafts and references.

My friends and colleagues, Lisa Hirschman and Antonia Meltzoff, have the warmth and generosity of spirit that I can always count on for support, intellectual stimulation, and loving concern. I am indebted to them for our early discussion of ideas and joint reading of the manuscript.

And to my dear old friend and fellow traveler, Froma Walsh, whose clarity of mind always helps me zero in on what matters, and whose caring, gentle persuasion gives me buoyancy and self-confidence. I also like to acknowledge Monica McGoldrick's generosity in being the first person who gave me the chance to publish on matters of culture, almost two decades ago.

My appreciation and love go to my three daughters, Tamara, Yael, and Anna, wonderful young women who make everything in my life worthwhile.

# Contents

# PART I

---

# Overview

---

Consistent with my belief that cultural contexts are far more varied and complex than belonging to an ethnic group, *Latino Families in Therapy* proposes a mosaic of cultural influences and steers away from essentialistic ethnic descriptions. The observations and ideas that comprise this mosaic are akin to cultural constructs themselves—they are informed by particular contexts. In Chapter 1 I introduce the "environments" (and their subsequent meanings) that contextualize this book. I touch briefly on the dilemma faced by psychotherapists in today's multicultural world—what is the therapist's role when "culture" is added to the therapeutic equation? Is there a way to apply a cultural-generalist approach that sensitively reveals both the idiosyncratic and collective cultural meanings in the lives of our clients? "MECA: A Meeting Place for Culture and Therapy" is presented in Chapter 2 and describes in detail such a generalist frame for approaching culture in therapy. It reflects issues of cultural diversity and social justice as well as the cultural borderlands, subjectivities, and complex, unique ecologies of each client and family. Throughout the book this way of thinking about culture is applied to a study of Latino families in therapy.

My focus on Latino families begins in Part II with an overview that contextualizes the migration background and the presence of the three predominate Latino groups in the United States: Mexicans, Puerto Ricans, and Cubans (Chapter 3). Chapters 4 and 5 address the tremendous impact of the migration experience on the lives of Latino families. These discussions encompass the remarkable strengths and resiliencies of immigrants, the particular dilemmas and challenges that arise over time, and a number of therapeutic approaches that help reveal and create migration narratives in therapy.

In Part III, I examine some of the most significant ecological contexts inhabited by Latino families. Chapter 6 addresses the experience of racism and discrimination, and its effect on cultural adaptation, socioeconomic status and social ills, family life, and contact with professionals. Chapter 7 highlights the domains of school and work, and looks to traditional beliefs, shifting ideas, and new programs—all of which alter how Latino families encounter the classroom and the job. Chapter 8 explores the interior ecology of many individuals and families. Folk beliefs about health and illness, formal religion, and complex blends of both may be closely tied to mental health issues and treatment. Similarly, styles of coping and ideas about control change the way clients and therapists view distress.

In Part IV, the Latino family in its myriad and ever-changing forms is the focal point. Chapter 9 looks at some of the concepts of family togetherness that underlie life for many Latinos. Relationships, roles, and hierarchies that may be commonplace are examined for both their strengths and vulnerabilities. Chapter 10 narrows the discussion to the world of men and women. Here the shifting meanings of gender mystiques are seen to touch the lives of most every Latino couple. Intergenerational and nuclear family ideals share the stage. Gender expectations and traditions of patriarchy are explored. Finally, I suggest ways of approaching these issues in the therapeutic encounter.

Part V presents a panoramic view of the Latino family life cycle. Beginning in Chapter 11 with an examination of childhood and adolescence and ending in Chapter 12 with adulthood across the lifespan, these discussions present predominate beliefs and practices, as well as changing realities, that meet Latinos from birth to old age.

In the conclusion I revisit notions about multiculturalism in mental health, and make both hopeful and problematic interpretations of the state of the art. I describe options that range from a universalist position, in which culture is considered tangential to therapy, to espousing an ethnic-specific way of doing therapy. I also suggest that it may be good to live with these and other dichotomous positions and take a "both/and" view, rather than asking therapists to choose one extreme position over another or end up with formulas to treat the "culturally different." Implications of these ideas, and of applying MECA to a broad array of cultures, completes this discussion.

Throughout the book I share many case studies and illustrations. Some of these may seem to reinforce stereotypes about "Latino culture." But others are atypical and thus raise questions about our assumptions about Latinos. Others may demonstrate striking similarities with clients and families of quite different backgrounds. This is how it should be. When it comes to the individual experience, there is no such a thing as a Latino culture, rather there are only approximations of patterns that appear in some cases and not in others.

By offering my own experiences as a therapist and supervisor, I attempt to underline the need to acknowledge the subjectivity of the therapist and to adopt a relational understanding of all cultural descriptions. This understanding is relational insofar as the therapist brings her own cultural "location" from clinical theories and practice models and from personal preferences.

Sometimes the cultural and personal stories of my client families stand alone, with my reflections and constructions. At other times the illustrations are interwoven with the evocative stories of characters of Latino fiction and poetry, which may be instructive and enlightening for therapists. Psychotherapy, like literature, is about individuals and their infinite complexity. And like literature, psychotherapy exists within a cultural context and a historical time.

I occasionally lace client stories with my own stories of migration and culture change. I am a Latino immigrant myself. I came from Argentina to the United States in the early 1960s and attended graduate school in Chicago. I learned new versions of the Spanish language and of Indo-Hispanic culture while working at the Institute for Juvenile Research on the west side of Chicago. For more than 10 years I worked there with Latino immigrant children, adolescents, and their families, many of them Mexicans and Puerto Ricans. Since 1980 I have worked in San Diego, California, in institutional settings where Latino immigrants seek help. I also have a private practice that serves a population of middle- and working-class Latino families, couples, and individuals. Some of the stories from these experiences are interspersed throughout this book in the form of brief vignettes, anecdotes, and commentaries. When I offer conceptualizations that are based on social science research about Latinos, I briefly provide the context and the information so that the reader can pursue it further to expand theory, clinical practice, and research. My opinions and biases are made explicit throughout, but they are also revealed in my selections, omissions, and oversights. At no time do I mean to imply that my views constitute the "truth" about Latinos in therapy. However imperfectly, I have tried to honor the ethics of inclusion that informs multiculturalism by staying away from either divisive separatism or from the sentimentalism of well meaning cultural outsiders. I am hopeful that MECA will help therapists avoid these pitfalls, and foster a meaningful and effective approach to cultural sensitivity.

# 1

## Introduction

### THE CURRENT DILEMMA

As a nation of immigrants, the United States has always faced the challenge of understanding and integrating racial and ethnic diversity. This challenge has never been greater than now. Increasingly, psychotherapists will provide mental health care to a wide range of clients of diverse ethnicities, races, socioeconomic levels, nationalities, and religions.

In attempting to provide culturally attuned psychotherapy, professionals face the dilemma of acquiring sufficient cultural literacy and competence to understand and to respect the cultural beliefs of the client, and yet not fall prey to stereotypical evaluations that rob clients of their individual histories and choices. An additional obstacle is that mental health providers are necessarily limited in the treatments they offer by the very concepts and methods they use—their training is imbued with the constructions and ideologies of mainstream American culture.

Psychotherapists are sometimes even unsure about what cultural heritage and present social/political context have to do with human suffering and mental health care. While they may acknowledge that clients are deeply connected to their cultural roots in ways that bolster their resources, clinicians also observe that cultural ideals may create conflicts and contradictions for individuals and families. Deciding how, when, and even why to introduce cultural and sociopolitical contexts in therapy is a difficult but necessary task. The following sections provide an introduction to the terms, ideas, and processes involved in that task.

## CULTURAL SENSITIVITY VERSUS CULTURAL ENCAPSULATION

Good therapists have always explored individual complexity with various degrees of sensitivity to cultural and social factors in their clients' lives. In fact, much of traditional social work training was about the inclusion of sociocultural factors. I don't believe, however, that there is a Latino therapy or a Latino way of doing therapy or that only Latinos can adequately treat Latinos. And it almost goes without saying that cultural sensitivity doesn't in itself ensure good clinical work. The therapist's theory and personal experience are also part of a particular cultural and historical context, as we shall see.

 Regardless of the therapist's cultural identity, some core principles of effective client care—the value of empathic listening and establishing a solid therapeutic alliance—are universally helpful. Therapists' given or acquired sensitivity to culturally diverse values and the effects of social stresses renders those general principles more effective in the evaluation and treatment of specific groups.

"Cultural encapsulation," a term coined by C. Gilbert Wrenn (1962), describes the narrow world view that psychotherapists may have when they allow culturally biased perceptions of reality to dominate. A culturally encapsulated therapist, unable to see others through a different cultural lens, may regard as pathological what is normal for the minority cultural group, as did the psychiatrist in Ricki's case. Conversely, a therapist who is not culturally encapsulated is aware of cultural differences, and accepts these when working with someone who comes from a different cultural background. Experienced, skillful clinicians of all cultures can become culturally attuned, which is the opposite of being culturally encapsulated.

## ECOLOGICAL NICHES AND CULTURAL BORDERLANDS

My own story, and the interaction between Ricki's family and the hospital staff (see Preface), illustrates that each of us participates in diverse and multiple contexts. These contexts span languages, places, preferences, and subjective experience. They create "cultural borderlands" (Rosaldo, 1989): overlapping zones of difference and similarity within and between cultures. Such points of contact and divergence can be both limiting and enriching. An awareness of these contexts can increase our capacity to recognize and respect the beliefs and practices of others, while building our tolerance for divergence and ambiguity.

Throughout this book, a partial solution is offered to the dilemma of how to take difference into account without reifying and stereotyping culture. In a pluralistic society like the United States, persons are multicultural rather than belonging to a single ethnic group that can be summarized easily by a single label (see, for example, Comas-Díaz, 1994).

Each person has a culture comprised of a number of collective identities—groups of belonging, participation, and identification that make up his or her "ecological niche." This ecological niche shares "cultural borderlands" or zones of overlap with others by virtue of race, ethnicity, religion, occupation, or social class. A middle-class Chinese experimental psychologist who is an agnostic democrat may have more in common with a similarly politically and religiously minded Jewish research psychologist than with a devout Catholic Chinese shopkeeper, because the first two share a greater number of cultural borderlands with each other. Rather than restricting ourselves to one cultural identity, we can talk about multicultural identities.

In a pluralistic society, we learn about cultural differences in myriad ways. As outsiders from distinct cultural groups, we rely on books, movies, radio, television, or first-hand contact at work, in the neighborhood, or at school. It is virtually impossible for Latinos not to know something about African Americans or for Catholics not to know something about Christians. Cultural exposure increases our capacity for social adaptation: a form of "adaptive multiculturalism." Mary Catherine Bateson, in her illuminating book *Peripheral Visions* (1994), makes a similar differentiation when she talks about an "identity multiculturalism," which supports individuals in their own ethnic or social identities, and an "adaptive multiculturalism," which increases everyone's capacity to adapt by offering exposure to a variety of other traditions.

## THE OBSERVER AND THE OBSERVED
## IN THE CULTURAL EQUATION

The basic assumption of this book is that the observer, in this case the therapist, is part of the cultural equation. The therapy encounter is really an encounter between the therapist's and the family's cultural and personal constructions about family life. The therapist as observer also becomes part of the ecology. He is no longer the privileged outsider looking in, perceiving patterns not apparent to those within the system. Edward M. Bruner's position, borrowed partially from Barthes (1974) and Foucault (1973), in which the sharp distinction between subject and object is dissolved, fits here because both therapist and client are seen "as caught in the same web, influenced by the same historical forces, and shaped by the dominant narrative structures of our times" (E. M. Bruner, 1986).

Rather than presupposing objectivism or the notion that reality can be grasped through direct knowledge and experience, the approach offered

in this book is based on a presupposition of "perspectivism" (Von Bertalanffy, 1968), that is, that one's views of reality depend on one's perspective,
which even organizes the observations themselves. A therapist's views about
families and family therapy stem from his or her ecological niche, which includes preferred brand of theory and professional subculture. These views,
in turn, restrict that which can be observed and that which can be named
(Nichols & Schwartz, 1995). The therapist's perspective is further affected
and organized by personal values, views, and preferences.

Perspectivism requires that we adopt a relational understanding of all
descriptions when working with culturally diverse clients. Edward Sampson
(1993) quotes the anthropologist C. Lutz as saying that when we describe
the child-rearing practices of another culture as being indulgent, we do so
by building a comparison with an implicit standard, hidden from our view
and provided by our own dominant culture. It is important to keep in mind
that "indulgence" isn't an essential or intrinsic quality possessed by the individuals of that culture. Rather, indulgence emerges as a result of comparison that includes the vantage point of the observer.[1]

## A GENERALIST FRAMEWORK FOR CULTURE: MECA

This volume is a first attempt to provide a "cultural generalist" framework
in which both client and therapist perspectives, including their cultural
similarities and differences, can be drawn out and used to enhance therapeutic work. In this text the framework is presented and then applied to
therapeutic encounters with Latino families.

The multidimensional ecosystemic comparative approach (MECA)
identifies four dimensions—migration, ecological context, family organization, and family life cycle—that can be used to describe and compare similarities and differences among cultural groups. It also enables the therapist
to integrate dimensions of culture with aspects of family interaction and
the therapeutic encounter itself. Through this approach, a therapist considers the multiple cultural contexts (race, social class, religion, occupation, language) in which the family and the therapist are embedded.

By examining these contexts, similarities and differences between family and therapist are identified and clarified. For example, family and therapist may have different ethnicities and religions but share educational level
and social class status. They may have both faced prejudice because of race
or political ideology, or they may belong to a cohort that witnessed the
same historical events or ideological shifts. In other words, a broader definition of culture opens the door for multiple ties of human connectedness.

This broader, multilayered definition also increases flexibility about
cultural matching between family and therapist. This is in contrast to the
more limiting (and often divisive) approach of "ethnic matching," which

encourages Latino therapists to treat Latino clients, African American clients to be treated by African American therapists, and so on. A therapeutic encounter between a white middle-class Jewish therapist in his mid-30s and a Mexican man of similar age, whose father came with a *bracero*[2] program, could seem doomed to misunderstanding and failure. Yet the MECA approach will help reveal that the therapist grew up in Los Angeles in a liberal family that lived close to Olvera Street where he met many Mexican vendors on weekends and many Chicano children in the schools. He knows a few words of Spanish and has learned to appreciate the strength of Latino families. He has shared in the many joyful aspects of the culture from the Mexican housekeepers and gardeners whom his parents hired. Sympathetically he remembers a powerful, late 1950s Mexican film titled *Espaldas Mojadas* (Wetbacks) in which jobless *braceros* crossing the Rio Grande are shot point blank by border patrol officers—those who survived went on to suffer great ignominies on the American side of the border. His daily reading of the *Los Angeles Times* tells him that in 40 years nothing has changed for the better for Mexican immigrants. In initial sessions, faint resonances can be felt between the Jewish therapist and the young Mexican man, resonances that are amplified as the two men discover their cultural similarities.

Upon examination, we all experience cultural borderlands and multiple cultural tastes and subjectivities. Belonging to a particular cultural identity group enhances self-esteem and engenders acceptance and respect for one's original groups of cultural reference. But an allegiance to cultural kin needs to be tempered with a multiculturalism that gives access to, and acceptance of, the culture of others.

## THE CHALLENGE OF DESCRIBING GROUPS

While writing this book I have wrestled with the dilemma of trying to say something general enough that might be useful for those interested in psychotherapy with Latinos, and the challenge to reflect continuous cultural transformations, new cultural blends, and cultural inconsistencies. I have always been opposed to static ethnic descriptions (Falicov, 1983, 1988b, 1995b) because they are more reflective of social science simplifications than of the true complexity of human behavior and experience. Indeed, static descriptions have never been more antithetical to reality than in the 1990s, when cultural movement is truly vertiginous and the interactions of class, race, gender, religion, and other cultural contexts have never been more complex.

At all points in this book a tension is maintained between making generalizations about Latinos (or about Puerto Ricans or Cubans as specific subgroups) that describe some aspect of a collective identity (e.g., "He is displaying Latino- [or Cuban] style *familismo*") while honoring cultural borderlands with other groups. Furthermore, cultural collective narratives should not be so tightly constructed that they rob people of their individuality. Recognizing and honoring subcultural and individual differences and probing personal interpretations, uses, or exceptions should become important parts of the therapeutic conversation.

## A WORD ABOUT TERMINOLOGY

Any attempt to describe and discuss ideas about culture and therapy is necessarily constrained by the vocabulary of psychological theories and social sciences, based as they are on the "universal" experiences of American and Western European populations. Yet when we apply a cultural lens to the usual constructions about family life, we gain a critical perspective of similarities and differences in beliefs and practices. This perspective becomes most clear when, in discussing conceptual constructions and technical interventions, we use a terminology that semantically attempts to capture the experiences of Latinos. For example, I use the new acculturation term "alternation theory" in addition to the dominant, linear discourse of acculturation and introduce the idea of using a "catching-up life narrative" to deal with separation and reunion issues in immigrant families. Established ethnic-oriented constructs such as *familismo,* "interdependence," *respeto,* and *personalismo* help describe the life arrangements and emotional atmosphere of collectivistic cultures. They are attempts to capture, qualitatively, the phenomenology of relational styles manifested in vivo. The intent is to portray a Latino collective narrative with a flavor of its own, rather than an accommodation of Anglo-American interactional styles to exaggerated versions of cohesion, enmeshment, or complementarity.

Likewise, constructions such as "proper demeanor" and "self-maximization" are brought into the realm of family therapy from comparative research about developmental goals for Latino and American children. Terms borrowed from medical sociology such as "somatization," or "cultural inversion" from educational anthropology are used to refer to special ecological issues faced by minority clients. The goal is not to create a separate vocabulary to deal with Latinos, but to respect, understand, and construct evocative descriptions of the nuances of cultural difference. A secondary goal is to avoid the reductionistic labeling of one culture as being either an exaggerated or a watered-down version of another.

By integrating this terminology in family work, my hope is to introduce some of the special characteristics of collectivistic cultures or of immigrant groups that merit particular descriptions and further study. With this caveat on semantics in mind, we can approach an in-depth look at MECA in Chapter 2 and move into the realm of the Latino family in Parts II through V.

## NOTES

1. Carlos Sluzki's (1982) analysis of the Latin lover further expands a similar observation in terms of how cultural stereotypes, on the part of "observers," trigger culturally predictable behavior in the "observed."
2. *Bracero* comes from *brazo*, which means "arm" in Spanish. A *bracero*, then, is literally somebody who works with his arms, or a hired hand. This was the generic term to refer to farm and industrial contract temporary workers recruited by the United States under labor agreements with Mexico from 1942 through 1964 (there have been similar programs with Puerto Rico and Jamaica) (see Novas, 1994; Portes & Bach, 1985).

# 2

# MECA: A Meeting Place for Culture and Therapy

> How comes it, after all, that, beginning with glancing experiences
> and half-witnessed events, one ends, as one sometimes does, with
> formed, written, recounted fact? Mainly, it seems, by way of *summary
> figures somehow assembled along the way: worked-up images of how matters
> connect.*
> — GEERTZ (1995, p. 18; emphasis added)

To develop summary figures about how "culturally relevant" or "socioculturally influenced" matters connect in family therapy, I devised MECA—the multicultural ecosystemic comparative approach—to transcend particular models of psychotherapy and reflect cultural variations that are especially relevant to family therapy theory and practice. Within this model, four basic areas of family life represent my own "account," assembled along the way in my work with Latinos and families of other cultures. The ideas expressed should not be taken as the "truth" about Latinos: doubtless there are other personal accounts and interpretations of the same reality.

In this chapter I introduce the most salient ideas and rationale that underlie MECA, discuss each of its components, introduce the four domains, and use a case study to illustrate MECA's application to assess and treat a family, as well as to describe the therapist's own theoretical and cultural position. In presenting this generalist framework, my hope is that therapists will find it both accessible and meaningful, regardless of theoretical orientation, in their work with individuals and families who represent an infinite variety of cultures and cultural blends.

## INSIDE MECA

Let's start with some examples that illustrate the thinking behind this emerging position. In most ethnic-focused descriptions, Mexicans are thought to uphold a conservative view of sexuality, given the strong influence of Roman Catholicism. The Mexican writer Carlos Fuentes (Day, 1992) relates an anecdote that illustrates the historical and ecological relativity of a traditional view of Mexican Catholicism and its influence on sexuality. In 1959, Fuentes went to see a French movie in Mexico City entitled *The Lover,* starring Jeanne Moreau. During a sexual scene (a close-up of her hand suggested an orgasm) that was then rather risqué, but today would be considered bland, an audience of 5,000 shocked, puritanical Mexicans screamed in horror. Now, let's advance the calendar to 1991. The acclaimed Mexican film *La Tarea* (The Homework) is about a young Mexican woman who chooses to film herself and her lover for her university assignment. They are naked. They make love with absolute frontal nudity. In the cinema audience there is not a whisper of disapproval. What happened? One answer is that Mexico, like many other countries, has undergone a sexual revolution during the past 30 years.

Are we to conclude that there are no differences in attitudes toward public displays of sexuality between Mexicans and Anglo-Americans? We emphatically cannot. Today, many urban Mexicans watch Cristina—the Cuban "Oprah Winfrey of Miami," whose show is broadcast in Mexico City—and feel both tantalized and outraged (*San Diego Union,* February 1993). Many viewers object to Cristina's bold discussions of taboo topics: homosexuality, AIDS, safe sex, extramarital affairs. They have been trying to get Cristina's program off the air. They find her offensive and vulgar, and they fear she will corrupt young people's minds.

Madonna's recent concerts in Mexico produced similar reactions (Dieterich, 1993). Many requested that her shows be canceled on grounds of obscenity. Should we conclude that these differences in meanings and underlying value systems represent cultural contradictions? Not necessarily. A simpler and probably more accurate explanation is that the Mexican people who watch daytime TV are different from those who go to arty movies at night, and Madonna opponents are more religious and puritanical than her supporters. While these groups share the same ethnicity, they belong to different generations and different social classes, and have different levels of education and different interpretations of Catholicism. To which group do the subject families of this book belong? Probably to all of the views described, and many others. The point to remember is that cultural evolution interacts differently with diverse segments of the society and the world.

To do justice to these complexities, we must go beyond the unidimensional "culture as ethnicity" framework toward a more comprehensive definition of culture, one that encompasses multiple variables, similarities and differences, the past and the present, and continuity and change in values, beliefs, and meanings over time. The three-part label, multidimensional-ecosystemic-comparative, summarizes the basic aspects of this expanded framework.

## Multidimensional

The following definition underlines the multidimensionality of culture:

> Culture is those sets of shared world views, meanings, and adaptive behaviors derived from simultaneous membership and participation in a variety of contexts, such as language; rural, urban or suburban setting; race, ethnicity, and socioeconomic status; age, gender, religion, nationality; employment, education and occupation, political ideology, stage of acculturation. (Falicov, 1983, pp. xiv–xv)

Cultural meaning systems have been defined as a set of premises about what is believed or thought to be preferable in human behavior and processes among people that share a similar subculture or ecological niche. These are cognitive interpretations of reality, but they have emotional components because of the convictions attached to them. They also have a motivational component because they become goals or ideals for behavior.

Perhaps this multidimensional view reflects more fairly the meaning of the word "diversity" than any one dimension alone. Families partake of and combine features of all these contexts. The contexts provide particular experiences and bestow certain values. It is the combination of multiple contexts and partial perspectives that shapes and defines each family's culture, rather than any of those separately. Nor does some monolithic "culture" exert an inexorable influence upon the individual. Each person is raised in a "plurality of cultural subgroups," that exert a "multiplicity of influences" depending on the degree of contact with each subcultural context. Culture can then be thought of as a community of individuals and families which partially share particular views, or dominant stories, that describe the world and give life meaning (Howard, 1991). Cultural similarities and differences reflect inclusion in or exclusion from various groups.

## Cultural Borderlands

An important derivative of a fluid multidimensional view is Rosaldo's (1989) idea of "cultural borderlands." As mentioned earlier, cultural borderlands are zones of similarity and difference within and between cultures. They give rise to internal inconsistencies, conflicts, and contradictions as well as commonalities and resonances among groups and individuals. Borderlands occur at the edges of "officially" recognized cultural groups, such as being an Argentine, a Jew, and a U.S. citizen. Other borderlands occur at less formal intersections—being raised a traditional girl (gender) in a family of poor immigrants (class and migration) of limited schooling (education), encountering a different world (and values) through advanced education, and acquiring higher social status through marriage. The idea of cultural borderlands captures more accurately the "encounters with 'difference' " or "communities of 'difference' " that now pervade modern everyday life in urban settings" (Rosaldo, 1989; West, 1993).

The Chicana poet Gloria Anzaldúa further developed and transformed the idea of people at the crossroads. She eloquently describes the potential of cultural borderlands for opening new forms of human understanding:

> The new mestiza [a woman of mixed Indian and Spanish ancestry born in the United States] copes by developing a tolerance for contradictions, a tolerance for ambiguity. She learns to be Indian in a Mexican culture, to be Mexican from an Anglo point of view. She learns to juggle cultures. She has a plural personality, she operates in a pluralistic mode—nothing is thrust out, the good, the bad, and the ugly, nothing rejected, nothing abandoned. Not only does she sustain contradictions, she turns the ambivalence into something else. (Anzaldúa, 1987, p. 79)

In making herself into a complex persona, Anzaldúa incorporates Mexican, Indian, and Anglo elements. In rejecting the classic "authenticity" of cultural purity, she seeks out the many strands of the borderlands. By sorting through and weaving together its overlapping parts, Anzaldúa's identity becomes richer rather than diffused.

## Ecosystemic

The definition of culture encompasses multiple ecological contexts. In fact, the unique combination of multiple contexts and partial perspectives that defines each family's culture can be thought of as their "ecological niche." A family's values form and evolve over time by their participation in these multiple contexts. The experience of dominant or marginalized access to resources, of entitlement and powerlessness, also derive from one's ecological place and experiences in various contexts. It is critical that therapists be aware of the family's simultaneous, holistic membership in these many, varied groups.

Edgar H. Auerswald, a pioneer of the ecological systems approach (1968), considers the total field of a problem and proposes moving beyond the individual and family to include interactions with outside systems, institutions, and agencies as an effective way to address the needs of poor families. This socially conscious approach is particularly relevant to Latino families, the majority of whom are poor and face discrimination. Developmental psychologist Uri Bronfenbrenner's "ecosystemic" model (1977) and family therapist Harry Aponte's "eco-structural" model (1976; Aponte & Van Deusen, 1981), Mony Elkaim's concept of "defamilization" (1982), Nancy Boyd-Franklin's multisystems approaches (1989), Evan Imber-Black's larger systems model (1988), and my own ideas (Falicov, 1988b) are all examples of approaches consistent with an ecosystemic view. Researchers in psychology also find promise in an ecological approach for understanding social issues. Steinberg, Dornbusch, and Brown (1992) allocated a large sample of adolescents to 16 ecological niches defined by ethnicity, social class, and family structure (biological, two-parent, and nonintact). They studied the phenomenon of ethnic differences in adolescent achievement by taking into account multiple, interactive processes of influence that operate across multiple, interrelated contexts.

In this book, all case examples utilize this more comprehensive ecosystemic definition of culture, which includes the multiple dimensions and cultural borderlands that compose a family's ecological niche.

## Comparative

A multidimensional, ecosystemic position doesn't focus on all the details of each culture or subculture being discussed. It emphasizes only those "differences that make a difference" to the family therapist's evaluation of and approach to clients. This requires a distillation and condensation of cultural information into "generic parameters" we can utilize in our work. Such parameters provide a map for comparing and understanding similarities and differences across cultures—a key element of MECA.

The comparative nature of this approach is demonstrated throughout this text. Thus the three Latino groups under discussion—Mexicans, Puerto Ricans, and Cubans—will not be treated in separate chapters. Rather the generic dimensions of migration, ecological context, family organization, and family life cycle are the central concern. Similarities and differences around the specific dimensions are treated comparatively so that their relativism becomes apparent. Comparisons include the meanings of accepted family therapy concepts such as individuation and connectedness, hierarchies, communication styles, and other subjects.

## THE KEY GENERIC DOMAINS

The first key generic domain—the journey of migration and culture change—attends to diversity in when, why, and how a family came to migrate. Latinos who immigrate to the United States share many issues with other immigrant groups. Among themselves they have similarities in language and cultural values, and manifest differences in countries of origin, motivations for migration, and adaptations they make to the host culture. Migration has significant mental health consequences for the internal and external workings of the family over several generations. This "psychology of migration" includes individual symptoms ranging from somatization to nightmares, family over- and underinvolvement caused by separations and reunions, and intergenerational conflicts between the immigrants and their parents or children. A number of clinical issues are tied to such pre-migration experiences as coaxed migrations or traumatic crossings. Other clinical issues, from cultural gaps between husbands and wives or parents and children to problems of cultural transition in individual and family relationships, emerge over time.

The second generic domain—ecological context—examines diversity in where and how the family lives and fits in the broader environment. To work with Latinos it is necessary to consider their total ecological field, including the racial, ethnic, class, religious, and educational communities in which the family lives; their living and working conditions; and their involvement with schools and social agencies. This domain sensitizes therapists to the "psychology of marginalization," those psychosocial and mental health consequences of marginalized status, discrimination due to race, poverty, and documented or undocumented status, and other forms of powerlessness, underrepresentation, lack of entitlement, and access to resources. A family whose community support networks resemble that of the native village may ascribe very different meanings to depression than a family that is isolated in a strange and unwelcoming new environment. The importance of natural and artificial support networks is underlined here, along with social and community programs that move the boundaries of therapy much beyond the private hour.

The constellation of beliefs about health, illness, religion, spirituality, and magic are relevant for understanding the preferred avenues and attitudes toward mainstream health care, psychotherapy, and folk medicine. Beliefs about personal responsibility and cultural styles of coping with adversity are of particular importance. This information is part of a "psychology of coping and healing," but it is included under exploration of the ecological context because often the spiritual and health resources provided by priests, church congregations, and folk healers are part of the immediate neighborhood and network setting.

The third generic domain—family organization—considers diversity in family structure and in the values connected to different family arrangements. Latino families tend to share a preference for collectivistic, sociocentric family arrangements that support parent–child involvement and parental respect throughout life. This is in contrast to nuclear family arrangements that favor the strength of nonblood relationships such as husband–wife. The crucial point for family therapists is that many family interactions are affected by this differential preference. Some of these relate to connectedness and separateness, gender and generational hierarchies, and styles of communication and conflict resolution among family members and outsiders. Families in rapid transformation often experience conflict and confusion over family models, obligations, and loyalties. It is common for a Latino couple to need help in balancing attachments to the family of origin and the family of procreation. These contradictions and dilemmas can be subsumed under a "psychology of cultural organizational transition."

The fourth generic domain—family life cycle—encompasses the dimension of time, and focuses on diversity in how natural developmental stages and transitions are culturally patterned. While the sequence of developmental events has universal biological aspects, many more are embedded in a cultural ecological fabric: the timing of stages and transitions, the constructions of age-appropriate behavior, various change mechanisms, and life cycle rituals and rites to name a few. Latino families share important similarities and differences, shaped in part by nationality, social class, and religion, regarding life cycle values and experiences. These are noteworthy for therapists who were trained to assess function and dysfunction based on an Anglo-American life cycle. A therapist may mistakenly assume a developmental delay in a 25-year-old married man who stops by his mother's to have a delicious *taquito* or *pastelito* and ask her opinions on many life issues. The impact of migration needs to be considered, too, because new values may emerge that affect developmental expectations. This information can be considered part of a "psychology of cultural developmental transition."

In short, the journey of migration and culture change, the patterned space of ecological context, the shapes of family organization before and after migration, and the temporal transitions of the family life cycle must always be present in the therapist's mind when working with Latinos.

## COMPARING CULTURAL MAPS: FAMILY MAPS AND THERAPIST MAPS

An essential component of the four comparative domains is the distinction between how the family and the therapist make sense of experience. In short, each participant in the therapeutic encounter brings with them a unique cultural "map." Awareness of these maps empowers therapists to work with families of different ecological niches—it raises consciousness about professional and personal biases, and underscores the "partial perspectives" and "situated knowledge" that color our therapeutic and cultural observations (Haraway, 1991).

By examining these overlapping maps, areas of dissonance and consonance between family and therapist become enriched as multiple contexts and cultural borderlands are revealed. For example, family and therapist may have different ethnic backgrounds and religions but similar education and social class; they may all have experienced prejudice and marginalization because of race, gender, or political ideology, or experienced relocation or migration; or they may share developmental niches, perhaps as parents of adolescents. This multidimensional, comparative approach builds cultural bridges of connectedness between family and therapist. And in areas of difference, interest in learning about the experiences and world views of others can forge new understanding and respect.

An ability to compare cultural maps relies on an attitude of close attention, curiosity, empathic understanding, and sociological imagination in the therapist. Paying close attention is the opposite of assuming that one knows about the culture of the family, and it is the best antidote for stereotyping. In fact, recent empirical evidence suggests that those who pay less attention and are in a position of power are more vulnerable to stereotyping others (Fiske, 1993). Another attitude is curiosity, a close ally of attention (Cecchin, 1987). Jay Lappin (1983) suggests using the family as a guide into their world, walking "the tightrope between risk and respect." Respectful questioning acknowledges that the clients know more than the therapist, and the questioning itself may stimulate new perspectives for the family. The concept of "sociological imagination" (Wright Mills, 1959) is similarly helpful in that it grasps connections between history, ideology, and biography for both therapist and client. Both parties in the therapeutic encounter become so aware of how socialization affects identity that personal problems can be approached as social issues and vice versa.

In developing a sociological imagination and cultural curiosity, the therapist is able to make cultural ideologies an important part of the therapeutic conversation. By sharing values, and comparing opinions about which behaviors would be adaptive yet culturally concordant (or deviant) with the family's goals, the therapist bridges meaning gaps with clients from other cultures. If a Latino family has moved from a setting in which the parents relied on extended family or others for parenting and household help but now are doing everything alone, articulating what can be "reproduced" and what must be "transformed" is important. For example, some of the old meanings about family life can remain as the couple relies on new networks of help *and* becomes more flexible toward the new values of sharing tasks between husband and wife.

To help the therapist navigate the Latino family's external and internal cultural landscape, a quick perusal of the four domains should happen during the first and second sessions. This facilitates decisions about what areas should be the focus of the therapeutic conversation. Exploring the family's migration history and acculturation, and its environmental re-

sources or constraints, including religious and health supports, will help locate both therapist and family in the family's "external cultural landscape."
Conversations about cultural beliefs and values, particularly those related
to family organization and life cycle markers and processes, helps a therapist enter the family's "internal cultural landscape."

The therapist might note similarities and differences between the
dominant discourse (and her own) and the family's cultural narrative,
while watching for possible dilemmas and enrichments brought about by
this meeting of two ideologies. Among these contrasts are collectivism and
individualism, hierarchies and egalitarianism, and communicative directness and indirectness. Therapeutic explorations of these and other similarities and differences should be conducted with respect, curiosity, and
collaboration as we attempt to understand the philosophical and behavioral consequences of a Latino way of life in the midst of American society.

In the extensive case study that follows, the therapeutic conversation
reveals data on each of the four domains, and the maps or ideologies of
family and therapist are compared in each domain.

## THE DÍAZ ORTIZ[1] FAMILY: A CASE OF CHILD ABUSE

The Díaz Ortiz family is composed of a 26-year-old mother, Isabel, a 29-
year-old father, Víctor, and two children, 6-year-old Yolanda and 2-year-
old Magdalena. Víctor had been accused of hitting Yolanda and was reported to Child Protective Services (CPS) by school authorities for
investigation. Because the evidence was inconclusive, CPS referred the
family for counseling at a local mental health center. There, the Díaz
Ortizes were seen by a therapist in training whom I supervised. Later I
interviewed the family at the request of the therapist, who felt overwhelmed by the task of accurately evaluating the presenting problem,
particularly because the family appeared to be uncooperative. Víctor
was articulate and very vocal about how upset he was by the school intervention and referral to CPS. He didn't deny hitting Yolanda, but justified it as a reaction to his, and his wife's, frustration with the girl's frequent whining and refusal to eat "her mother's food." He was indignant
at what he considered a violation of his rights and the intrusion of
strangers into his family life. His wife, Isabel, was quiet and appeared
tacitly to support Víctor's position.

### The Family's Maps

#### Circular Journeys: Migration and Culture Change

Seven years ago, Mr. and Mrs. Díaz Ortiz migrated from a small town near
San Luis de Potosí, Central Mexico, to San Marcos, California, a small town

north of San Diego, in search of a better economic future. Their migration narrative—the story of their migration experience—revealed that Víctor had initially come to Orange County, California, on his own. There he found a number of small construction and gardening jobs that paid him less than minimum wage. Nonetheless, Víctor felt that, over time, he would be better able to support a family in this country than in his own. He returned to Mexico to marry Isabel and then came back to the United States with his new wife. At that time, he poignantly described to her how comfortable the couches seemed to be in America, and how the TV programs advertised many wonderful household appliances that could be bought in easy installments. He assured Isabel that some day they would be able to afford a good couch, and other commodities, for their home. Isabel, who was only 19, worked as a maid the first year and became pregnant soon after. The couple was concerned that, without the help of their extended family in Mexico, they would be unable to manage financially and emotionally once the new baby arrived. They returned to Mexico where they lived with Víctor's family (as will be seen in Chapter 5, this is a common pattern) for 10 months. But their economic situation became worse, spawning a desire to return to the United States.

For practical and economic reasons, Víctor urged Isabel to leave their baby, Yolanda, in Mexico with her paternal grandmother. Isabel was uncomfortable with this idea, but Víctor argued that without the responsibility of caring for Yolanda, his wife could continue to work in the United States. Víctor also feared that because Isabel was so young and did not speak any English, she would not be able to handle any emergency involving Yolanda in this country. With intense pressure from Víctor (and Víctor's mother), Isabel finally acquiesced. The arrangement was a common one from the standpoint of Mexican culture—children often remain behind with extended family during the initial stages of migration and are reunited at a later date.

Four years later, when the couple was expecting another child, Isabel decided she would stop working and bring Yolanda back to San Diego. The grandmother resisted. Yolanda resisted. The girl and the grandmother prevailed (with a little help from Víctor, who continued to value his mother's wishes over his wife's). A year later, as the time approached for Yolanda to start elementary school, Isabel renewed her campaign to fetch her daughter. Arguing that her child would get a better education in the United States, Isabel's choice prevailed.

The family came in contact with the mental health system 4 months after Yolanda's own difficult migration and reentry into the Díaz Ortiz family. As soon as the child arrived from Mexico she began throwing tantrums during meal times. She disliked many foods and often refused to eat. She also resisted calling her parents "mother" and "father," for she had learned to call her grandmother "mother" and believed her parents to be her siblings.

Among the therapist's first hypotheses was that Yolanda must be missing the flavors of her grandmother's home-cooked Mexican food. This assumption turned out to be incorrect. On the contrary, Isabel was a superb Mexican cook, while the grandmother indulged Yolanda's sweet tooth with commercial candy.

## Space: Ecological Context

An investigation of the present ecological context served to aid in understand the presenting problem, the reactions to the problem, and the family's constraints and resources in the search for solutions.

The Díaz Ortiz family lived in an isolated trailer park on the outskirts of San Diego with a few Latino neighbors and other working-class families. Given their precarious economic position, Isabel's wish to stay home was not possible. She found a job at a factory that had a nursery to care for her youngest, Magdalena. But Isabel and Víctor had trouble finding after-school child care for Yolanda. Both parents were working, and neither was able to pick up Yolanda at 5 P.M. Víctor was angry at the indifference of school authorities who told him there was a long waiting list for after-school care and that he had applied too late. The couple said in therapy that they suspected discrimination because of language difficulties and their race. In fact, they felt the school wanted to get rid of them. The report to Child Protective Services confirmed the Díaz Ortizes' feeling that school authorities "had it in for them." Unfamiliar with American laws, they believed that a child abuse allegation was a ploy to invade their privacy, to close doors on them, and to send them back to Mexico. Feeling scared, isolated, ashamed, and unaccustomed to asking for institutional help, the Díaz Ortiz family felt they had nowhere to turn. The therapist was initially seen as in cahoots with the school officials, aiming to find fault so as to "get rid of them." Feeling very defensive and suspicious, the parents united to fight off the "invaders"—Víctor challenged the young therapist, asking her why and how she expected them to disclose so much personal information when she was unwilling to reveal anything about herself. The "attack" was an uncharacteristic deviation from customary cultural politeness: the family was clearly reacting to a perceived threat. At this point the therapist asked for my help and I interviewed the family.

## Family Organization and Transitions in Structure

When asked about the meaning of his decision to leave his daughter in Mexico, Víctor Díaz's responses opened the door to an exploration of the family's organization. His answer to that question was, "There is no greater love than a mother's love, blood of her blood." At first he confused the therapist and myself with what we thought to be a contradiction—he had worked hard to convince the child's mother, his wife, to leave Yolanda behind. The mother he was referring to, however, was not his wife, but his own mother. For Víctor, the direct blood line was between his mother and his daughter, without recognition of his wife. His allegiances and definition of mother (perhaps with a capital "M") revolved around his own mother, not Isabel. By virtue of his Mexican ethnicity and his Roman Catholic upbringing, his family had been organized such that loyalty to intergenerational bonds, particularly between mother and son, were stressed over marital allegiances.

Actually Isabel understood the guilt and distress Víctor felt leaving his mother to come to the United States. She explained empathically that Víctor was worried his mother would *morir de tristeza* (die of sadness) had he refused to leave Yolanda with her. This strong intergenerational bond typifies many extended family arrangements in which family connectedness is valued over individuation, interdependence over autonomy, and compliance with authority rather than assertion of individual needs or rights. In addition, this extended family lifestyle promotes a high reliance on the family network for support rather than on help from institutions.

After a few years alone in this country, however, and perhaps because Isabel was working outside the home, the Díaz Ortizes' conception of family was slowly transforming into an arrangement that focused more on the husband–wife tie and on egalitarian views and desires. For example, they began to socialize with others as a couple rather than separately with same-sex friends as was common in their native village. They also began to rely on each other rather than an extended family network for emotional support.

## Family Life Cycle Transitions

For the Díaz Ortiz family, migration precipitated a dramatic change in family organization. This change intersected with the normative life cycle transitions of early marriage, creating a troubling combination of stressors. Víctor and Isabel were a very young couple, still steeped in family of origin norms when they married and left Mexico. A sense of responsibility toward their families and guilt for leaving tormented the couple, creating insecurity and a need for parental approval. This was especially true for Víctor, who was the prime initiator of the migration. Had they stayed in Mexico, it is likely that both Víctor and Isabel would have remained tied to their families of origin even after marriage. Greater autonomy and personal authority (relative to their parents') would have come when the couple was considerably older, if ever. Víctor's loyalty to his mother would have been manifested differently and somewhat more subtly, perhaps by paying daily visits, helping out financially, and bringing the baby to visit her grand-mother at least every weekend.

Leaving a child behind at the time of migration may have ensured some continuity of presence, a symbolic offering of family loyalty, in spite of the distance and the separation. The Latino grandparents also live these stages differently than those in an American middle-class family because in-volvement with grandchildren and associated caretaking is much more intense. An Anglo-American middle-class grandmother would seldom dream of having her grandchild live with her and her husband, and away from the child's own parents. Nor would the "ideal" Anglo-American grandmother take such a tremendous amount of work and responsibility upon her shoulders unless she was forced to help her children for health or economic reasons.

In the Díaz Ortiz family, migration truncated a stage of the life cycle that is shared collaboratively or conflictually, but almost always together, by the three generations in the country of origin. Both young parents, but more so Isabel, attempted to retrieve Yolanda during developmental transi-tions, such as the pregnancy and birth of the second child. Isabel was un-successful for several reasons: lack of support from her husband and the forcefulness of his attachment to his mother, with which his wife empa-thized; Isabel's own initial guilt and ambivalence about leaving extended family for a second time after the failed attempt to return home; practical and economic limitations; and the grandmother's and the child's own resis-tance. At a later point in the life cycle two natural developmental transi-tions legitimized Isabel's renewed attempts to reunite with Yolanda: first, the birth of another baby had already consolidated the Díaz Ortizes as a family unit and established Isabel as even more of a mother than before; second, the forthcoming entrance to primary school for Yolanda supported the immigrant's dream for their nuclear and extended family—education and a better future for their offspring in a new country.

## The Therapist's Maps

Before considering the therapeutic process in detail, let's look at the thera-pist's maps, which include her perspectives of the four key domains, her in-teraction with the family, and hypotheses she began to formulate, based on the unique interaction of what she and the family both brought to the therapy.

The therapist was a 24-year-old social work trainee, a first-generation Mexican American whose parents had migrated about 30 years earlier and had raised six children before her in California. Her Spanish was laborious, but acceptable. She was definitely more comfortable speaking English. She understood the values that shape family life for Mexicans and for Americans, but had incorporated the mental health model in which she had been trained, namely, that which values autonomy over interdependence and symmetry over complementarity, particularly in relations between men and women.

Out of these world views, the therapist had developed three psychological hypotheses: first, the parents and Yolanda were insufficiently bonded with each other given the history of separation at a critical developmental time; second, the father had a "pathological" attachment to his own mother and lacked empathy for his wife; third, the wife was subservient to her husband and needed to become more assertive. As constructions they were all possible, and could certainly become part of a conversation with the family.

The first hypothesis seemed to be the most promising place to start because it involved the three family members and even the baby. It also had the most positive, blame-free emotional tone and could be easily linked to Yolanda's eating problems and to her parents' polarized, punitive, and protective reactions. The other two constructions were based, at least in part, on stereotypes (and the therapist's personal feelings) about Mexican men's relationships to their mothers and wives, and the women's reactive or complementary responses. These two latter hypotheses were charged with considerable irritation and disapproval, manifest in the trainee's judgmental attitude toward Víctor.

In supervision, the trainee was encouraged to practice her "sociological imagination" about this family's culturally patterned life (particularly in terms of their family organization, developmental expectations, and ecological context) had they remained in their native village. The trainee was also asked to imagine the nuclear and extended families' state of mind then, and now, based on the couple's migration narrative. This imaginative stance opened up an avenue for a more flexible, more empathic, more curious, and less critical view of the two young parents.

## The Therapy Process

When the therapist encountered what had felt like an "attack" by Víctor, she worried that an impasse had been reached. How could she make a useful appraisal of the family situation given what felt like a standoff? The therapist told me about the family's feelings of isolation, anger, and vulnerability, and requested that I meet with them. Following a brief review, I expressed my understanding of the Díaz Ortizes' outrage and fear. I explained the child abuse laws of California, stressing that these applied to people of all ethnicities and social classes. I gave examples of American parents who were undergoing even more severe scrutiny from Child Protective Services, cases in which children would most likely be removed from the home. Hearing this, and learning about the state's interpretation of "the best interest of the child," Isabel and Víctor visibly relaxed their guard. This enabled them to be more open to taking the steps necessary to comply with the legal requirements. The latter included attending parenting classes and family therapy sessions geared to help Yolanda's integration in the family.

The therapist and I were uncertain as how to interpret and deal with Mr. Díaz's physical disciplining of Yolanda. We felt that a better connectedness for the couple would require a shift in the husband's ability to empathize and support his wife, even at the risk of disappointing his own mother. As it turned out, the abusive episode was the first time the father had intervened forcefully on his wife's behalf against the whining child, who was undergoing her own unrecognized trauma of recent migration and despondency over the loss of her beloved grandmother. Though poorly handled, the husband had good intentions to help his wife establish her influence over their daughter because, as he put it, "She [Yolanda] is ours now." This attempt to develop a stronger parental alliance could be construed as a move toward a husband-wife model of family organization.

We were also concerned about Mr. Díaz's anger, and wondered if Mrs. Díaz, and perhaps even Yolanda, could be concealing the extent of physical abuse for either of two reasons: to protect the family against outsiders that might deport them, or intimidation into silence by Víctor's possible retaliation. We explored these issues by interviewing each family member separately, and although the private sessions did not unearth new information, they gave the wife and child a chance to freely share their concerns. Individual sessions also improved the relationship between each parent and the therapist, who later used the information she had gathered to comment on many positive aspects of the family: their care for and interest in one another, their pride in their family, and their desire to do what was right for all members.

We labeled the parents' problems with Yolanda, the school, and child protection authorities as issues of "cultural transition." We openly supported Víctor's attempts to help Isabel get Yolanda to eat. Using a cognitive approach, both parents were helped to co-develop, list on a blackboard, and discuss other possible reasons for Yolanda's eating problems and to move away from feeling that Yolanda was simply "bad" or "spoiled" by the grandmother. Alternative explanations were that Yolanda could be *nerviosa* (nervous) and upset, reacting to the trauma of recent migration, which included the loss of many familiar faces, places, and objects, but especially her grandmother. Indeed, an eating disorder could be seen as a somatization for psychological stress, a connection that is culturally congruent and that the parents could easily understand. Yolanda's parents became more sympathetic toward their daughter's situation. In addition, Isabel began to disentangle her relationship with Yolanda from a web of rivalry with her mother-in-law.

The Díaz Ortiz family faced another common dilemma of minority parents. The state orders most families to take parenting classes after they have had encounters with Child Protective Services, but the therapist could find only English-speaking classes in the area where Víctor and Isabel lived. Surprisingly, Mr. Díaz became interested in turning this upsetting experience into a useful cause. He figured other Spanish-speaking parents were unaware of state child protection laws and the psychological reasons behind them. Víctor and Isabel asked us to find a Spanish-speaking expert to begin a group with other parents. They offered to help develop this group by inviting parents they met at work or at their trailer park. The therapy trainee working on this case facilitated the group, which met at a local church. The family's empowerment came from understanding the parameters of their ecological niche and the potential resources of family and community that could emerge from this difficult experience within the family and with outside agencies.

## MECA APPLIED: WHAT MAPS REVEAL

Within a multidimensional ecosystemic definition of culture, each case represents a unique combination of cultural influences. The case study becomes a fundamental avenue for the family and therapist to discover the interplay of cultural forces and family processes. Cultural meanings are explored through dialogue and conversation, not based on presuppositions, a priori categories, or any other formulaic "knowledge" about the culture of a family. The approach is like that of Geertz (1973), who suggests that cultural understanding is similar to social understanding—an approximation achieved through dialogue, a cultural understanding via mutual corrections by each party (clients and therapist) in conversation.

In spite of this exploratory stance, it can be very helpful to go into the uncharted territory of a family's culture armed with a few guidelines. Without any sort of map, one might get lost and miss completely what could have been just around the corner. Hence MECA's generic cultural maps and its four domains. In the chapters that follow, I delve more deeply into each of these four domains, offering the constructs and the techniques that I have developed or found helpful for focusing with greater complexity on each domain.

It will also become clear in the case descriptions that each family is dealing with universal issues, with idiosyncratic experiences and solutions, and with religious, class, or ethnic-specific views and constructions, all of which emanate from the multiple contexts that comprise each family's ecological niche. Auerswald (1990) further illuminates how these multiple contexts are experienced when he says that culture occurs in two very different realities or domains. One is the realm of rational thought, of "making sense." The other is the irrational realm of feelings, experience, creativity, and play, which of course is often nonverbal. He suggests the term "explicate culture" to designate the construct culture when it is linked to sensible objective reality, reserving the term "implicate culture" to designate the experienced, but difficult to describe, nonobjectifiable culture as the patterned connections in a domain of relations.

The descriptions that follow about Mexicans, Puerto Ricans, and Cubans are attempts to make sense, by moving to an explicit reality something that most often occurs as an implicit, felt, and hard to describe reality. The implicit level is more analogic and qualitative than it is digital and quantitative. Culture occurs more in the realm of beliefs and myths, customs, language, and modes of communication than in the realm of behavior or rational explanation. The translation from one level to the other is inherently limited by the different nature of these two different orders of things.

An analogous reference might be read in the painter René Magritte's well-known canvas of a smoking pipe, cautiously titled "This Is Not a Pipe." Even in an attempt to represent a simple object such as a pipe, the artist can only come up with a two-dimensional drawing, a flat and lifeless representation that falls short of the real pipe: a complex, three-dimensional object replete with texture, smell, taste, color, and age, all of which evoke history, associations of pleasure, relaxation, and other, more personal, subjective and emotional memories and meanings.

Likewise, readers of this book are cautioned about what follows—this is not Latino culture. Any discussion about Latino culture and Latino families is only a simplified, schematic representation of an exciting, rich confluence of meaning and identities, of worlds of words, sounds, sights and flavors, ideas and emotions of which these pages are very pale mirrors indeed.

## NOTE

1. Latino families, and even more so Mexican families, almost always use two last names. The first one is the paternal surname. The second one is the maternal surname. Although there is a tradition of Hispanic formality behind this custom, there are also practical reasons. The great majority of the population in the country of origin uses a relatively limited number of common Spanish surnames. Therefore, it is very likely that many people will have the same last name. The only way to avoid confusion is to add the maternal surname in almost every transaction, but particularly so in those that involve institutions. A family may insist on adding on a second last name if the therapist has not acknowledged it. However,

for a therapist to insist intentionally on securing the second surname from a family who has not volunteered it may raise fears if family members have an unclear documented status or they are distrustful of American stereotyped attitudes toward Latinos.

*PART II*

---

# The Latino Experience: Movement and Change

---

In a decade in which human migration has reached an all-time high, Spanish-speaking people rank as the most mobile group of all. The sheer number of Latinos in the United States compels attention to this minority group. United States population projections show that by the year 2000 more than one-third of the total population will be racial and ethnic minorities. The Latino population will reach 55 million and will constitute the largest minority group by the year 2025. Over the past decade, the Latino population increased by 67% in California alone.

As mental health professionals strive to reach this burgeoning group, they are required to go beyond the confines of familiar Anglo-American theory and practice and examine the immensely rich and complex meaning systems of their Latino clients. Essential to this endeavor is an understanding of why Latino individuals and families are on the move, and how their experiences as immigrants (whether first- or second-generation or beyond) affect the ways they adapt, change, and maintain continuity in what, to many, is initially viewed as a promised land.

Migration is a massive ecological transition in time and space. It begins before the act of relocation and goes on for a long time, affecting the descendants of immigrants for several generations. Even when freely chosen, the experience of migration is replete with loss and disarray—there is loss of language, the separation from loved ones, the intangible emotional vacuum left in the space where "home" used to be, the lack of understanding of how jobs, schools, banks, or hospitals work. Immigrants are rendered vulnerable, upset, and susceptible to physical and mental distress.

Yet not all is dislocation, trauma, and crisis. Migration can also be an adventure that opens possibilities of living a better life and provides an opportunity to prove oneself capable of hardiness and survival. Immigrants may gain self-confidence by learning a new language and finding work. They learn to form new bonds while constructing new lives and partially reinventing themselves. Indeed, the study of the immigrant experience offers fertile ground to look at what helps people stay healthy as well as what makes them ill (Portes & Rumbaut, 1990b).

Viewed over time, migration follows a somewhat chronological progression. In Chapter 4 I look at the first stages of the experience: (1) premigration and entry, and the bidirectional impact of migration on those who stay and those who leave; (2) the uprooting of meaning across physical, social, and cultural domains; and (3) the dismantling and reconstructing of family ties. During these early stages the therapist often becomes a "social intermediary," helping the family translate and negotiate their contacts with institutions and networks, as well as a facilitator in answering the family's need to preserve and recover continuity in the face of massive change. The "migration narrative" is described as an especially helpful tool in helping families manage these tasks.

Clearly, change of cultures reverberates across time and across generations, and narratives about migration extend far beyond the initial consequences of uprooting, migration distress, and culture shock. These initial consequences recede as immigrants gain cultural and language competence, while other challenges gradually emerge in the internal and external landscapes of family life. Social science, including psychotherapy, has considered "acculturation" or "assimilation" as key to the adaptive processes of immigrants, especially during the latter stages of migration. The assumption that this mode of adaptation benefits an immigrant's mental  health is now under serious question. In Chapter 5 I examine this debate and consider more recent ideas such as "alternation" and "hybridization," which may provide more meaningful, viable, culturally congruent, and adaptive options for immigrant clients. We also explore the role of therapist as cultural intermediary during later stages of the migration process.

Before launching these discussions, some significant historical facts and figures are presented in Chapter 3. While migration experiences share certain similarities, the history of the three Latino groups presented in this book—Mexicans, Puerto Ricans, and Cubans—vary considerably. Further, the reasons and timing for various waves of migration from Latin American countries and the sociopolitical mood of the United States deeply affect how Latinos perceive, and are perceived by, the people of their new home. The implications for psychological distress and help seeking are a natural corollary to these historical events, and part of this discussion.

# 3

# Mexicans, Puerto Ricans, and Cubans: An Overview

It is the imposing flow of reality with its hallucinating proposal of newer, furiously conquered spaces. It is the relentless flow of a people who float between two ports, licensed for the smuggling of human hopes.

—LAGUNA-DÍAZ (1987; cited in Flores, 1992, p. 201)

Latinos in the United States are a varied, heterogeneous population of immigrants from many different countries, settings, and cultures. The forces that spurred them toward migration vary widely, from escape from political change to a search for better economic or educational opportunities. Latinos are a diverse group, not only from one nation to another, but from one cultural group to the next. In their Latin American homelands they share a unique blending of Hispanic values and lifestyles with many indigenous languages and cultures. In fact, in most Latin American countries one can find at least three major groups: the indigenous groups that may still speak their own native languages and preserve beliefs and traditions from their native culture; a large *mestizo* group which represents a mixture between the indigenous and the Spanish blood and culture; and the "pure" descendants of the Spanish colonizers. Along with these three groups one finds a smaller number of descendants from other countries in Western and Eastern Europe, and an even smaller number of immigrants from the Middle and Far East. Latinos can belong to any of those Latin American groups.

This book focuses on the experiences of therapists working with three prominent groups of Latino immigrants: Mexicans, Puerto Ricans, and Cubans. Although this choice represents an oversimplification of the actual similarities and differences among Latinos, it has become a matter of convention to consider these to be the three major groups in the United States.[1]

## WHY "LATINOS" AND NOT "HISPANICS"?

Although many call Spanish-speaking immigrants from Latin America and their descendants "Hispanic," politically correct–minded groups prefer the term "Latino" because it reaffirms their native, pre-Hispanic identity. It is difficult to understand how the term Latino was chosen because the indigenous groups of the Americas did not speak Latin. Spanish is a language derived from Latin, and it was first spoken in the Americas by the Spanish Conquerors. Contradictory as the term may be, the intentions are praiseworthy. "Latino" is a more democratic alternative to "Hispanic" because Hispanic is a term strongly supported by politically conservative groups that regard their Spanish European ancestry as superior to the "conquered" indigenous groups of the Americas. Latino is also geographically more accurate, since it refers to people from Latin America rather than to people from Spain, which excludes the native-born Indian ancestry. Despite its limitations (e.g., "Latino" may not describe many other immigrants who came to Latin America from Africa, Asia, and around Europe), the term provides a generally accepted way to differentiate groups that have migrated to the United States from those that remained in their Latin American countries.

Earl Shorris (1992), journalist and author of the influential book *Latinos: A Biography of the People*, prefers the term Latino for linguistic reasons in addition to political, economic, or geographic accuracy of representation. According to Shorris, "Latino" has gender, which is Spanish, as opposed to "Hispanic," which follows English, nongendered rules of grammar. Indeed, as he claims, the Spanish language may be the most clearly unifying characteristic of Latinos in spite of different degrees of proficiency in second- and third-generation immigrants.[2]

Shorris (1992) begins his book with an anecdote. He relates how he asked a Mexican grandmother what she called her generic cultural group. She answered, "I belong to the 'Mejicanos.' " He insistently probed further offering her "Hispano, Latino, Latin, Spanish, Spanish-speaking" and the grandmother, amused but unruffled, maintained that she belonged to the "Mejicanos" group. The point of this anecdote is well taken, because, as Shorris says, to lump cultures together under one rubric is to take away the name and erase with one stroke the individuality of the group. Indeed, the best names for Latin Americans are their own countries and cultures: Chileans, Bolivians, Venezuelans, Puerto Ricans, and so on.

Still, Latinos speak a common language, a fact that inevitably shapes affinities of mind and heart. Augenbraum and Stavans (1993) offer a broad, poetic description of how language structures explain, in part, the contrasting world views between English- and Spanish-speaking peoples:

> Language is useful in contrasting both worldviews. Spanish, labyrinthine in nature, has at least four conjugations to address the past; the lone future tense is hardly used. One can portray a past event in multiple ways, but when it comes to one of tomorrow, a speaker in Buenos Aires, Lima, Mexico City, and Caracas has little choice. The fact is symptomatic: Hispanics, unable to recover from history, are obsessed with memory. English, on the other hand, is exact, matter-of-fact—in Jorge Luis Borges's words, "mathematical," a tongue with plenty of room for conditionals, ready to seize destiny.
>
> Spanish makes objects female and male, while in English the same things lack gender. As if one were not enough, Spanish has two verbs for *to be:* one used to describe permanence, another to refer to location and temporality. Thus, a single sentence, say Hamlet's famous dilemma, *To be, or not to be,* is inhabited in Spanish by a double, never self-negating, clear-cut meaning: to be or not to be alive; to be or not to be here. English simplifies: to be, period— here and now. Again, Spanish has two verbs for *to know:* one used to characterize knowledge through experience, the other to designate memorized information. To know Prague is not the same as to know the content of the Declaration of Independence. Much less baroque, English refuses complication. (pp. xi–xii)

The English language itself may place limitations on how mainstream American therapists think about and work with diverse, non-English-speaking groups. Many social science concepts, including those that describe human behavior and therapeutic processes, are prey to the limitations of the English language. All too often, what therapists uncritically consider to be universal psychological processes, that is, beliefs in the future, in the simplicity and rapid speed of change, in inalienable individual rights and such ideas as the right to "privacy" (a word which has no Spanish translation), may in fact be cultural narratives semantically summarized in the words and construction of the English language.

The challenge for therapists is to critically examine and understand their own and their clients' contexts, including language and culture-based differences that impact our work. Only then can therapists do justice to the uniqueness of each family in each cultural group and still recognize that many Latin Americans share many values and customs.

To address these cultural contrasts, I compare the three largest Latino groups with mainstream Anglo-American voices.[3] Reviewing the migration history and cultural backdrop of Mexicans, Puerto Ricans, and Cubans provides a necessary initial context.

## A BRIEF HISTORY OF LATINO MIGRATION

### Mexicans

> Poor Mexico, so far from God, yet so near the United
> States.
> —Popular refrain attributed to a speech by
> MEXICAN PRESIDENT PORFIRIO DÍAZ (1912)

This refrain captures a popular Mexican sentiment about the complicated relationship of mutual and uneasy dependency between the United States and Mexico, and the sense of exploitation experienced by Mexico. Unbalanced interaction between the two countries has gone on for centuries.

The conflict between Mexico and the United States over Texas led to the Mexican War (1846–1848) in which the United States gained most of the land that is now Arizona, California, Colorado, Nevada, New Mexico, Utah, and Wyoming. More than 75,000 Mexicans who lived in those areas became instant U.S. citizens. To this day, many people within this ancestral group consider the Southwest to be Mexican, if not politically at least culturally. These people don't think of themselves as immigrants. In fact, many claim to be the proud descendants of Spanish conquerors and deny any blood ties with Mexico.

After the discovery of gold in California in 1848, miners and prospectors from the eastern United States poured into the West. Racial, religious, language, and other cultural differences created much conflict between the Mexican people and the newcomers. Through discrimination and injustice Mexicans became low-paid workers in a land that now belonged to English-speaking Americans.

Throughout the 1900s, complementarity of market needs between Mexico and the United States resulted in an economic roller coaster ride for Mexicans: during periods of labor shortage north of the border, the United States recruits workers, encourages relocation, and legalizes immigration; when American unemployment is high, Mexican immigration is discouraged, made illegal, and punished with deportation. In fact, the "Bracero program" not only brought Mexican laborers legally to the United States, but ironically it facilitated the social networks that began to support undocumented migration when the program ended in 1964.

The allure of better opportunities in the United States has been a magnet for Mexicans throughout this century. Although Mexico has a variety of landscapes and climates, most of its present territory is dry, rocky, and unsuitable for agriculture. Industry and technology are growing much more rapidly than in the past, but these changes are not reflected in higher employment rates. More than one-third of Mexican people work very hard and live in extreme poverty, while the population grows about 3% per year because of the high birth rate.

Most frequently immigrants come from the northern bordering states and central rural areas of Mexico (i.e., Jalisco, Michoacán). More recently, lack of employment opportunities has prompted immigration from large urban centers like Mexico City and Guadalajara. Immigrants settle everywhere in the United States—many have settled in the Midwest, but the usual choice is California and other southwestern states.

Although some Mexicans have lived in the southwestern states for several generations, the majority currently living in the United States are immigrants, either born in Mexico or born to parents who were born in Mexico. Most specify Spanish as their native tongue and as the language spoken in their homes as children. The predominant religion, practiced by more than 90% of all Mexican Americans, is Roman Catholic. In border areas like southern California, Jehovah's Witnesses, Pentecostal and other evangelical faiths, and even Judaism (see *San Diego Union,* July 21, 1995) have gained recent followers among Mexican Americans.

Some Mexican Americans define themselves as "Chicano," and a word of clarification should be said about this commonly used term. Chicanos are people of Mexican descent who were born in the U.S. They see themselves as outsiders to both mainstream United States *and* Mexican cultures. Most speak better English than Spanish. They identify with the indigenous roots of Mexican history, and they see the Southwest as intrinsically Mexican. The term Chicano came from the nationalistic political and labor movements of the 1970s, exemplified by Movimiento Estudiantil Chicano de Atzlán (MECHA) and the United Farm Workers led by Cesar Chávez and Dolores Huerta. (For an excellent account of Chicanos up to the present, see the book *Anything but Mexican* by Rodolfo F. Acuña (1996) and an older representative collection edited by Edward Simmen (1972) titled *Pain and Promise: The Chicano Today.*.

Mexicans comprise the largest Latino group in the United States, nearly 64%. The population has risen steadily, in spite of immigration restrictions that began in 1960 and the denial of legal alien status to most immigrants. Fear of detection, a sense of anomie, and social alienation permeates the lives of these nondocumented immigrants. In an anti-immigrant political fever, California voters approved Proposition 187 in November 1994, which requires publicly funded health care facilities to deny care to illegal immigrants and to report them to the INS (Immigration and Naturalization Service). The threat of enforcing Proposition 187 has set in motion many negative consequences for the utilization and the delivery of mental health services (Falicov & Falicov, 1995; Ziv & Lo, 1995).

Migration has become so much a part of Mexico's everyday, everywhere life that men between the ages of 15 and 45 are few and far between in many small towns. These men return frequently for visits, and for vacations, or to fetch wives and children. The families accept this situation because the men send money regularly, and in many cases they make it possible to build a modest family home, a cherished dream of many poor people, particularly women, in Mexico.

Migration has also assumed a quasi-mythical meaning as part of the masculine mystique—some might even consider migration as an expected life cycle stage. Many young men have come to think of the journey north as a rite of passage, a way to prove their manhood, and to go through a "life experience that has to be lived" (Bronfman et al., 1995).

A number of resilient young men, as young as 13 or 14 years old, see migration as a way to escape harrowing life conditions and to prove their independence, while also sending aid for their families. They often fail in this endeavor, continuously caught in a cycle of apprehension by immigration authorities, incarceration in jail, and rapid deportation. They wait again at the Mexican side of the border to dart across once more, only to be sent home again in a never-ending cycle (Berry, 1996).

Undocumented Mexican immigrants face dangerous and traumatic experiences to circumvent border detection—creeping over hills, hiding in sewers, crossing rivers, crawling under barbed wire, paying "coyotes" (experienced border crossers or "people smugglers") who promise safe conduct, but often abandon, rob, or abuse their customers. The bitter reward awaiting these brave men and women, after conquering enormous obstacles, may be a rude awakening to the realities of exploitation and discrimination in large U.S. cities. Rose, the Guatemalan heroine of the movie *El Norte,* sums up the predicament of many illegal immigrants: "In Mexico there is only poverty. There is no place there for us. In the North we are not accepted. When are we going to find a place?"[4]

Migrant workers who come north to pick crops in rural areas suffer their own hardships. A recent film (1995) based on Tomas Rivera's book *. . . And The Earth Did Not Devour Him* (1987) is a compelling portrayal of a proud, migrant worker family's indefatigable search for social justice and a better life in the face of hunger and exploitation. The film, directed by Paul Espinoza and distributed by the Public Broadcasting System, stands out from others because of its multiple voices and nonstereotypical renditions of Mexican migrant workers.

Although Mexicans "choose" to migrate, the experience isn't necessarily positive. True, they are voluntary refugees from a bad living situation, but most likely they would prefer to stay within the emotional familiarity of their own country, farms, and villages. But models for mobility abound— Mexican immigrants' coping skills for exiting the old and entering the new may be enhanced by the prevalence of migration in their hometowns, and by relatives or friends that await them at their destination.

In addition to the thousands of poor and working-class immigrants who struggle to make new homes in the United States, a number of middle-class and wealthy Mexican families live in the southwestern states, attracted there by economic and political stability. These families maintain close ties with their relatives and businesses in Mexico and travel back and forth frequently. In addition, many Mexican American children and grandchildren of immigrants have moved up the educational and financial ladder and so have gained economic power. These two groups make use of private psychotherapy services and usually speak English well. Yet they appreciate therapists who speak Spanish or at least understand *nuestra mentalidad* (our mentality).

## Puerto Ricans

> Nuyorico, so far from paradise and no longer close to possibility.
> —Popular refrain

The relationship between Puerto Rico and the United States began in 1898 when the United States won the war with Spain and acquired that lovely island. Puerto Rico was particularly attractive to the United States because of its strategic military location and rich coffee plantations. The United States then faced the dilemma of what to do with one million Puerto Ricans who spoke only Spanish—a dilemma that has never been fully resolved. A series of legislations, passed over many years, only compounded the problem by leaving Puerto Ricans in limbo about their identity. The island residents are U.S. citizens, subject to military duty, but they don't pay U.S. income taxes, aren't full beneficiaries of federal social service programs, and are prohibited from voting. It's as if they were suspended in thin air, neither citizens of their own independent nation, nor full citizens of the United States. The future of Puerto Rico, whether it will continue to be a territory of the United States become the 51st state, or become an independent nation, remains a vital issue for Puerto Ricans.

The fierce pride Puerto Ricans have for their land and Afro-Spanish heritage may, in fact, be partially compelled by their limited civic rights and economic resources. Many Puerto Ricans living in the United States are deeply involved in the politics of their homeland and may return to vote when the island's political status is resolved. (Their attachment and identification with the politics of their homeland creates commonalities with the Cuban émigré community.)

As a commonwealth, Puerto Rico isn't a federal state, nor is it a colony or incorporated territory. It is actually autonomous in some ways, but subject to federal control in other ways that limit its ability to deal with internal sociopolitical problems. Those who favor independence, or at least statehood, point to many forms of exploitation and colonialism on the part of the United States, with psychological effects on Puerto Ricans' self-esteem and sense of despair.

American influences are greater in Puerto Rico than in any other Latin American country. The United States is everywhere on the island. Puerto Ricans have two languages, two cultures, two flags, two national anthems, and two basic philosophies of life—dichotomies that did not exist to the same extent when Spain was in possession of the island (Ramos-McKay, Comas-Díaz, & Rivera, 1988). The uneasy, tense, and resigned coexistence of the two cultures and languages has had many confusing consequences for family interactions, not only between the generations and between men and women in the same nuclear family, but between family members who live on the island and those who live on the mainland.

The Anglo-American presence in Puerto Rico significantly altered every aspect of life on the island. An oppressive relationship between colonizer and colonized developed quickly, and one of the first psychological consequences was the importation of a racist disdain for black people. Light-skinned Puerto Ricans, *criollos*, quickly became allied with commercial American interests, cutting down the number of small independent farmers, the *jíbaros*, who became disenfranchised. Without a subsistence economy, and facing scant labor wages, Puerto Ricans began their exodus to the mainland as early as the 1920s. Their migration continues today.

When European migration to the United States ceased after World War I, the opportunities offered to Puerto Ricans were similar to the seasonal farm work offered to Mexicans. Puerto Ricans appeared mostly in the East and the Midwest, but also in Arizona and Utah. During World War II, railroads and a variety of industrial employers attracted Puerto Ricans to the United States once more. The greatest immigration occurred at the end of the war when surplus airplanes and low airfares from Puerto Rico to New York boosted the diaspora movement. Dense colonies formed near workplaces on Manhattan's Lower East Side, Harlem, South Bronx, and Brooklyn. Other major Puerto Rican settlements sprang up in Chicago, Miami, Los Angeles, and Philadelphia.

Although by the 1950s it became evident to Puerto Ricans, and Mexicans, that mainland cities were cold and hostile and did not offer the economic opportunities they had dreamed of, the back and forth flow of migrants has continued, sometimes reaching two million people a year. Periods of high unemployment in Puerto Rico propel islanders to the mainland to look for jobs. When they accumulate small amounts of money on the mainland, Puerto Ricans go back to the island to see their loved ones and nourish their cultural roots. These motivations are similar to those that propel Mexicans back and forth across the border. Although Puerto Ricans, unlike Mexicans, can legally and freely stay on the mainland, return to visit, transact with institutions, or retire back on the island, they remain the poorest of Latinos and suffer even higher unemployment than Mexicans—most likely the result of a long history of pervasive exploitation, discrimination, and institutional racism like that endured by African

Americans. Research shows that Puerto Ricans who migrate to parts of the country other than New York, Texas, or California do better educationally and economically than their counterparts in other centers (Novas, 1994).

Perhaps Puerto Ricans represent more than other Latinos the idea of "transmigrants"—sustaining multiple familial, economic, and social relations that span geographic and cultural borders, aligning their countries of origin with those of settlement. It is a culture of commuting, of constant back and forth (*¿allá? ¿acá?*), a border culture of transfer and doubt between two intertwined zones. The paradox is that although Puerto Ricans are not technically considered immigrants, their uprooting and relocation to the mainland is equivalent to the adaptation experiences of other Latin American, Spanish-speaking groups.

## Cubans

Oh Cuba, so near and yet so unreachable.
—BEHAR AND LEÓN (1994)

Cubans are ideological refugees, seeking to preserve their economic resources and lifestyle. The majority escaped the economic and political changes brought about by the Cuban Revolution in 1959. Previously, around 1930, some Cubans came to the United States in connection with the cigar manufacturing business, but it was really the economic reforms imposed by Fidel Castro's regime in the late 1950s that sent a flood of immigrants from the shores of Cuba to the shores of Florida.

The immigrants who left first in 1959 were those most affected by the new economic regime. This group of upper-class and upper-middle-class Cubans, unlike the economic immigrants from Puerto Rico or from Mexico, came with plentiful educational and occupational resources. Their many assets insured a favorable reception: upper-class financial and political resources, middle-class entrepreneurial skills, privileged (white) skin color, and dissention from Castro's regime that was looked upon favorably by the United States. Thus this group of immigrants was welcomed into Anglo-America with open arms and backed by financial, educational, and job training from the federal government. In fact, Cubans were thought by some to be "model" immigrants because of their economic success in small businesses in such centers as Miami, parts of New Jersey, and New York (Bernal, 1982; Bernal & Gutierrez, 1988).

In spite of those ideal conditions for "Americanization"—assimilating U.S. values and lifestyle—the resettled aristocracy and middle class, old and new, have tried fiercely to re-create traditional Spanish values and the status lifestyle of prerevolutionary Cuba in their Miami enclave. These Cuban exiles are sometimes called *los tenía* (the I-used-to-have people) because they often speak with heartbreaking nostalgia about what they used to have before Castro came to power.

In 1979, in a moment of euphoria, a dialogue began between Castro and a group of Cubans living abroad. This dialogue opened the doors for Cuban U.S. residents to visit their families on the island. The romance ended when thousands of islanders demanded political asylum in the United States and Castro "solved" the problem by ordering the Mariel boatlift, which brought to Miami in 1980 more than 100,000 Cubans. These refugees were more representative than earlier groups of Cuba's full spectrum of race, including a large number of Afro-Caribbeans and Cubans of various social classes and levels of education. Many looked to the United States to improve their economic lot or to reunite their families. A smaller group was composed of gay men. Another group comprised antisocial persons who had been incarcerated in Cuba but came to the United States with the strong, "good riddance" encouragement of a Cuban government that considered them to be the "scum" of the revolution.

A distinctive feature of Cuban migration may have been unwittingly advertised in a 1930s tourist poster that read, "Cuba, so near and yet so foreign." Although Cuba is only 90 miles away from the tip of Florida, it is nearly impossible for its countryfolk to reconnect and update ties with home. As is true for many political refugees, those who left found the doors of their country closed. Divergent ideologies further separate those who stayed and those who left. Compatriots back home call those who left first *gusanos* (worms), because they are regarded as defectors who rejected their country. In reality, the connection of refugees with Cuba has remained and taken different forms during different historical periods.

Azieri (1982) described the Cuban-American experience in two phases. The first one extends from 1959 to 1978; he calls it "de-Cubanization" because of the cutoff with the culture of origin. It prompted vigorous attempts to reconstruct a pre-1959 Cuba in the United States or, in some cases, an uncritical embrace of U.S. values. A second phase, dubbed "re-Cubanization," refers to the brief period of dialogue in 1980 when travel to Cuba temporarily opened up and facilitated the Mariel immigration. These contacts and the new influx of Cubans revitalized cultural roots and exposed old immigrants to contemporary Cuba.

Polarizations between Cubans in their country and Cubans who live elsewhere stem in part from the Cold War mentality of both governments. But today a different dialogue between intellectuals, activists, and artists on both shores is providing a ray of hope. These second-generation Cuban Americans are reclaiming their roots by rejecting their parents' injunction that the bridges between Cuba and the United States be burnt and broken (Behar & León, 1994). Cristina Garcia's novel *Dreaming in Cuban* (1992) is the first novel written in English by a Cuban American that spans borders and gives voice to Cuban women as it tells the tale of three generations of women separated by revolution and exile.

Tensions and hostilities between the United States and Cuban governments continue at full blast in the late 1990s, fueled in part by the U.S. boycott of all imports, exports, and other commerce to and from Cuba. The boycott increasingly strangles, isolates, and starves Cuba's people, with dire emotional consequences for Cubans on the island and their polarized conationals on the mainland.

Cuban, Mexican, and Puerto Rican immigrants have all endured an unpredictable waxing and waning of contact with their homelands, though for different economic and political reasons. These ruptures and renewals have a tremendous impact on psychological well-being and on the ways Latino families seek and experience therapy.

## MIGRATION, PSYCHOLOGICAL DISTRESS, AND HELP SEEKING

Latinos are, by definition, immigrants, and their migration has tremendous psychological consequences. It precipitates multiple losses of deep attachments to family and to supportive networks. The remarkable dissonance between the cultural codes of the old and the new countries is disorienting. While many books, both fiction and nonfiction, have been written about Latinos in the United States, very few address the emotional upheaval and family disruption experienced by these people. The need for such a focus is evident. In fact, the World Health Organization (1979) identified "uprooting" as the common factor in a number of high-risk stressors such as migration, urbanization, resettlement, and rapid social change. Uprooting is associated with substance abuse, depression, crime and delinquency, family conflict and violence, school dropout, and other forms of individual and family breakdown.

In spite of clear links between migration and psychological distress, Latino immigrants rarely seek health care services except for very severe symptoms and emergencies (Rumbaut, Chávez, Moser, Pickwell, & Wishik, 1988; Wells, Hough, Golding, Burnam, & Karno, 1987). Latino families may be reluctant to seek psychological help for less severe symptoms for several reasons: language barriers, lack of money, geographical distance from services (and limited access to transportation), fear of detection by immigration authorities (for those with undocumented status), and fear of being misunderstood culturally or discriminated against racially.

Two different theories suggest why Latinos underutilize social services (Rodrigues, 1987). The "barrier" theory posits that this population may want and need services but has language and cultural difficulties with the impersonal, bureaucratic nature of agencies. In this respect, it makes sense that acculturated Latinos are more likely to use services than the less acculturated (Wells et al., 1987). The "alternative-resource" theory assumes that clients want and need help but turn to their own conational support system with their emotional problems. This may include nontraditional healers like *curanderos, espiritistas,* or herbologists. Sometimes Mexicans take their health, mental, or behavior problems for treatment or support back to their towns in Mexico.

Once offered and accessed, family therapy is easily accepted because it fits with Latino theories about emotional problems, which are regarded as largely due to family conflicts and financial difficulties (Moll, Rueda, Reza, Herrera, & Vásquez, 1976). Even folk or indigenous illnesses are attributed to such interpersonal problems as infidelity or jealousy. To be effective, therapists trained and practicing in the United States need to incorporate specific information about cultural differences and take into account the connections between the social strains suffered by Latino minorities and psychological distress.

As we have seen in this chapter, movement and immigration are part of the cultural narrative of most Latino families, whether that movement is a recent event or part of a family story that began two, three, or more generations ago. MECA provides a flexible, generalist framework to locate and work with subsequent connections between these narratives and a family's distress. As we will see in the next two chapters, the domain of migration is especially key in understanding the experience of many Latino families.

## NOTES

1. With a growing number of Central American refugees entering this country, it seems likely that in the not too distant future more statistics, more research, and other studies focused on Central Americans will emerge. The comparison of three cultures in this book reflects my concordance with Mary Catherine Bateson's (1994) observation that comparing two cultures leads all too readily to regarding one as superior; it is richer and less polarized to compare at least three. Actually, because of the broad comparisons with Anglo-American, middle-class ideals, one might say that there are four cultures being considered in this book.
2. One should note that Brazilians are also Latin Americans and should be thought of as a Latino group, but perhaps because they speak Portuguese rather than Spanish they are seldom thought of as Latinos. Needless to say, this is another unexplained inconsistency (since Portuguese also derives from Latin).
3. The term "Anglo" or "Anglo-American" is used throughout to describe white individuals of non-Hispanic, European ancestry. Terms such as Americans or Euroamericans ignore the fact that Central, South, and other North Americans could just as legitimately be called Americans, as U.S. citizens are commonly called. In fact, Puerto Ricans are U.S. citizens, yet they are not called Americans—most likely because they are not white. The term "white" is also problematic, however, because most Latino racial backgrounds have considerable "white"

in their mixture, and many have considerable European ancestry, but not of Anglo-Saxon origin.

4. There have been many movies made about the immigrant experience on both sides of the border. For a listing and annotated commentaries about independent and Hollywood produced films, consult Maciel, D. R. (1990). *El Norte: The U.S.-Mexican Border in Contemporary Cinema*. San Diego, CA: Institute for the Regional Studies of the California, San Diego State University.

# 4

---

# Journeys of Migration:
# Opportunity and Continuity

"Ay," she says, she is sad.
"Oh," he says, "not again."
"Cuándo, cuándo, cuándo?," she asks.
"Ay, Caray! We are home. This is home.
"Here I am and here I stay. Speak English. Speak English. Christ!"
And then to break her heart forever, the baby boy who has just
begun to talk, starts to sing the Pepsi commercial he heard on TV.
"No speak English," she says to the child, who is singing in the
language that sounds like tin. "No speak English, no speak English,"
and bubbles into tears. "No, no, no," as if she can't believe her ears.
— CISNEROS (1994, p. 78)

## THE MIGRATION NARRATIVE

The process of leaving one's home country and encountering a new one
constitutes an overlapping of events, developmental changes, and existential tasks that render a very unique "phenomenology of migration." This
subjective experience can best be understood and shaped by the family
through a "migration narrative." The construction of such a narrative in a
therapeutic setting reveals the personal meanings of migration events and
processes for each family and for individual family members.

Starting with a migration narrative with recent immigrants establishes
a frame of reference and provides an invitation to explore the premigration experience, the migration proper, and encounters with cultural transition. Therapists can begin by asking how long the individual or family has

been here, who immigrated first and who was left behind or came later, and who is yet to be reunited.

While addressing questions about the premigration and entry experience, the migration narrative provides a tool to explore the motivations behind the move, the sense of responsibility of the people who initiated the process, their hopes and regrets, their choice points, the ordeals suffered to get here, the attachments to those family members who stayed and those who had already left, and the reception by those who were already here. Questions about how family members are learning the new language and culture can provide an avenue to tap interpersonal synchronies, discontinuities, imbalances, or injustices. The next sections present salient phenomena of clinical relevance to this stage such as coaxed migrations, ambivalent or unprepared migrations, posttraumatic stress following migration, and the impact of family members and friends on the lives of immigrant clients.

## THE PREMIGRATION AND ENTRY EXPERIENCE

### Coaxed Migrations and Rebalancing Contracts

Often there is a subtle, gendered, and generational line between voluntary and coaxed migrations. Many immigrants are not equal participants in the decision to migrate. Coaxed participants may include children, the elderly who come to join their adult children, or women in asymmetrical marriages who reluctantly follow their husbands. These individuals may experience many more difficulties in adjustment than those who actively choose to migrate. When it is possible to distinguish "leader" from "follower," the party responsible for initiating the migration may need to exert extra effort to help make the reluctant immigrant's situation more emotionally desirable and comfortable.

In my own experience, getting a higher education was the most ambitious, cherished goal of my youth. Education wasn't part of my growing up. In the Eastern European ghettos of their childhood, my parents had not gone to elementary school. And they did not think a girl needed to be educated, in the old or the new land. I was fiercely determined that my life would be different. Yet, ironically, with a very heavy heart, I left my university studies at age 19 to get married and dutifully follow my husband wherever his life, or in this case, his postgraduate studies, took him.

Just prior to the wedding and sailing off to the States, I had a huge emotional crisis. It seemed to me that no man and no wedding could be so important as to abandon many years of so solitary and unsupported an effort that was so close to fruition. I refused to go on with the wedding and migration plans. My fiance was beside himself. He took it as proof that my love for him was less than complete, or as evidence of a cold-heartedness he had not detected before. Yet he did not join forces with my family, and instead pleaded directly with me. He willingly accepted a compromise and we secretly wrote a prenuptual agreement: I was to follow him to do his medical internship in Chicago for 1 year, but he would not recontract to start a medical training residency after that year unless I agreed completely to do so. And I would agree to the continuation of his training only if I had certainty that I too could continue my own studies in the United States. If the latter was not feasible, we both would return to Argentina where I would complete my degree. Or, if we could not reach an agreement, we vowed to part amicably. I worked full-time as a file clerk in the hospital medical records department during the day. Within 4 months I began attending night school and "moonlighted" as an electrocardiogram technician. My husband worked more than full-time as a medical intern. After 6 months I became a graduate teaching assistant with full-time tuition paid. Although it meant the loss of my income and living on my husband's intern salary, we both agreed to honor the plan we'd made of my resuming my study.

Over the years, this story has helped me to understand that an alternative, clearly thought out, and agreed upon plan for staying or returning is empowering, even if those plans are "as if" and never materialize. Such plans help family members who feel coaxed into migration and who have reservations about the move. Further, plans help assuage the guilt of the "brave ones" who are seemingly ready to take the plunge. Indeed, it helps them to think more carefully and to have a way out in case their dreams fizzle.

A contracted, "conditional option" to return home can be beneficial in therapy cases involving wives who migrated reluctantly, mostly to follow their "fearless" husbands. While these situations were already under way (the migration had already taken place), the newly devised contract can still create a trial period for everyone. Paradoxically, permission to feel and even indulge in one's obsession to return or not return "home" helps create stability during a period that is unstable and transitory by nature. The idea of both partners making an effort to acquire a more favorable—even temporary—life situation for the wife in this country usually becomes part of the agreement. This migration "rebalancing contract" may involve clear-cut efforts on the husband's part to support the wife's needs, as shown in the following therapy case.

Three months after her husband prevailed in his efforts to have her join him in the States, Remedios, a young mother of two, developed intense tingling throughout her body, particularly in her extremities for the first time in her life. Physical tests ordered by her physician to detect possible organic disease were negative. Finally, a psychiatrist ventured a diagnosis of "somatizing delusions," a DSM-III classification, and referred Remedios to me.

The migration narrative revealed that Remedios was feeling anxious and guilty about having left Socorro, her younger sister, unsupported back home in Patzcúaro, Michoacán, Mexico. Socorro had just had a baby as the result of a sexually abusive relationship with an intimidating uncle, a violent relationship Remedios feared might continue in an even more uncontrolled fashion after she left. Remedios had felt dragged into migration and her tingling only abated when her husband agreed to her request that he go back in person to fetch Socorro and her baby.

In this case I assumed a psychoeducational role, first discussing the different psychological consequences between voluntary migrations that had a great deal of certainty and decisiveness behind them and coaxed migrations that were accompanied by doubts and reluctance. Gender differences in relational and task orientations were also discussed because the husband tended to minimize Remedios's loyalty obligations toward her sister. The husband's empathy was enlisted more readily when going over the steps and feelings involved in his own migration story. This recounting with an emphasis on feelings revealed how lonely he felt and how worried he had been in the past about Remedios and the children.

Latinos generally balk at task-oriented therapeutic techniques such as homework assignments, contracts, behavioral experiments, or communication exercises. Perhaps this type of approach is too impersonal or too pragmatic or contrived rather than spontaneously stemming from the flow of a relationship. However, a "rebalancing migration contract" is usually readily accepted, perhaps because, like other immigrants, Latinos understand the monumental effects of migration on a person who is asked to embrace the journey when they are not quite ready for it. In fact, the person who initiated the migration may feel somewhat relieved of guilt with an agreement that emphasizes shared responsibility. The contract also provides a sense of security with its mutual contingency plan. Reparations help redress the unevenness of the migration decision and are accepted as part of the rebalancing plan—such was the case when Remedios's husband returned to Mexico to fetch her sister.

## Ambivalent, Unprepared Migrations

Ambivalent and unprepared migrations share some similarities with coaxed migrations. Many older immigrants experience a confluence between premigration events and life cycle stresses such as illness, old age, or the loss of a spouse. This often creates confusion and ambivalence over readiness to migrate, even if it is for the joyful purpose of joining their adult children. Sometimes this uncertainty is exacerbated by an ambivalent reception by some of the host country family members, which creates a very difficult, shameful situation.

An illustration is the case of Mrs. Santos, who arrived in San Diego via a complicated set of circumstances outside of her control. Although she had lived all her life in Puerto Rico, she came to New York to be close to her daughter, Juana (51), when Mrs. Santos's husband retired. A year later Juana married for the third time. Juana's husband, John, was Canadian and wanted to return to Canada. Shortly after they settled in Toronto, Juana moved her parents to Canada. A month after this move, Mr. Santos died suddenly of a heart attack. Juana wanted to have her mother come live with her and John, but he refused. He said it was stretching his generosity too much. In his cultural view of family organization he believed that having his wife's mother in the same house was a likely formula for destroying the new marriage, regardless of how pleasant Mrs. Santos might be.

Juana, feeling protective of this relationship and following her own cultural views of relying on family help, asked Maggie, her single daughter, to take Mrs. Santos to live with her in San Diego. Maggie was a dutiful daughter and she loved her grandmother, but Mrs. Santos was difficult to care for. Although she was very sweet and accommodating, she spoke no English, did not drive and, having migrated so late in her life, did not understand how anything worked, from home appliances to transportation. Mrs. Santos appeared to be in culture shock, forgetful and disoriented, grieving, often weeping and calling for her husband.

The second migration in Mrs. Santos's life, from New York to Canada, had taken place shortly after the one from Puerto Rico to New York. This second move abruptly intersected with a major life cycle change, the death of her lifelong companion. This devastating loss aggravated the fact that as an elderly person she already had very limited alternatives for acculturation. Nonetheless, a medical consultation was necessary to rule out organic components of her symptoms and to consider antidepressant medication.

As a single woman, Maggie needed help in carving out some space and time for herself. The therapist helped her develop network and neighborhood resources that could relieve her from being her grandmother's sole caretaker and sole translator, of both language and culture.

Close attention to premigration family dynamics and events throws light on the unique meanings and psychological readiness of various family members for the momentous, all-encompassing journey of migration. By listening carefully to the details of each migration experience—before, during, and after the move—we gain clues to the meaning of symptoms and the impediments to adaptation.

## Posttraumatic Stress and *Testimonio*

Most Latino immigrants are men who come alone to explore the territory and save or send back some money before they bring their wives and children. Increasingly, more women, often heads of households, are making the journey alone. They plan to work and send money home for their children, hoping to reunite the family in this country in the future.

Posttraumatic stress has been observed in both men and women, particularly if migration involved trauma. Many Mexican women (and some men) are raped and robbed while attempting to cross the border, often by smugglers (*coyotes* or *polleros*) who promised to help them for an agreed-upon sum of money (Zamichow, 1992). Cases have also been reported of women being physically and sexually abused by employers, usually an older man who pays for a woman's transportation after promising to employ her as a domestic. But upon arrival he exploits her by making her work without pay and by abusing her sexually. Recurring nightmares, dreams, feelings of guilt and shame, phobias, or panic attacks may appear shortly after these entry experiences or at some later date.

Consequently it's important to obtain a migration narrative that includes details of the crossing, transportation, and entry, even from people who have been in this country for several years. The narrative tool called *testimonio* (testimony) involves a first-person oral or written (perhaps by the therapist or another family member) account focused on validating personal experiences of loss, trauma, and abuse. It is extremely valuable in dealing with the consequences of traumatic migrations for women, men, and children. Testimony is an avenue for reworking the painful experiences, but also for regaining *dignidad* (dignity) and *respeto* (respect) (Aron, 1992; Comas-Díaz, 1995).

## THE UPROOTING OF MEANING

My own "root" metaphor for migration, survival, and adaptation is that when we pluck a plant from the earth, some residue of soil always remains attached to the roots. Gardeners replant the plant in the new soil with this residue included, and perhaps this small amount of soil contributes to the success of the transplantation. Although immigrants no longer have the depth and the expanse of the native soil to nourish their roots constantly, the little bit of original native dirt is represented in the type of household one creates, the children one raises, the language one speaks, the foods one cooks, and the friendships one cherishes. When indulging in occasional sentimental moments, I believe these little bits of old soil eventually mix and integrate with the new soil to give its particular fruits and flowers.

Perhaps the most fundamental and disruptive consequence of migration is the uprooting of cultural meanings. Peter Marris (1980), an urban ecologist, suggests that the closest human counterpart to the root structure that nourishes a plant is the structure of meanings by which people sustain relationships to a physical, social, and cultural reality that provides familiarity and stability. With the disruption of lifelong attachments and stabilities, meanings are uprooted internally and externally. For immigrants, even voluntary ones, such as most Mexicans and Puerto Ricans, a complex involvement in those contexts is disrupted, uprooting large areas of physical and emotional stability.

Migration involves at least three forms of uprooting of meaning systems: physical, social, and cultural (Shuval, 1982). Each of these has psychological implications and potential clinical manifestations.

## Physical Uprooting

Physical uprooting entails living without the familiarity of people's faces and the sound of their voices, without the feel of the streets and the comfort of the houses, without the odors of the foods, the myriad smells, sounds, and sights, the cold and the heat of the air, without the color of the sun, or the configuration of stars in the night sky. The landscape that had been internal as well as external—a very part of the immigrant's soul—is gone. All is changed now. Imagine the move from a sleepy little rural village in Latin America to a bustling American metropolis. Even if you could reinvent yourself, how do you reinvent a whole physical, social, and cultural landscape?

I remember one of my first therapy clients, a newly married young woman who had come from Puerto Rico to accompany her husband. He was a new graduate student at the University of Chicago. She was very depressed and missed her home and her country very much. She kept repeating that it was like starting all over again, having to learn everything from scratch, to read, write, bank, shop for food. I felt her pain as we explored details. I told her that, for me too, when I first came to this country, it was so much like starting all over again. Even simple behaviors were no longer automatic. I felt, for example, I had to learn to walk from scratch. I was accustomed to Buenos Aires's streets—the large tiles, full of bumps and cracks. Growing up there, I had found over the years exactly the right angle that allowed me to look both up and down simultaneously to avoid either falling down or bumping into something or somebody. The streets in the States were too flat and smooth, too clean and intact. There was no need to look down. I missed the bumps.

And then there was the Chicago weather. My body resisted the extreme conditions. I remembered standing one night, for what seemed an eternity, on a corner waiting for a bus in minus-18 degree temperature. In my mind I said goodbye to everyone I knew, certain that death would overtake me right then and there, before the bus could rescue me from a cold I never fathomed could exist.

As I relayed these anecdotes to my client, she cried for a long time. I could not help but join her. Later she told me that the memories of that session made a difference for her. She felt she had received permission to feel her feelings. Up until then she had told herself that something was wrong, that she was too weak and dependent, that she was having too much sadness, too much difficulty liking it here and finding a way to adjust, that she should get over it already, as her husband had told her to do on so many occasions.

It may be important at this early stage of migration to recover physical aspects of the familiar within the home—searching in the stores of the new city for the ingredients to cook typical dishes, listening to music typical of one's land, writing to and receiving letters from family and friends, keeping diaries, concretizing life memories to be woven and embroidered into the new, developing tapestry. These forms of memory re-creation are not only healing, they also represent the beginning of developing a bicultural lifestyle.

In *The Teachings of Don Juan*, Carlos Castaneda (1972) gives a poignant example of the primary need for a "home" and how often this elusive experience is attached to some concrete element that evokes security for the traveler. When Castaneda visits Don Juan to begin his spiritual journey, Don Juan tells him that he is not ready to begin yet. Disappointed, Castaneda insists on being told what he needs to do. Don Juan responds that he must find a spot he can call home, and this would be revealed in a clear feeling or an unmistakable sensation. To Castaneda, it proves to be a daunting task. Determined to find "home," he goes inside and outside the house hoping for revelations at every step and turn, day and night. Frustrated to the point of despair, Castaneda finally falls asleep upon a rock that had been warmed by the sun right outside Don Juan's house. The following morning he approaches Don Juan and tells him about his failure and his feeling that he must move on to find "home" elsewhere. Don Juan exclaims that there is no need for any more searching: in letting go of his vigilance and trusting the rock that supported his sleep, Castaneda had found "home."

## Social Uprooting

Social uprooting from a human network of relationships compounds the sense of physical alienation and intrapsychic confusion. Social marginality and social isolation (Johnston, 1976), which relates to decreased self-esteem and depression (Warheit, Vega, Auth, & Meinhardt, 1985), are part of the immigrant's lot. There may be numerous breaks in the immigrants' social attachments with compatriots in the country they left (Sluzki, 1989). Or the new immigrants may have migrated into an already settled network of family and friends. Some immigrants may have left a difficult, oppressive family environment, unfair work conditions, or a societal situation that was very stressful, and the immediate feeling of relief, of being free and unencumbered may be stronger than the sense of loss. In some cases, the separation from kin, particularly for young people who feel engulfed or controlled by their parents, is experienced as exhilarating initially, yet it may become disturbing after a period of time or after experiencing difficulties establishing new social ties.

> Such was the case of a young Jewish Mexican middle-class woman, Raquel Bolsky, who gladly followed her husband when he came to California to open a water filter business. Two years later she felt very lonely and depressed and wanted to return home. She described her migration as having been partially motivated to free herself from the smothering love and controlling involvement of her parents. Raquel actually made a remarkably fast, positive adaptation to San Diego. This adaptation had been greatly aided by her participation in a new social network of neighbors. These were all young mothers who had formed a mother-child play group. After 18 months of continuous involvement in this group of four women, who were all immigrants from different countries, Raquel had a nasty falling out with one of them. Apparently Raquel had made a comment about the dark skin color[1] of one of the babies. The other young mothers considered it a racist remark, and Raquel felt she had to leave the group. When this crucial support and modeling peer network was cut off, Raquel felt she would never be accepted or have a solid sense of belonging. She began to feel desperately homesick for her lifelong family and friends.

Helping clients mobilize themselves to find support groups among people with common interests or needs—such as child care, church, sports, reading, cooking, either in the ethnic neighborhood or the larger culture—can ease the loneliness and provide valuable information. English as a second language classes (ESL) are often a first avenue to meet other immigrants in similar situations.

## Cultural Uprooting

Cultural uprooting is the third experience in which meanings are changed or lost. Personal stories and views of reality are anchored in the lived experiences of one's gender, race, ethnicity, and social class as they were infused with meanings in the cultural settings of origin. The uprooting of established ways of thinking and doing, and the massive, abrupt exposure to a new language and new way of life precipitate psychological distress, usually subsumed under the generic term "culture shock" (Furnham & Bochner, 1986; Garza-Guerrero, 1974).

Culture shock is a reactive process that results from the coexistence of two factors: the disconcerting, stressful, anxiety-producing encounter with a new culture, paired with a painful mourning for the loss of every physical, social, and cultural aspect of the old culture. Stress is always involved in migration if one considers that "stress occurs when an individual confronts a situation where his usual modes of behavior are insufficient and the consequences of not adapting are serious" (House, 1974, p. 12).

## Psychological Consequences of Uprooting

Anxiety related symptoms such as bioendocrine stress, acute psychoses, panic attacks, agoraphobia, and alcohol- and drug-related problems and dissociative conditions may occur during these early phases of culture shock (Westermeyer, 1989). Somatizations such as palpitations (*piquetes*), dizziness, nervousness, and insomnia are common. It seems possible that these symptoms have accompanied immigrants at other times and places. In the 16th century, the physician Maimonides coined the term "nostalgia," from the Greek *nosos* (knowledge) and *algia* (pain), to denote a malady or syndrome that he observed in immigrants and that in his opinion could be fatal. It consisted of heart palpitations, weeping, moaning and lamenting, sweating, shaking and other nervous tics or symptoms, writhing and rolling in pain, and crying for home. The cure? Return the patient to the "known" (home) immediately.

It's difficult to ascertain whether Latinos, and Puerto Ricans in particular, may be culturally inclined to express emotional problems somatically. A social stress theory suggests that the emotional stresses of poverty and migration are difficult to articulate or beyond awareness. It may also be that emotional pain is more difficult to admit to strangers than complaining about a health problem (Canino, Rubio-Stipec, Canino, & Escobar, 1992).

Nevertheless, therapists shouldn't be too eagerly reductionistic about the psychological consequences of migration, as the following case consultation illustrates.

A psychiatrist diagnosed a woman who was experiencing persistent unbearable itching as suffering from a conversion disorder—a psychosomatic, "pruritus-like" delusion—that was posttraumatic to migration. This is a rare symptom that has been found in some immigrants. The woman was a Cuban, middle-class married professional who had been able to leave Cuba with her family 5 years before. During her evaluation, she had several "culturally" flavored theories for her symptoms.

Her preferred theory was that her Salvadorean maid[2] was giving her the evil eye out of envy and was purposely washing her sheets and towels with abrasive irritants. Another theory was revealed to her through the lips of a statue of her patron saint while she was praying. The saint had hinted that the itching was punishment for her sinful thoughts. As the medical team began to wonder if incipient psychosis might be involved, a dermatologist sent her to an internist who was the first to discover that this Cuban woman had gotten silicon breast implants as part of her "new life" when she first arrived in this country. The implants had recently broken and the fluid had entered her bloodstream, causing the itching.

*GROSS*

In securing a migration narrative that includes the three types of uprooting—physical, social, and cultural—it is best not to get bogged down by contradictions about dates or places or events about the time or place of entry. The family's vagueness may be an attempt to conceal their illegal entry or status, or the extent of their hardships back home. Talking about the first weeks and months in this country generally elicits no inhibitions or hesitations, but rather welcome relief. The therapists' reading of the family's emotional response to these questions, plus collaborative decision making with the family, should determine how far to go and when to stop the process of narration. For some families it may be too soon and too painful to review the experience of physical, social, and cultural uprooting, for others it may prove cathartic.

## Uprooting and Family Polarization

Immigrants often arrive with a set of preconceived notions about what the new culture has to offer. After the initial culture shock, those notions are either confirmed or exploded. Disillusionment is commonplace. Depression often sets in, and the old culture is likely to become idealized. Material connections with the past may be sought, sometimes for prolonged periods —familiar foods, music, clothing, the native language. But an opposite reaction can occur as well. That is, aspects of the old country may be rejected, denigrated, viewed as inferior, deficient. These reactions may be divided between family members, often husband and wife, who assume opposite views with respect to the new country (Sluzki, 1979). These polarized, conflicting positions are usually reactive and temporary but sometimes become rigid and chronic, persisting far beyond the initial adaptation phase. They appear as truncated mourning processes that get in the way of integrating emotional identifications with the old and the new cultures (Grinberg & Grinberg, 1989; Shuval, 1982). The polarization of emotional reactions to the uprooting is a common clinical presentation.

When emotions and views about the uprooting become polarized, parts of the self appear to be dissociated or denied and often projected onto another person. These polarizations deserve special attention for relational therapists because they may involve two or more family members who play out their denied or suppressed internal processes in their external relationships. The distress of the uprooting often inclines family members to take sides, either idealizing or denigrating the native and the host countries or supporting decisions to stay or return home. These problems may present as runaway escalations between husbands and wives, or may be discovered in conjunction with other symptoms, such as a behavioral problem in a child or depression in one of the spouses.

Juanita and Nemesio had been married for 3 years when the husband's business in the small town of La Parguera, Puerto Rico, suffered a serious setback and he decided to immigrate "temporarily" to improve their economic situation. Like many of his countrymen, he came alone first to explore the situation before bringing Juanita and their two young children. When they arrived, Juanita took an instant dislike to the United States. She adamantly refused to learn English, because, as she put it, she wanted to "create a barrier" with this country. She was afraid that if she learned the language or got used to living here, they would never go back. Juanita waited anxiously for daily letters from her mother and sister.

The more Juanita disliked this country, the more Nemesio tried to make her see that she was exaggerating the differences between the two countries and the happiness they could have back home. Money matters became another focus of the conflict. The couple blamed each other for not making enough, or for spending too much. They told me that in the midst of one of those symmetrical escalations, Juanita had gone back to Puerto Rico for a short visit and ended up staying for 3 months before returning to the United States.

As the therapist, I faced a dilemma. It was clear that the couple was immobilized, unable to reach common decisions because any course of action toward collaboration or toward continuous conflict by one would be construed by the other as proof of commitment to, or alternatively, to lack of commitment to acculturation. I felt equally torn as to what would be best for them (in my own subjectivity, the wisdom of people's decisions about voluntary migrations, including my own, has never come to a resting place). But, of course, I did not conceive my role as to favor their staying or returning. I could only elaborate on the dilemma. To overcome this impasse, I suggested a "moratorium" in the form of a truce and trial period of 1 year. (Only later did I realize that this was the same solution my husband and I had attempted years earlier.)

Juanita and Nemesio agreed to experiment with this moratorium, during which all the behaviors engaged by husband or wife could be cooperatively negotiated on the basis of their potential benefit for "human adaptation and enrichment" in any country. For example, if the wife were to learn English, or take on a part-time job, these could be regarded as useful skills (or "money in the bank")—in any country, all important experiences for a young woman to have. On the other hand, if the husband was to spend more time with his isolated wife, and learn to participate in household chores and child care, this could be construed as gaining the experience of acting as a "modern" husband, an important practice for a young man.

The importance of maintaining necessary continuities, the wisdom of "no change," and of not overburdening an already unstable or taxing situation with quick solutions or more suggestions for permanent "adaptive" change, even if it means to continue to be "in limbo" somewhat longer, has been illustrated with clinical examples elsewhere (Montalvo & Gutiérrez, 1989; Falicov, 1993).

Immigrant couples can profit from temporarily anchoring one side of their ambivalence about leaving or staying, adapting or not adapting, learning or not learning. Interventions include suggesting the client practice or "pretend" to stay or to leave; or suggesting they purposely do some things "as if" they were in the old country, even at the risk of being seen by others as old-fashioned; or suggesting they practice doing things in the way of the new country, even at the risk of being thought of by conationals as disloyal or too Anglo.

The odd days/even days technique of the Milan group (Selvini Palazzoli, 1978), which "prescribes the symptom" by alternating both sides of the polarizations, is another option. In cases of polarization where it's clear that one family member has been pressured to migrate (or to stay behind), rebalancing contracts that make restitution are suggested also. All these interventions highlight the need for continuity while encouraging an experimental attitude about change. This situation creates a *both/and* mindset and win/win assets.

## PLAYERS IN THE MIGRATION DRAMA: RUPTURE AND RENEWAL

Migration is not an experience that belongs solely to the immigrant, nor does an immigrant move in isolation from the attitudes and influences of family and friends. Indeed, migration has repercussions and implications for several groups: those who leave their homes, the relatives left behind, the relatives already waiting in the new country, and the people of the host culture. A migration narrative necessarily includes attention to the complex interactions of these players.

### Those Left Behind

Most discussions of migration focus only on the immigrants, but those who are left behind are not untouched by this momentous transition. The reactions of those who remain behind are diverse. Inevitably there is a sense of loss when loved ones migrate. The sadness may be compounded by anger toward the departing persons because they may be emotionally, if not rationally, perceived as abandoning their parents, siblings, and friends. One should expect a mourning process to occur in those who are left behind as well as in those who leave. It's even possible that given their forced passivity, those who stay may suffer with greater intensity than the immigrants themselves, who are busy with the adaptations and the novelty of the new land and life. Some feel envy, yet hope to benefit from the gains of the departed ones. For others, envy may take the form of hostility or depression, increasing the guilt already felt by those who have left.

Occasionally those who remain, particularly parents, are the ones overtaken by self-reproach, attributing to themselves or their spouses' responsibility for the decision of the son or daughter to leave. At a recent workshop I gave in Athens, Greece, I was surprised by the intensity of the emotional reactions of participants who had lost relatives to migration to the United States. Many were grieving the loss, which often represented an irrevocable end to a complete family group, a counted-upon shared life. The stresses brought about by these losses are often connected to somatizations, illnesses, or hypochondriacal reactions that appear shortly after a loved one's departure, and sometimes represent attempts to maintain contact or control over those who leave. Grinberg and Grinberg (1989) give the most comprehensive account of these processes, including those involving children.

## Separations and Reunions of Family Members

A common pattern of Latino migration that dismantles family organization involves separation of one or more children from their parents and siblings during migration. These could be younger or older children left behind for economic or practical reasons, but also for less conscious motivations that involve guilt, loyalty, or separation anxiety with the family of origin of one of the parents.

For practical and economic reasons, a father often migrates first, and as a consequence his wife reorganizes into a one-parent unit supported by the extended family back in Mexico or Puerto Rico. When the couple reunites they must undergo a second reorganization, analogous in some ways to the incorporation of a stepfather. Or father may become increasingly more rigid in his attempts to recover his authority.

Disruption and reconstitution of family structures also come about when single mothers migrate alone. They often employ themselves as domestics to send money to support their children, while their own mothers and/or sisters remain back home as functional parents for the children. When she returns for visits, the single mother may be treated like an older sibling by her children and by her own mother. If she manages to bring them to this country after monumental efforts, she may be the distant stranger in the family, or alternatively, enter into intense overt or covert conflicts both with her mother and her own children.

The separation of an immigrant parent and child has several common consequences. Children who are left behind by their immigrant parents may react with symptoms of depression, nightmares, school failure, eating problems (under- or overeating, vomiting), or somatic complaints. Or they may show symptoms for the first time upon reunion, often an attempt to become the focus of the parents' concern and affection once more. Separation of parent and child also tends to solidify the child's ties with the new caretaker, and by extension, with the entire maternal or paternal line, but weakens the attachment with the biological parent. Family separation often calls for careful planning and much more continued contact in the care of children than is realistically possible for many immigrants.

Reincorporation of the child is often traumatic for all involved, and integration of the "new" family may be slow and protracted. As we saw in the case of 6-year-old Yolanda Díaz Ortiz, who was separated from her parents from the age of two, Yolanda refused to eat her mother's food for the first few months after she reunited with her parents, a behavior which prompted her father to hit her. The following case of Puerto Rican Juan Sandoval bears strong similarities. It is described extensively here because it illustrates the construction of a "catching-up life narrative," a therapeutic tool that is helpful in dealing with transitions by highlighting the emotional consequences of the ruptures and renewals of family ties.

## The Construction of a Catching-Up Life Narrative

Juan Sandoval, a 7-year-old Puerto Rican boy, had suffered a mild problem of encopresis from a very young age in his native country. The family never became concerned about this issue. In the past 6 months, however, the soiling had increased from once a day, to five or six times a day. His postural tension about elimination had also increased. (His 2-year-old sister, Jazmín, was fully toilet trained.) While his father, Mr. Sandoval, appeared stern and distant from the boy, the mother, Mrs. Sandoval, was very attentive and affectionate. She regularly tied Juan's shoes, cut his meat, helped him with homework, and lay down in bed with him to help him fall asleep.

At the same time, Mrs. Sandoval had long harbored resentment toward her husband. When Juan was 2 years old, Mr. Sandoval had yielded to his own mother's insistent request that Juan remain in Puerto Rico with her because "she loved him so much." In going along with her wishes, Mr. Sandoval was complying with hierarchical norms that discourage challenging one's own mother, at any age. Mrs. Sandoval did not want to leave Juan, but she could not oppose her husband's family, which also had better resources to take care of Juan than they themselves would have at the time of migration.

About 3 years later, Juan was brought to the United States to join his parents. Juan did not recognize his mother and continued to call his grandmother "Mamá." To win back her son, Mrs. Sandoval became a "super Mamá." Juan was aware of the power he had over his mother. Whenever father tried to discipline the boy, or suggested that mother should punish him (i.e., for soiling his pants), the boy would weep and ask his mother if his father did not love him and preferred his sister Jazmín instead. An upset Mrs. Sandoval would then reassure Juan of their love for him and criticize the father. Cultural support for viewing a good mother as the children's protector against the father made Mrs. Sandoval feel justified in her behavior. Mr. Sandoval also saw nothing unusual and did not complain about this protective stance by his wife. (His own father had been very strict, and his mother had acted as the mediator between father and children, a culturally sanctioned pattern that we will revisit later in this book.)

During the second session, the Sandovals mentioned that a few months prior to therapy they had been planning a Christmas visit to Puerto Rico to see the paternal grandmother. Through these conversations, the parents became aware for the first time about the traumas of separation and reunions for Juan. It seemed possible to me that the recent dramatic increase in Juan's symptoms could be related to anticipatory anxiety about visiting his country and family, a common experience of immigrants.

The future trip provided an avenue for a "catching-up life narrative," co-constructed with Juan and his parents. The story was geared to weave the elements of Juan's life during the first two years when his parents were living in El Yunque beaches, then reviewing and relating Juan's move to his paternal grandparents' home when his parents left, and eventually getting to his arrival and adaptation to the mainland for the past one and one-half years. This was done through drawings of the houses Juan had lived in, while developing a story that I wrote down paragraph by paragraph,[3] repeating the basic facts and relevant details, beginning with "Juan Sandoval was born on the 3rd of September of 1988 in El Yunque, Puerto Rico. Present at the time of his birth were . . . He lived in a house with two bedrooms . . . Juan's parents, Edmundo and Sarita Sandoval, left for the United States to find work. . . . " I read the entire story every time, and I added two or three paragraphs every time, asking if everybody agreed with the contents and phrasing. My questions explored descriptions, comparisons, and meanings of what happened inside the houses room by room, including public and private spaces, such as toilet rooms. We all learned together, for the first time, that in Puerto Rico grandmother had taken Juan regularly to sit on the toilet while she stood by him. Migration had changed that familiar routine.

As it turns out, Juan had lived in six houses, two with his parents when he was an infant, then two more after they left for the United

States (Juan had lived temporarily with an uncle to relieve the grand-mother, who had to take care of her sick husband, and at times had lit-tle patience with Juan's rambunctiousness), and then two more since he had arrived in the United States. In our conversations, clear deline-ations were made of external motives (to dispel a meaning of rejection) as to why Juan was moved from one home to the next. This narrative construction went on until we got to the motives behind and expecta-tions of the planned trip to Puerto Rico.

Juan seemed very unclear about why they were all going, other than that it was Christmas. It seemed possible that Juan feared being left back in Puerto Rico again, a threat sometimes hurled by his father when he got angry, so I suggested we continue the storytelling, future forward, and writing until the beginning of the new year in California when the family would have returned from their visit. Among other events, we talked about preparations for Juan's first Holy Communion, a ritual with many important developmental implications. This scenario included talking about all the feelings, and the objects, and other me-mentos they would bring back with them from Puerto Rico.[4] Slowly Juan's fears and generalized anxiety decreased and he regained much better control of his bowels.

Several healing transformations were involved in the storytelling for this family. The father's empathy and tenderness for Juan increased tre-mendously, the mother's competitiveness with her mother-in-law dissolved, and the parents seemed to gain a better existential perspective by recapitu-lated their own migration story. The child's life narrative somehow seemed to consolidate the Sandovals as a foursome with the parents working to-gether. Each person was more in charge of themselves, less fragmented. In our last session together, Mr. Sandoval said: "This is our home now, maybe we can have our whole body here now, rather than one piece, one foot there and one foot here . . . we do not have to leave a trail everywhere we go anymore . . . we are going to deposit ourselves here." One could hear these words as being strangely evocative of the issues behind Juan's separa-tion, and perhaps even his soiling.

When families reunite, other problems arise from the contrasts in childcare routines and styles between the biological parents and the grand-parents, aunts, or uncles entrusted with caretaking, which may result in confusing messages for the child. The case that follows illustrates this di-lemma and the reshuffling of family roles at the time of reunion.

Margarita Alonso was a 31-year-old woman who came to therapy with her mother, Alma Alonso, 68, her sons, Cristóbal, 10, and Raymundo, 8. The children called their revered grandmother *abuelita* and their mother, Margarita or Maggy. One year ago they had all been reunited in San Di-ego. Eight years prior, Margarita had left Guanajuato, Mexico, to find work in the United States, and had entrusted the care of her children to her mother. After several jobs as a housemaid, Margarita found a full-time position at a large laundry facility and was able to find work in the same place for her mother. At the time of their consultation, both women were working different shifts and caring for the children. But Margarita could not handle Cristóbal. He was provocative, disobedient, and behaved like a stereotypical masculine tyrant, demanding to know of his mother's whereabouts.

The therapist, who was a Latina single mother like Margarita, had assumed that a Latina grandmother with her familistic orientation would be very happy to have the family reunited. The assumption was quite incorrect. Not only had Alma lost all her cherished places and her home in Mexico, she had disapproved of Margarita's migration all along. In her view, good women have no business living alone, having the freedom to go out with men unsupervised. Although Alma had never told Margarita directly how she felt (in order to preserve harmony), she would often bitterly unload these thoughts onto the children, particularly Cristóbal, who was the most receptive.

The therapy provided an open forum for communication between Alma and Margarita about their past 10 years, as two women taking care of children, each with her own function and both bridging two countries. Margarita recognized that although she loved her children, her lack of experience and skills made her vulnerable to not being respected as an authority. Alma, meanwhile, was elevated through the therapy to the same importance she had had in the village; she was designated as the only person who could coach Margarita on dealing with her children by catching up with anecdotes and details about the children's development and personalities.

As the case above illustrates, the adults experience their own share of tensions and stresses. Grandmother's ability to cope with the stresses and multiple burdens of raising several children may be limited, but she may feel many cultural and economic constraints against refusing to perform the caretaker role. Thus she may express her stress only indirectly, by complaining about her nerves or about health problems, often to the children left under her care. (For further description of this case, see Chapter 9.)

While grandmothers and sisters deal with responsibilities of substitute caretaking in the countries of origin, immigrant mothers search for ways to deal with the anxiety and sadness associated with separation, displacement, and their own loneliness. They may use medical facilities and medication frequently for symptoms of insomnia or for "heartache."

## Coping with Absences: No Pensar

One common psychic mechanism for coping with worries about absent children is *no pensar* (not to think too much). The avoidance of thinking about sadness is closely related to other culturally based forms of dealing with emotion such as *aguantar* (to bear, or to suffer in silence), *sobreponerse no need to deconstruct the defense?*

(overcoming oneself), or *controlarse* (control of the self). These various coping styles are described in Chapter 8. This culturally influenced pattern of
coping with anxiety by attempting to avoid disturbing thoughts (which may
be a form of cognitive control or even denial) is sometimes successful, but
not always. Other symptoms may appear in the same women who claim not
to think much about the situation they left behind (Cohen, 1980). Therapists need to be sensitive to this culturally common psychological defense
of the lonely mother (or father) and respect her wish not to enter into the
details of her emotional pain about the past and the present. If this is the
case, a catching-up or migration narrative may not be indicated: A future-
oriented approach that helps gear present efforts to eventual reunion can
provide welcome relief and reality testing about issues to be resolved in pav-
ing the way for reuniting family members.

Immigrants are often all too aware of the changes in family organization set in motion by migration, but they may not know how to integrate,
negotiate, or alternate disparate family forms: the one they had, the one
they acquired during the course of migration, and the one they are evolving toward. Therapeutic conversations that include this temporal triple
lens of past, present, and future help sketch these evolving forms.

*good*

## Losing and Finding Networks

In an article about the impact of relocation on an individual or a family's
social network—including family, work or school, friends, and community
and religious-based relationships—Carlos Sluzki (1989) describes the shifts
of social networks before and after the transition. Networks are smaller and
less dense for a long time, have a much narrower repertoire of functions,
and are less reciprocal and intense. Needs and expectations are greater,
but there are fewer people or relationships to fill them. This poverty of relationships must be a contributing factor to signs of individual and interpersonal stress such as marital breakup, domestic violence, and greater in-
cidence of disease following migration.

Two large studies of Mexican immigrants in California, conducted by
William Vega and his associates (Vega, Kolody, & Valle, 1988; Vega, Kolody,
Valle, & Weir, 1991), underline the tremendous impact of support networks in the ecological context the immigrant finds upon arrival. In the
first study, migrant workers were at a much higher risk for depression than
the general population, most likely because of their isolation in a rural,
transient context. The second study of almost 2,000 Mexican women in San
Diego revealed a much higher number (41%) with depressive symptoms
than in the general population. However, the number of depressed immigrant women was much higher among the poorly educated and unemployed than among those who were married, had higher income, and
greater resources, such as transportation or savings. The presence of ex-

tended kin and friends, or even just the financial possibility of eventual reunion with them, was highly correlated with psychological well-being.

The study highlights the value of coethnic networks of support that provide continuity of language and customs, and sometimes even coaching in the new culture. Networks of assistance by conationals are crucial to the adjustment of Puerto Ricans and Cubans too, and even influence help-seeking behavior and the use of mental health services, which are usually introduced to new immigrants by their more knowledgeable compatriots who have already used or heard about them. These contacts may provide sympathetic and supportive networks, or they may be resentful or fear job displacement. Siblings or cousins may offer a place to stay or give a hand with the children. They may also be upset, having counted on the newcomer to stay back home to take care of parents or aging relatives. Inquiries about these issues should be included in the migration narrative. Over time, circumscribing relationships to extended networks or conationals may curtail adaptation to the new setting or create excessive cultural distance with offspring born in this country, but initially these connections seem to be crucial to successful adaptation.

Clearly an exploration of the uprooting of meanings will often uncover the immigrant's lack of information about the workings of institutions such as schools, hospitals, and job settings. Where conational networks are lacking or are still being developed, the therapist may need to act as a "social intermediary" between clients and often meager institutional resources. This role requires a balancing act in which the therapist must be careful not to take over or be too helpful in finding all the external resources for the family. As a "rescuer," the therapist may inadvertently increase the low self-confidence, passivity, or isolation the immigrant may already be experiencing. Alternately, immigrants who are encouraged to take charge of their lives, making their own contacts and finding their own services, experience a sense of personal agency and control which, in turn, positively influences other areas of their lives.

## The Role of the Host Culture

The road from being a newcomer to becoming a veteran in a culture is seldom smooth. Attempts have been made to articulate some expectable regularities in the process of migration over time. In his classic work, Carlos Sluzki (1979) adapted the curve of performance under stress, used in biology and experimental psychology, to migration. Other research has focused on the relationship between health and migration (Portes & Bach, 1985; Portes & Rumbaut, 1990b; Rumbaut et al., 1988). Whether newcomer or veteran, many of the immigrant's experiences reflect the attitudes and actions of the host country. The reception by the individuals and institutions of the host country, whether covert or overt, affect adaptation and even performance by immigrants. Social constructions about Latino immigrants in the host culture have suffered the vicissitudes of historical pro- and anti-immigrant agendas. Depending on these contexts, immigrant strengths may be emphasized by describing them as hardworking, dependable, courageous, and exceptionally resilient to stress. Or deficit-oriented theories may prevail, which regard immigrants as uneducated, lazy, unskilled, and trying to escape from a life of failure or mental pathology in their own countries. Both types of messages are inextricably and circularly tied to economic opportunities, sense of belonging, and entitlement for the immigrants.

Therapists, too, become participants in shaping the migration experience of their clients. They are influenced by political, ideological, and sociohistorical constructions about migration and need to become conscious of their own idealized or denigrated views of Latino immigration. The aim is to treat each family with openness and curiosity and to discover the strengths and vulnerabilities in each individual experience of migration.

This chapter has focused on constructing a migration narrative as a powerful therapeutic means of helping clients assign meaning to their experience of uprooting, recover some semblance of continuity in the face of change, and incorporate positive gains along with the many losses. In Chapter 5 I take a look at the ongoing story of migration and the many models of culture change through which to view a family's ultimate adaptation.

## NOTES

1. The occurrence of insensitive, racist remarks among Latinos is discussed in Chapter 6.
2. "Blame-the-maid" theories for problems experienced by the employer usually invoke envy as the culprit for the maid's wish to harm. These "theories" occur particularly from *la patrona* (the lady of the house) to the maid more frequently when stressful events arise for which there are no immediate or apparent explanations.
3. The technique of drawing the outline of each house a child has lived in chronologically and sequentially, while developing a written and read story about the child's life in the third person was suggested and beautifully illustrated in a presentation by the Norwegian family therapist Wencke Seltzer (1995). I followed a very similar course of action as Seltzer's in this Puerto Rican child "catching-up life narrative."
4. More "concrete" narratives can be healing for the whole family through the use of objects, photographs, music recordings, or audiotapes of familiar voices. In the case of an immigrant girl who had been separated from her immigrant parents from age 3 until age 7, I suggested the child request and collect mementos and decorations from her previous room and home in Mexico to decorate her American room and home.

# 5

## Journeys of Adaptation: Options for Change

> While living always in a world that builds them, families live also in the worlds they build themselves, as they always have.
> —HANDEL (1967, p. 79)

Some of the challenges immigrants still face after a decade or so in this country are often by-products of earlier solutions to the initial dilemmas of migration and adaptation. Salient among these are the fragmented families that never reunite physically or emotionally, and the parentified, compliant children who become resentful of helping dictatorial or uneducated immigrant parents. Intergenerational and gender-based conflicts also loom, the result of having U.S.-born children who more and more embrace the new language, new cultural meanings, and gender expectations as they grow older.

A number of models attempt to make sense of these processes and experiences, which are ubiquitous during the immigrant family's establishment in a new country. Such models are important because they have very different implications for psychological well-being and for theories about education and childrearing. They also influence the position of the therapist when treating internal conflicts or interactions between first- and second-generation immigrants. Indeed, therapists are encouraged to critically examine their own ideologies regarding acculturation and assimilation as they work with immigrant clients.

This chapter provides a description of these models and their implications for mental health theories and therapy. We then present therapeutic approaches that address dilemmas of cultural meaning, often manifested in gender and generational conflicts and in the ideologies of nuclear and extended families. While we stressed in Chapter 4 the need to preserve continuity in the face of overwhelming change, the emphasis in this chapter will be on the opposite goal, promoting change by creating the flexibility needed at later stages of adaptation to cultural change.

The following case illustrates the complex interplay of responses to old experiences and new adaptations:

Mabel Ochoa was 15 years old when she emigrated with her parents from Cuba to Los Angeles. At 31 years of age, she was still resentful toward her parents for separating her from her most cherished family member, an aunt who died some years later without ever seeing Mabel again. She also felt unforgiving of her parents for the abrupt change from a carefree adolescence to the overly strict supervision they imposed on her in the United States. Mabel learned early on to be obedient and respectful and never opposed or fought with her parents, not directly at any rate.

Mabel's intelligence and industriousness enabled her to learn English quickly, and within a year of moving to the United States she became a tremendous asset to her family as an intermediary with the new culture. She would type letters, look for jobs, answer adds by phone—"the Ochoas' perfect administrative secretary," as she put it sarcastically. In fact, she had become fiercely competitive at school and later at work to show that "Hispanics are somebody too."

Mabel's first rebellious act of "cultural resistance" was to marry an older, left-wing American. Her parents disapproved of him because of his age, his nationality, and his political leanings. The Ochoas threatened to cut off relationships with the young couple. The romance and the marriage were short-lived, and Mabel returned to her parents' home.

More "mature" and apparently "culturally conforming," at age 28, Mabel married Jorge, a Cuban American, right-wing conservative—an acceptable candidate in her parents' eyes. However, Mabel and Jorge regularly engaged in fiery political (pro-Castro/anti-Castro) and ethical arguments over just about everything. This marriage provided a setting for the presence and continuity of old values and the simultaneous expression of new values. In her arguments with Jorge, Mabel voiced the opposition she had always wanted to express toward her authoritarian father, hoping for validation of her "modern" values. Mabel's depression over the impending failure of this second marriage brought her to therapy.

To understand the individual and family turmoil experienced by the Ochoas, let's turn to existing theories about the processes involved in culture change across generations.

# MODELS OF CULTURE CHANGE

## Acculturation/Assimilation Models

Theories about migration and acculturation processes and their psychological impact have undergone considerable debate and evolution over the past 60 years. Beginning in the 1930s, a number of theorists (Kerchoff & McCormick, 1955; Johnston, 1976; Park, 1928; Stonequist, 1935; Goldberg, 1941) laid the foundation for *marginality theory*, which suggested that individuals who are born in one culture and raised in another belong to neither, and thus are marginal to both. Marginality was linked to such psychological stresses as identity confusion, a divided self, low self-esteem, and impoverished social relationships.

The idea of marginalization became closely tied to *acculturation theory*, which was a focus of literature between the 1950s and 1980s. This theory posited that immigrants suffer from "acculturative stress," manifest as anxiety and depression, feelings of marginality and alienation, psychosomatic symptoms, and identity confusion (Williams & Berry, 1991). Faced with the one-way influence of a powerful majority upon a weaker minority, the immigrant gradually acquires the values of the dominant culture, and his acculturative stress diminishes.

The underlying assumptions of acculturation theory include notions of adaptive "fit" and an *inevitable* transformation in the direction of the dominant culture. The original shapes become less sharp and increasingly more blended with the new background, which is itself shaped.

Under the rubric of acculturation, theorists have distinguished between degrees of "fit." Some argue that immigrants "assimilate," losing or rejecting the original culture and identity in order to adopt the values and behavior of the majority. Following the parallel of acculturative stress, the immigrant is thought to suffer from alienation and isolation until she or he acquires a new identity, specifically one that is congruent with the dominant culture. Acceptance by the majority culture follows. Other theorists argue that assimilation is an impossibility. Those who subscribe to the concept of acculturation without assimilation note that, despite competence in the new language and culture, the immigrant will always identify himself as a member of the minority culture, and the majority culture will assign him that status as well.

To what degree can immigrants make choices about these issues? The old concept of marginalization provides one answer. Studies indicate that Mexicans, Puerto Ricans, and Cubans suffer racial and ethnic discrimination and are often relegated to a lower status within the majority group. Under these circumstances, acculturation can indeed be a stressful experience and total assimilation an impossibility, reinforcing "second class citizenship" (LaFramboise, Coleman, & Gerton, 1993). Thus assimilation may not be a matter of personal choice. Race and poverty may inhibit an immigrant from identifying with any group other than his culture of origin, in spite of shared cultural borderlands.

Despite this, a common belief was that the faster the process of acculturation and the greater the assimilation to the dominant culture, the healthier a person would be (Williams & Berry, 1991). And while studies indicate that immigrants do acquire many behaviors and values of the dominant culture, the simultaneous exclusion or loss of old cultural ties can be costly. Consider the following case:

Rafael Ponce was a successful 44-year-old sociologist and head of a private research firm. He was the son of an Anglo father and a Cuban-born mother who spent her childhood in Puerto Rico and her adulthood in Mexico. He was born and raised near Monterrey, Mexico. He had gone to San Francisco in his mid-20s to attend graduate school with the intention of settling in the United States. Because his father was an American citizen, he had no trouble getting citizenship himself. But Rafael could never "pass" for Anglo. He was short and robust, moustached, dark-haired, and dark-skinned, and had a strong Spanish accent. His adaptation to California and his social acceptance and status were greatly helped when he married statuesque Elizabeth, an American woman of Swedish and Swiss descent. Elizabeth was well educated, blond, tall, and beautiful. She had impeccable taste. They lived in a gorgeous house in an upper-middle-class suburban community with their two teenage children, who went to a private, predominantly white school.

Elizabeth brought Rafael to marital therapy because he had grown distant and "estranged," much less attentive to her and the children, and completely uninterested in sex. When I interviewed him alone, Rafael revealed that he was in a total state of confusion. He was at the career and personal pinnacle he had always strived for, but instead of feeling ecstatic over his successes, he was "destroying" everything by carrying on an affair with Carmen, a Mexican American woman. Rafael described her as dark-skinned, with a most "tacky" taste in clothing, jewelry, and hairstyle. But Carmen was vivacious, uninhibited, and very affectionate with him.

Much to his dismay, Rafael had begun thinking of Carmen as the love of his life. He sought individual therapy to alleviate his confusion. Rafael had always assumed that rejecting his language and his culture provided more advantages than holding on to them. This rejection seemed to be connected at a deeper level with his intense shame over his Latina "flamboyantly overprotective, affectionate, talkative" mother, and the disdain he had perceived in his own Anglo father's treatment of her. Rafael also seemed prey to an early perception that the United States had "better-quality everything," including people.

Many of our therapeutic conversations revolved around the need to reclaim lost parts of his ethnicity and externalize his own internalized racism (see Chapter 8). I often asked him how and by whom, to use Michael White's (1993) words, was Rafael "recruited" into self-prejudice? He needed to replace devaluation and denigration with respect, pride, and enjoyment of his heritage rather than love Carmen as an ambivalent representation of the Latino language and culture "outside" of him. The challenge for Rafael was to achieve some measure of balance rather than choose between two polarized positions: either an ethnic affirmation encapsulated in the minority culture; or an assimilationist "recruitment" to the dominant culture.

A year later, Rafael divorced Elizabeth, married Carmen, had a baby with her, and adopted Carmen's youngest orphaned brother who had recently arrived from Mexico. He continued as a successful professional and was devoted to all his children. His work and time with children comprised, in his words, an "American lifestyle"—work was his most time-consuming preoccupation and he followed a limited and controlled schedule of visiting his children. He also recovered many of the Latino preferences in his life with Carmen but continued to feel that it was too late to recover Spanish as his primary language.

Rafael Ponce learned that alienation can follow a precipitous assimilation, and most recent observations confirm the risks of abandoning one's old culture and opting exclusively for the new.[1] A number of studies (Griffith, 1983; Portes & Rumbaut, 1990b; Warheit et al., 1985) suggest that Mexicans who attempt to "Americanize" or assimilate in this way actually have more rather than fewer psychological problems and drug use. The best outcome seems to be for those who retain their language, cultural ties, and some indigenous rituals while simultaneously learning the new language and customs (Burnam et al., 1987; Ortiz & Arce, 1984). Similar findings for Puerto Ricans and Cubans point to the importance of enduring attachments to language, identities, and old meanings.

In recent years research has discovered the limitations of traditional acculturation theories, devised new versions, and has even questioned the distinctions between an immigrant's original culture and that of the dominant majority (Berry, Trimble, & Olmedo, 1986; Padilla, 1980; Ramirez, 1984; Rogler, Cortes, & Malgady, 1991). Harwood (1994) notes that many immigrants who enter the United States today already participate in a global culture, by virtue of growing international migration, information dissemination, and technology transfer. In varying degrees, people around the world are exposed to American culture from U.S.-made movies and TV programs, and manufactured goods. According to Harwood, we can no longer assume which behaviors or values will be perceived by an ethnic group as typically American, or for that matter, typical of their own ethnic group. The next section explores two new concepts that reflect these changes in theory and provide mental health interventions that better answer the adaptational needs of immigrants in a postmodern world.

## Alternation Models

The alternation model assumes that it is possible for an individual to know and understand two different cultures—old cultural meanings persist while new cultural modes are acquired. An individual can use this knowledge and understanding to suit different purposes, at different times, and in different places or social contexts (Ogbu & Matute-Bianchi, 1986; Rashid, 1984; LaFramboise & Rowe, 1983).

The alternation process is far from the neat progression proposed by acculturation theory. Some old cultural themes are blown up very large, others shrink out of sight, while still others remain the same. Cultural themes meet and mix, with no need or desire to choose between old and new. Rather, one can know two perspectives, languages, and cultures, be traditional and modern, conservative and liberal, depending on the context or the topic.

The alternation model assumes an individual can have a sense of belonging in two cultures without compromising his or her sense of cultural identity (LaFramboise et al., 1993). Unlike the classic acculturation/assimilation model in which the dominant culture is experienced passively by the immigrant, the alternation schema proposes a bidirectional, mutual influence between the culture of origin and the adoptive culture. A personal example illustrates this coexistence of meanings and behaviors:

> Even after I had been in this country long enough to learn all the basic social conventions, my automatic tendency was to do what had been ingrained in Argentina: to greet all the people connected to family and friends with a firm kiss on the cheek. Although it always meant that I was happy to see them, some Anglo friends and acquaintances were disconcerted—the gesture was rarely reciprocated in earnest.
>
> My children's friends had the most negative reaction. One day I complained to my children that I had kissed more kids' ears (which is where my lips landed after they tried to avoid me by turning their heads!) in this country than I ever had before. Did I smell so bad? What was so disgusting about my kisses that they had to turn away so abruptly? Were they afraid of my germs? When I asked these questions my children were kind. They didn't say, "All of the above, Mom." They simply said, "You have to learn to be less mushy . . . people don't know what to do with that here . . . we've told you already that you're too sentimental . . . save it for when you go to Argentina."
>
> Their advice wasn't a linear prescription toward acculturation. It was a suggestion for *alternating* adaptive greeting behaviors according to the social context. Yet that didn't completely extinguish my social kissing in the United States. I became selective and reserved kisses for long-term Anglo and Latino acquaintances, including those Latino clients (especially children and grandmothers) who had taken the initiative to kiss me or where the kissing flowed spontaneously when saying goodbye until the next session.

In recent years, to my pleasant surprise, many of my Anglo friends offer light pecks on the cheek. Perhaps their own cultures have incorporated the modes of so many immigrants around them, or maybe they do it just to please me.

A number of factors make the alternation model well suited and empowering for Latino clients in treatment. An ability to move or alternate between two cultures is especially beneficial for Mexican immigrants who maintain multiple connections with their original homes. First, Mexico is very close to the United States, with five border cities joining the two countries. Increased travel by land and air and improved telephone systems enable regular contact, which epitomizes the circular (Bustamante, 1995) nature of "transnational" migrations (Schiller, Basch, & Blanc-Szanton, 1992), or what Turner (1991) calls the emergent two-home, "transcontext" lifestyle.

Puerto Ricans also update and invigorate old connections with the help of inexpensive airfares between Puerto Rico and New York. A Puerto Rican client of mine called his mother in Puerto Rico twice a week from San Diego, and his wife and children were able to spend 2 months in Puerto Rico every summer. Cubans have a harder time experiencing their country firsthand, but its proximity allows for updating through short-wave radio, magazines, and newspapers.

An additional factor favoring the alternation model for Latinos pertains to language. The proximity of the country of origin, coupled with the growing number of Spanish speakers in the United States, makes it possible to alternate culture and language easily. Latinos must, and do, learn English, at least enough to successfully adapt to this country. Yet, for many, Spanish continues to be the language spoken in the home, full of emotional meanings and reinforced by frequent trips back to the country of origin, interactions with local countryfolk, Spanish TV and radio, and relatives' visits to the United States. Indeed, research supports the positive psychological effects of bilingualism (Lambert, 1977; McClure, 1977). LaFramboise et al. (1993) found that biculturally competent individuals who can alternate behavior between two cultures are less anxious than those attempting to assimilate or acculturate.

Anthropologist Roger Rouse (1992) makes a similar argument for what he calls "cultural bifocality," or the capacity to view the world alternately through different lenses. He noticed that Mexican immigrant laborers in Redwood, California, learned new values and beliefs, but also retained old ways of interpreting and evaluating the world. For example, many of the men shared complaints about their lives in the United States that ranged from the tyranny of clocks and supervisors in this culture to feelings of disempowerment from having their authority challenged at home (reinforced by the protection of women and children by the State), to the lack of moral guidance provided by the schools, which they saw as connected to the children's vulnerability to drug addiction and prostitution. Rouse observed that these criticisms were closely tied to the normative frames acquired in the mens' native towns. Their complaints focused on areas in which the native culture stressed a man's responsibility as head of the household to control, protect, and discipline. The men feared annihilation of their cherished cultural preferences by American values that were already permeating the behavior of their wives and children. Yet these same men learned to speak English and adapted to the American work ethic.

## Hybridization

The alternation model implies a sort of cognitive, cultural know-how—one knows intuitively or learns purposefully when to use one cultural code or another, depending on what fits better at the time. But immigrants, especially children, sometimes blend rather than alternate cultural meanings. For new immigrants, differences between the old and the new are fairly clear, but those differences may become blurred for offspring who regularly move in a world that combines the two. The result is a kind of hybridization of culture in which affective and cognitive frames are enlarged by a more complex and diverse view of work, gender socialization, and interpersonal boundaries.

The term "hybrid cultures" was coined by noted Argentine anthropologist Nestor García Canclini (1995) to reflect cultural situations in which traditions are not quite past and modernity is not yet wholly present. Similarly, as the world becomes a smaller place cultural products and ways are less frequently "pure" or "authentic," but comprise a complex confluence of traditions and modern beliefs.

The large urban metropoles of today provide a rich context for hybridization. Immigrants in these centers live in a world of movable contexts that provide simultaneous access to different cultures. Widely diverse models exist for doing just about everything, from living in close proximity to one's parents to moving away and seeing them once or twice a year, from having many friends to living a private life, from having some relationships based on dominance to others based on partnership. While first-generation immigrants were guided by the stable social controls of group norms, their children interact in a pluralistic, multiethnic environment where they have, if they choose, greater anonymity and freedom to invent themselves.

Choosing to use an Anglo first name and keeping a Latino last name is a good illustration of hybridization, or the blending of influences. In another form, the Puerto Rican teenager who invents rhythms that blend rock music with salsa isn't consciously taking elements of both cultures. He is simply able to hold multiple descriptions simultaneously in relation to the same activity. And so is the peasant from Oaxaca who goes to a *curandero* (folk doctor) when he is ill, but would like his daughter to go to medical school.

Such hybrid individuals form a complex "collective" identity, invoking various cultural aspects (voluntarily or involuntarily) in different social situations. Harwood (1994) points out the importance of these situations for defining ethnic identity. For example, a person may define himself as an urban Puerto Rican immigrant to differentiate himself from his countryside compatriot. Among Latinos, he may be fiercely Puerto Rican. At the national political level, he may affirm his Hispanic identity. In his work, he may define himself as an American.

Just as individuals create unique blends of cultural identity, so do immigrant families represent mixtures of old and new. A culture's influence on family members is uneven. Montalvo and Gutiérrez (1989) present compelling clinical evidence of earlier roots of a culture finding expression in some members and not in others and stress the importance of therapists' differentiated understandings. While families often benefit from the increased flexibility and adaptability that hybridization can bring, emotional challenges abound for them as well. The following sections explore these challenges and some of the ways therapists can approach culture change issues.

## Biculturalism: The Emotional Benefits and Pitfalls

Immigrants, especially those in the second generation and beyond, make "bicultural choices" when they alternate or combine language and behavior. Alternation and hybridization models increase our understanding of how these choices are made and what they mean. Choosing to speak English outside the home and Spanish inside, or to use English to discuss money and work and Spanish to discuss family matters, or to read only in English but think only in Spanish, is usually based on emotion, both recognized and unrecognized. Hybridization may also represent choosing what one judges to be best from each culture.

Clearly, hybrid families usually have more alternatives to cope with the complexities of a changing environment than a family that rigidly adheres to old ways or uncritically adopts new ones. But symptoms of distress in "hybrid" individuals or families may be a manifestation of unresolved conflicts regarding cultural meanings. Developing a hybrid identity is no easy task, as the case of Celia (Sally) Juárez demonstrates:

> Celia, alias Sally, Juárez insisted that she married a Jewish American man because in her view, all Mexican men, including her own father, were unfaithful to their wives. She promised herself she would never allow this humiliation to happen to her. The best insurance, she thought, was to marry a man from a cultural background that had a reputation for producing faithful husbands. In her view, Jews didn't have "anachronistic" meanings of what it is to be a man. Now she was weeping in my office, deeply hurt and humiliated by her unfaithful Jewish husband.

She was adamant about divorcing him. Her reactive conceptualization of a "modern Latina" was of one who would never tolerate any infidelity by a man. Ironically, among the bitter arguments she gave for not deserving such treatment was the cultural list of things she had in common with her own mother, a very good Mexican wife. The list included dutifully starching and ironing her husband's shirts, never letting him go without a delicious hot and spicy meal, always being there for him physically and emotionally. She had never thought of these traditional meanings of being a woman as "anachronistic."

As we have seen, biculturality raises a set of continuous emotional issues and adjustments that are always relevant to an individual's mental health (Harwood, 1994). The meanings and concomitant feelings people attribute to their biculturality need to be explored in each case.

## MODELS OF CULTURE CHANGE AND THE THERAPIST'S POSITION

The different theories described above about the processes involved in culture change have important and quite divergent implications for therapy. Therapists, following the lead of social scientists, have been biased toward a linear acculturation framework in which the life struggles of immigrants are assumed to gradually resolve by increasing acculturation or assimilation to the dominant culture. Within this model the therapist's role becomes that of a cultural mediator or a translator who helps the family adapt to the new country, the new trend, or the new values (i.e., individualism, feminism, democracy) of the dominant culture. Therapists become acculturation agents. The adaptational value of maintaining relational styles and cultural traditions is minimized in this approach.

Good intentions notwithstanding, acculturation-oriented therapists may create more, rather than less, emotional distress by stripping the family too quickly of the protection of the old culture. By emphasizing adaptation to normative structures of their own ecological niche in the dominant culture, therapists may come to believe that they're favoring the objective truth rather than personal cultural biases, and may unwittingly commit a form of cultural imperialism. For example, it's not unusual for Latino and non-Latino therapists to be critical of Latino parents who hold on to "old-fashioned standards" in control of children or adolescents, and thus become automaticallly "inducted" into the children's defense.

At the other extreme (of acculturation-oriented therapists) are those who assume an indigenous or ethnic reaffirmation position. This ideology is based partly on a belief that adhering to one's original culture provides access to its sacred and healing aspects, resulting in positive identities and mental health. This position encourages families to find health and healing by returning to, or adhering to, their ethnic or cultural roots. Such cultural reaffirmation requires practicing "cultural resistance" against definitions of family and individual life implied in the dominant culture (Prilleltensky, 1990; Waldegrave, 1990).

Despite the value of reaffirming culture, life in a pluralistic, multiethnic society requires a modicum of external acculturation. Some competence in language, "American" work habits, and institutional know-how are necessary for scholastic achievement, economic success, and of course the ensuing mental health benefits these accomplishments can bring. Furthermore, individuals and families in cultural transition may find certain aspects of their original cultures oppressive. Changing and even embracing some of the alternate values provided by the dominant culture may feel liberating.

Presenting problems can often be linked to dilemmas of cultural transition, but the choice to move toward acculturation, alternation, or hybridization should be the client's, with the therapist acting as a facilitator. In doing so, therapists must be aware of their own ideologies and personal leanings—do they regard assimilation, or some version of acculturation or perhaps ethnic reaffirmation as the ultimate goal for immigrant families, be they Latino or other? Or is their preference for alternation or hybridization? In addition to answering these questions, therapists should be able to articulate opinions about culture change to the clients as just that, opinions, rather than "truths." If the therapist isn't aware of her ideologies and values, she may fall into unconscious maneuvers that support one side of a polarized family or larger system subgroups over the others.

## DILEMMAS OF CULTURAL TRANSITION

Culture change doesn't occur only at the interface of the family and the new social environment. These complex adjustments and reactions also happen as precipitously and dramatically within the family—different members and groups (spouses, siblings) adapt at different paces and represent different aspects of old and new customs. They often encounter the most common of cultural conflicts or adaptational impasses: dilemmas tied up in language choice, generation gaps, and gender role conflicts.

### Language Choice and Conflicted Loyalties

As immigrants remain in this country, they may develop fluency in English, and with it, new cognitive structures for articulating ideas. But the ultimate choice of language goes beyond fluency or comfort in the new tongue—language is symbolic of memory, affect, places, family alliances, and intimate and public situations. While bilingual competence and alternation (and even the hybridization represented by "Spanglish") represent an invaluable resource for adaptation, the use of both languages can become entangled in family conflict. Family members often differ widely in language proficiency and in their positive or negative regard for Spanish or English. Those differences sometimes compound and symbolize loyalty conflicts between past and present, or between polarized stances on the decision to remain or to return to the homeland.

Among the linguistic manifestations of an adaptational impasse is elective mutism, the refusal of a young child to speak in certain contexts (often at school) despite competence in the second language. Elective mutism, which is not uncommon in bilingual families, may provide a way to denounce cultural conflicts between family members or reinforce such conflicts by perpetuating the polarization of cultures and languages.

In a most interesting chapter titled "The Sounds of Silence: Two Cases of Elective Mutism in Bilingual Families," Carlos Sluzki (1983) describes double-binding circumstances for two 9-year-old girls who refused to speak in school, in spite of being otherwise adequate students. Both girls came from families plagued by an ambiguous organization between old and new family structures, between their migration as provisional or permanent, between allegiances in which one parent valued English and the other Spanish. These conflicts had become stagnant due to injunctions against communication, such as rules of silence or secrets about the past and present. In one case, Sluzki provided positive connotations of each family member's behavior, with an emphasis on the symptom-bearer for bringing the dilemmas between cultures and family members to light. He framed the child's muteness as a sacrifice of silence, one that assured her father she was not betraying him by speaking the language of a country that brought him so much bitterness. Similarly her performance as a good student also proved the child's loyalty to her mother's wishes for the education offered by a country that had been so generous to her. When Sluzki turned to the parents to ask them casually how long it would take them to make a final decision about staying or returning, the answer came promptly: "2 months," a decision that had been postponed for almost 10 years. The therapist then recommended that the girl continue her elective silence in order to give her father time to make his decision while reminding him of the need to do so. At 3 months, a follow-up revealed the girl had become quite talkative. The parents' impasse over migration, manifested in the girl's elective mutism, had resolved.

## Generational and Gender Conflicts

Generational conflict emerges from a number of factors. First, cognitive maps collide—views about gender roles, work, leisure time, sex, marriage, religion, and family of origin ties may be called into question—and disagreements roil between family members. Further, contexts outside the family lead to generational rifts within it. The immigrant parent and head of the household who initiated the migration, perhaps considered a "hero" at one point, may find himself displaced. As Latino immigrants tend to occupy a low level in the hierarchy of jobs and social status, dreams for advancement are thwarted, the hero loses his status in the family. This shift displaces fathers, grandfathers, and even mothers from their leadership positions in the family, often to be partially replaced by an acculturated son or daughter or by a profound lack of leadership and guidance. The displaced adult often feels anger, sadness, and vulnerability, which can lead to self-criticism or complaints about spouse and children (Haour-Knipe, 1989).

Generational conflicts such as displacement and parentification are further complicated by the normal stresses of adolescence and the ubiquitous disparity in gender role ideals between immigrant parents and their teens. Gender roles are changing woldwide, including in Mexico, Puerto Rico, and Cuba, creating a wide array of views about the balance of power between men and women. These positions range from traditional hierarchical structures to various intermediate arrangements, to egalitarian balances in gender roles (Gutmann, 1996; Padilla, 1994; Vega, 1990). These tensions are manifested most intensely in the father-daughter, mother-daughter, and husband-wife family relationships.

Father-daughter conflicts that escalate cycles of rebellion and restriction often focus on manner of dress, dating, curfew, parties, smoking, drinking, and premarital sex. These conflicts may lead to emotional distress, behavioral problems, and even suicide attempts (Zimmerman, 1991). (See Chapter 11 for further discussion and case illustrations regarding adolescence.)

Immigrant mothers seem to be somewhat more inclined than fathers toward "Americanization" in the form of greater freedom for their adolescent daughters. But immigrant women of both generations often share heart-wrenching tensions and hidden ambivalence over traditional gender roles—a reality they have in common with other immigrant women from patriarchal societies (Akamatsu, 1995). Older and middle-aged women often attempt to incorporate some of the new expectations (greater assertiveness for women, more liberal attitudes toward sex for the younger generations) that their daughters are promoting and perhaps have wanted for themselves. And yet the older women also express pride about aspects of their belief systems that have worked for them, such as the territoriality of women's housework or the considerable power afforded by the culture's reverence for mothers. Such contradictions may lead a mother to send double messages to the adolescent: "Exceed the limitations of my life but maintain our traditional selflessness."

Zimmerman (1991) wrote eloquently about how Hispanic women can make a "shared crossing" that maintains connections with old and new cultures, while respecting the unique voices of mother and daughter. Further,

Latina women may share a long-standing cultural resistance to their subordinated positions (see A. R. Del Castillo, 1996). A sensible new self-help book bravely takes on the challenge of counseling Latinas to find compromises between the new meaning systems about womanhood and the cherished traditions of their mothers and grandmothers' cultures (Gil & Vasquez, 1996). These represent both/and formulations that endorse alternation and hybrid solutions over either/or choices.

While parent-child relationships encounter the double dilemma of generational and gender role conflicts, interactions between husband and wife also undergo gender-related transitions. These transitions are evident in the slowly changing roles of men and women in Latino immigrant cultures, as demonstrated in the following example. Matthew Gutmann, an anthropologist from Berkeley, recently published a book titled *The Meanings of Macho* (1996) based on a study of changing definitions of what it is to be a man in a neighborhood of Santo Domingo, Coyocán, in Mexico City.[2] According to Gutmann, in 1995 the majority of 5-year-old boys were happy to participate in a game called *lavando la muñeca* (washing the doll), although in 1982 young boys thought this game was only for girls or "sissies." In 1995, boys also swept the floor, watered the plants, and picked up the garbage. This change is taking place because young boys see their fathers and older brothers helping with housework more than ever before. Yet older men who live in the same place, but were raised with a different meaning system about gender, remain uninvolved in these activities. Interestingly, most men of all ages have absolutely nothing to do with cooking, perhaps because the kitchen space is such a strong ancestral territory of Mexican women's pride and identity, as the popular 1992 movie *Like Water for Chocolate*, based on the book by Laura Esquivel, so clearly depicts.

In the countries of origin these cultural transitions in gender roles occur against a rich backdrop of strong traditions. The process of cultural evolution is more measured and allows for greater complexity. In sharp contrast, new immigrants face or are exposed to the issue of gender imbalance while they are struggling with many life transitions in a daunting, alien environment. The new contextual setting for Latino immigrants makes these conflicts even more jarring. For a detailed discussion of gender issues and therapeutic approaches to gender-related conversations, see Chapter 10.

## THERAPEUTIC APPROACHES TO CULTURAL TRANSITION

### Identifying Cultural Transition

A straightforward way to begin dealing with cultural dilemmas is to frame a family's trials and opportunities as precipitated by a process of "cultural transition." This label is usually comforting because it allows the family to exist in an unfinished and suspended state, which paradoxically relieves some of their anxiety. (For an extensive discussion of the use of this concept in cross-cultural marriages, see Falicov, 1995a). A state of cultural transition can best be discussed in terms of legitimate and necessary double discourses (or even triple discourses if one includes the client's future personal hybridizations) that encompass the cultural codes of the old and the new, the indigenous and the industrialized, the traditional and the modern, the ethnic and the acculturated.

> A very Catholic Latina mother was despairing to control the premarital activities of a 19-year-old daughter with her steady boyfriend. In a family therapy session, after I empathized with the mother's anguish, I offered that this "transitional situation" was among the best I had seen because it encompassed dignified aspects of both cultures. The daughter was experimenting with becoming a modern (American) woman, but she was doing so in a rather traditional, conservative, and judicious Latina way that focused on only one long-term boyfriend. This probably occurred, I ventured to say, thanks to the messages about seriousness and loyalty transmitted by her mother's cultural and personal code. I praised them for their ability to strengthen themselves by blending cultural influences.

## The Therapist as Cultural Intermediary

Moving toward a view that considers and respects the *meaning systems* of all participants—whether acculturated, indigenist, or mixed, family and therapist included—requires the therapist to take a collaborative role rather than a hierarchical one in which she directs acculturation. As a family intermediary, she helps to clarify similarities, differences, and philosophical and practical implications, and tries to comprehend the underlying assumptions and societal logic behind each cultural system. The therapist can play an intermediary role in a number of ways, from commentator on philosophies of life to educator (Falicov, 1982; Falicov & Karrer, 1984).

Landau-Stanton (1990) described the innovative approach she calls "link therapy," which mimics life by relying on the most acculturated family member to create bridges inside and outside the immigrant family. She also discusses other useful cultural transition methods such as "transitional mapping" and "transitional sculpting," methods that permit family members to see their positions relative to each other in terms of life cycle, culture, ease or difficulty of transition, and so on.

Other pragmatic approaches have emerged that support the mental health benefits of bicultural competence, such as the Bicultural Parent Effectiveness Training (BPET) program (Szapocznik, Santisteban, Kurtines, Perez-Vidal, & Hervis, 1984) and Family Effectiveness Training (FET) (Szapocznik, Santisteban, Río, Perez-Vidal, & Kurtines, 1986) which teaches communication skills that incorporate old and new value systems in working with Cuban immigrant parents and their American-born adolescents.

Therapy with immigrants is, in many ways, about finding creative solutions to dilemmas that come about as families try to merge, split, or integrate dissonant (and sometimes complementary) sets of meaning systems. Therapists can reduce conflicts between meaning systems in one family by legitimizing contextual flexibility and alternation. Families may honor the intergenerational bond demands in one setting, perhaps during a visit to their home village, and still respond fully to the companionship needs of the marital dyad in the new, adoptive home.

The following section presents a method for working with conflicting cultural views in families, with an emphasis on integration of meaning rather than acculturation.

## Building Bridges between Cultural Meanings

The following case illustrates how family problems in a rapidly evolving, multicultural society may be related to several conflicting cultural experiences and perspectives. The therapeutic method outlined here is an adaptation and elaboration of ideas from Turner (1991), who suggested steps for co-construction of new immigrant narratives for families who are struggling with cultural differences. The case describes a family living in a border or contact zone and thus in the midst of intersecting cultures. Their borderland existence provides a metaphor for hybridization and biculturality.

The Olmeda Garcías are a middle-class family from Tijuana, Mexico, which borders San Diego, California. They have two children, Diana (14) and José (9), and they are expecting a third child. Mr. and Mrs. Olmeda García sought psychological help for their son, José, who was underachieving in school in Tijuana, was very quiet and often silent, and had developed total mutism when taking English lessons in San Diego. He did not actually refuse to attend these lessons, but he became paralyzed when asked to read or speak. His teacher noticed that José was very nervous and stressed, and recommended a psychological evaluation.

Mrs. Olmeda García, who is 8 years younger than her husband, comes from a small, educated, and liberal family. Mr. Olmeda García comes from a very large, less educated, and more religious family. Mrs. Olmeda García is dedicated full time to her children and home, and has full-time household help. Mr. Olmeda García is a partner in an auto repair shop, where his brother and brother-in-law also work. The mother and her two children, Diana and José, would often go to San Diego to shop, for doctor and dentist visits, and for swimming and English lessons. Mrs. Olmeda García and Diana spoke acceptable English, while Mr. Olmeda García and José did not. The husband would visit his parents several times a week and stay in Tijuana for recreation, where he played billiards with a group of male friends. Mrs. Olmeda García would see her family in Tijuana, but not as frequently, and the visits took up less of her time. She had two Mexican friends who lived in San Diego.

The father minimized José's school problems while the mother maximized them. Mrs. Olmeda García, somewhat led by the English teacher, believed that José possibly had a serious problem. For Mr. Olmeda García, the boy's reluctance meant that "José was a boy and preferred soccer to poetry." He was more worried about Diana's flirting and night outings with friends, while Mrs. Olmeda García saw these activities as part of normal teenage exploration.

Mrs. Olmeda García and Diana were very close. In fact, Diana regularly accompanied her mother to San Diego for Lamaze classes in preparation for childbirth. When asked about this decision, the wife explained that she did not even ask her husband to attend the classes because she knew he would refuse, a prediction he did not deny.

There was tension, alienation, and a twinge of mutual contempt as family members asserted the "correctness" of their individual views. The mother and daughter represented striving to incorporate American ways, while father remained loyal to his homestyle values and his large and busy network of parents, uncles, and siblings. Although the Olmeda Garcías were not immigrants, their proximity to the border dramatizes a "two homes" or transnational lifestyle and the cultural bifocality that often leads to polarized values.

The therapist, a young woman born of Mexican parents, was raised in California. She valued English and spoke it more fluently than Spanish. She could not imagine any parent not helping a child learn English. As a feminist, the therapist approved of the wife's attempts to give the children the best bilingual education and to modernize the daughter by allying with her against the husband for more freedom. The therapist stirred conversations in ways that challenged the father's views and the tone between the two of them became quarrelsome.

The therapist viewed the husband's resistance as resulting from his patriarchal entrenchment. However, in conversations with me as her supervisor, she soon realized the dangers of being inducted into marital polarizations, as had happened to the children. Consequently she was able to neutralize her negative reactions with the father by exploring her own cultural and personal meaning systems. She also tried to understand the family's meaning systems relative to areas of conflict, including family organization, family life cycle, ecological context, acculturation, and health/religious belief systems.

Therapy with this family encompassed the steps listed in Table 5.1, which outline a method for the therapist and family to explore, situate, and integrate different cultural meaning systems.

1. The first step is to **draw attention to differences** in ideologies or meanings. In the Olmeda García case, some of these included education, including differences in language and location (English/Spanish, Tijuana/San Diego) and its possible connection to social class differences; life cycle markers that indicated differences in timing for dating and childbirth; family-of-origin organization, which highlighted considerable differences between the husband's and wife's frequency of visits, closeness, and sharing of information with their families of origin; family size, which addressed the spouses' very different experiences growing up; and gender socialization, which touched on the father's control over his daughter's dating as opposed to the mother's idea that adolescent girls need freedom to experiment, as well as the father's "boys will be boys" philosophy compared to the mother's views about the boy's socialization and scholastic achievement.

This initial conversation about each person's views attempts to be as accurately descriptive as possible, but contextual links are underlined by the therapist as the conversation unfolds. For example, when Mr. Olmeda García's wife complained about his reluctance to go to San Diego, the contextual issue of race entered the conversation. Mr. Olmeda García revealed that in San Diego he felt discriminated against because of his color and pronounced Mexican features. He also feared his son was probably seen as a *morenito* (darkie) or a "dumb Mex," an experience the father thought might contribute to José's inhibitions. Mr. Olmeda García felt that his wife and daughter were treated respectfully as *güeras* (white, or blonde ones). Mrs. Olmeda García, who had always been aware of the unspoken difference in color and appearance between herself and her husband, had never thought of racism or dared to speak of discrimination as part of her husband's dislike for the American side of the border. (For many Mexicans, race may be alluded to or joked about, but it is shunned as a topic of serious conversation.) With this revelation, Mrs. Olmeda García could now feel emotionally closer to her husband and acknowledge why he wanted to avoid experiences in San Diego, rather than continue to attribute his reluctance to a personal trait or limitation.

Thus these links provide a cognitive lens that paves the way for the second step: an appreciation that a person's constructions about life can be partially understood in terms of his or her ecological niche—that combination of institutional contexts or social settings (family structure, school, church, occupation) from which the person has been included or even excluded.

2. Once differences are identified and described, the second step is to **contextualize the differences.** Those taken-for-granted, "correct" views that family members hold as truths or fixed realities become central to the conversation. Some "truths" for members of the Olmeda García family included "education is the road to success," "children need a lot of undivided

TABLE 5.1. **Integrating Meaning Systems**

1. Draw attention to differences.
2. Contextualize the differences.
3. Reframe problem as dilemma of coexisting meanings.
4. Preview future family patterns and cultural blends.

attention," and "medicine is more advanced in the United States," which were voiced by the mother; and "boys will be boys," "education can wait," and "girls need to be controlled and protected," as voiced by the father. These "universal" views become less fixed and more relative and socially situated when discussed in terms of the cultural and familial contexts that helped generate them.[3]

Contextualizing of differences relates to the awareness of how our lives, thoughts, and preferences are influenced by our experiences in sociocultural and family settings. This process has two outcomes:

A. It decreases mutual blaming and character assassinations. In the Olmeda García family, the combativeness between husband and wife dissipated at this stage, perhaps because they developed more justification and respect for each other's views.
B. It opens up a space for personal choice similar to what narrative therapists call a space for separation–externalization. Viewing their experience from outside as well as inside the family, family members can choose to protest, combat, or resist certain acquired cultural values and critically reflect upon the norms and values they have been "recruited" by society to accept.

In my opinion the outcome of this step need not necessarily be "cultural resistance," for example, opposition to cultural definitions. After deliberation, a person should also be free to embrace those values from his original culture, or the dominant one that he views as part of his collective identity, regardless of their popularity or "political correctness" relative to the therapist's values. Any manner of cultural choice helps organize one's life, whether it entails embracing a group culture that values tradition and continuity, or asserting one's critical uniqueness in an individualistic setting. Both are legitimate, as are the myriad combinations in between.

3. The third step focuses on **reframing the presenting problem as a dilemma of coexisting cultural meanings.** Here the therapist asks how family members' differences about gender socialization, educational ambitions, recreation, language, and inclusion of kin pose dilemmas for the adults, the children, the males, and the females in the family. The therapist then

explores a number of hypotheses about the presenting problems: Could José's refusal to become bilingual and bicultural reveal a dilemma of polarized paths or divergent decisions? One could imagine that if José learned English and gladly came to recreational and educational activities in San Diego, he could feel that he was betraying his father's wishes and definitions of manhood. On the other hand, if José did not learn English and did not do well in San Diego he would betray his mother's desires that he learn a language which she highly regards. The therapist suggested that José had found a compromise, an attempted solution to his dilemma: he gladly went to San Diego (to please his mother), but he would not learn English (to support his father).

4. The fourth step, that of **previewing future family patterns and cultural blends,** introduces a future-oriented dimension. What kinds of alternations or blends of meaning systems are possible? Can all cultural ways of being be honored and retained? Can one be valued over another, depending on the context? Are there any overarching meanings, what Turner (1991) calls "meta-texts," that can span two cultures or transcend specific contexts? For example, could transcultural or universal meanings about manhood and fatherhood provide Mr. Olmeda García with a culturally congruent way to be involved with both his wife's pregnancy and his son? Asking about these ideas can orient the family toward a future in which multiple cultural meanings can either coexist or be integrated, depending on what makes sense to them.

> The therapist for the Olmeda García family went on to positively frame the presence of two sets of values as allowing for a complex and rich blend, though one that sometimes could present challenges. With regard to José's education, the father said he never intended for the son not to be schooled, and in fact, he offered to be more involved in José's education. He preferred to first talk to the teacher in Tijuana about helping José with school work before continuing with the English tutor in San Diego.
>
> But it was the impending birth of the baby that provided the greatest opportunity to explore future-oriented questions. What kinds of decisions might be made about the child's upbringing in terms of language, schooling, forms of discipline, and gender socialization? Would the baby pioneer a new era of solutions to the dilemmas posed by living in two cultures? Would solving the dilemmas of raising José in Spanish and English, and Diana as both a traditional and liberal young woman, pave the way for the education of the baby-to-be?
>
> Mr. Olmeda García opted for an in-between, traditional solution; to be the chauffeur and take his wife to Lamaze classes. Mrs. Olmeda García chose to go with her mother-in-law rather than with 14-year-old Diana. Mr. Olmeda García dropped them off and waited patiently outside for the two women, who kept him up to date with the progress of

the class during the drive back. This gesture was as much as Mr. Olmeda García could do since he found the whole idea of assisting in the labor and witnessing the birth too culturally dissonant. Self-mockingly he said he needed two strong women in case he did attend the birth, because both of them would be needed to catch his fall when he fainted. "Just more proof," he said, "that for all of our bravado, we macho men are really 'chicken' underneath it all."

The parents found ways of bending toward each other and of blending, sometimes smoothly, sometimes awkwardly, the different cultural influences and meaning systems brought from their families of origin and their diverse experiences in Mexican and American cultures.

Each family will discover and develop its own manner of living with two cultures, whether through acculturation, alternation, hybridization, or combinations of these. But dilemmas can be articulated and creative solutions found if the therapist shows an intense interest in understanding cultural influences and can "read" some general maps about the contexts that generate different meaning systems.

The Olmeda García family and other case studies presented so far demonstrate that the domains of MECA are interrelated, if not interdependent. Although this chapter focused mostly on the later stages of adaptation, it should be clear that other issues—family life cycle, family organization, and ecological context—are significant no matter what "stage" of migration or acculturation family members represent when they arrive at your office. In the next section I examine how several specific contexts—from the "exterior" exposure to racism to the "interior" experience of religion—deeply affect individuals and family members as they navigate in the dominant culture of a new home.

## NOTES

1. With the evocative book titles of *Hunger of Memory* (1989) and *Days of Obligation: Conversations with My Mexican Father* (1992), writer Richard Rodriguez renders an anguished autobiographical account of the painful family disconnections that followed his forced childhood choice of English over Spanish.
2. These are poor immigrant families who moved from the countryside to this metropolitan site in 1971 and have never been anywhere else. But women work outside the home much more than they ever have.
3. This process of examining taken-for-granted realities, those so-called truths that are split off from the conditions or contexts of their production, is similar to what Michael White calls "deconstruction." It renders strange or alien everyday taken-for-granted realities. White uses what Bourdieu, a sociologist, calls "exoticize the domestic," that is, make exotic the domestic. If we become aware of how certain modes of life and thought shape our existence we might then be in a position to choose to live by other modes of life and thought (White, 1993).

*PART III*

# The Crossroads of Inner and Outer Worlds: Ecological Contexts

One of the greatest risks, and subsequent tragedies, of using facile ethnic explanations to interpret the behaviors and beliefs of minority clients is its failure to account for their ecological context, those often bitter realities that are part of everyday life for Latinos and other minority groups. Therapists cannot, in good faith, understand the complex processes in the lives of these families without a careful analysis that includes race, class, and gender, and considers the psychological impact of subordination and social injustice.

A further risk and common outcome among so many professionals who proclaim multiculturalism is the confusion of social class with ethnicity. When cultural differences are cited as explanations for economic failure, the larger, negative effects of poverty and racial discrimination are downplayed. "Culture" becomes a troublesome dimension that distracts from the social inequities of an increasingly hopeless class stratification. An example of this confusion (in spite of good intentions to consider cultural differences) is found in a review of a book by Phillipe Bourgois based on interviews about selling drugs in a Puerto Rican neighborhood of New York (*The New York Review of Books*, February 1, 1996). The reviewer, journalist Michael Massing, tells us that Puerto Rican youngsters miss their chances for upward mobility because of conflicting "cultural codes." He gives two examples that involve Primo, a young Puerto Rican. First, when Primo is required to work extra hours at his job he demands to be paid overtime, "not realizing," according to Massing, that in the American cultural code he is hurting his chances for a promotion. The second example occurs when Primo is asked by his boss to come to her apartment to help with a last-minute mailing. Rather than expresing gratitude, Primo acts *offended* (emphasis added) because "in *El Barrio,* an unmarried woman never invites a man to her house." This "cultural code" hypothesis fits the ethnic stereotype of the Latino emphasis on protecting the virginal honor of women.

Frankly I do not think this young man is so culturally obtuse. If Primo is "overreacting" to being asked to work overtime, his behavior must be understood in the context of mistrust of employers who may exploit and trample him and his doubts about his access to the American dream. Likewise, Primo's reaction to being invited to his boss's apartment could have alternate meanings that are less ethnically based. I doubt that Primo is really offended by his boss's invitation. He might feel that way if he "caught" his unmarried sister in the act of inviting men to her apartment. As a Latino he is likely to appreciate that there may be two, three, or more sets of cultural codes or explanations for the same behaviors.

If we look again at Primo's position, could it be that his insecurity about his social status gets the better of him when his boss asks him to work overtime and to come to her apartment? Many psychological processes may be at play. He may fear that his white female boss is taking advantage of him because he is the Puerto Rican low man on the totem pole, or that she may humiliate him in some way. He might wonder why she doesn't appear to be afraid of his manhood. Or, it could be that when Primo shows some offense at his boss's request, he is taking the only avenue he has to secure some dignity for his own culture. Or, could Primo be wearing an ethnic camouflage in front of his interviewer, using his culture as an excuse and not revealing deeper injuries to his self-esteem? The point is that we should not dismiss complex processes that are closely tied to one's ecological niche with simple cultural stereotypes.

A primary goal of this book is to help therapists move past ethnic stereotypes by applying a comparative, multidimensional model of culture. In doing so, one comes to understand the role of social marginalization in the lives of most Latinos in the United States. Gender and social class are intertwined with variations in migration, family organization, and life cycle, but nowhere are socioeconomic class issues more evident than in a Latino's interaction with the institutions of their ecological context.

Mainstream social studies have tended to treat cultural differences among Latinos mainly as a product of their ethnicity. The crucial effects of ecological context as shapers of individual and family life are often left out. The pitfalls of excessive emphasis on specific ethnic styles and traditions without acknowledging the interactions of the minority family with macro-system institutions—school, work, social service agencies, or hospitals—have been amply illustrated by family therapists Braulio Montalvo and

Manuel Gutiérrez (1983, 1988, 1990). Kenneth Martínez (1994) suggests that "sociocultural blindness" leads people to ignore the effects of institutional and intracultural racism, unemployment, and subsistence living on self-esteem and achievement motivation for Latinos. By overlooking social influences and interactions and focusing on solutions from a specifically ethnic perspective, therapists can inadvertently work against the family in therapy.

Moving past a "culture-equals-ethnicity" stance relies in part on acknowledging that most of America's 50 million Latinos comprise a subjugated component of a racial and class hierarchy (Baca-Zinn, 1994, 1995), with one out of four in this group living at or below the poverty line.

Focusing on a client's ecological context sensitizes therapists to the psychological effects of marginalization—the mental health consequences of marginalized status, discrimination due to race, poverty, immigrant status, and other forms of powerlessness, underrepresentation, and lack of entitlement and access to resources. While there is no question that racism and prejudice influence social status, Latino clients who struggle with marginalization may come from middle-class and wealthy settings as well as lower-class and poor environments. The ecological context of marginalization is especially "heavy with meaning" (Seltzer & Seltzer, 1983) and can become part of a therapeutic conversation about cultural symbols, personal representations, and the daily stresses of coping with hard social realities.

While racism and discrimination comprise common experiences for minorities across social class, many find interior strength and external social support in a wide variety of religious and spiritual beliefs and practices. Because most psychotherapies are basically secular endeavors, they have purposely kept matters of spirituality and religion out of the therapy session. A trend is under way, however, to incorporate these often critical meaning systems into therapeutic work. The notion that religion and spirituality are an important part of a family's ecological niche is particularly valid for the majority of Latino individuals and families for whom Catholicism (the most predominate affiliation) and various forms of indigenous and folk beliefs about health and illness often play a significant role. In Chapters 6, 7, and 8 we examine the ecological contexts of race, education, work, and belief systems in detail.

# 6

---

# The Impact of Racism
# and Discrimination

America is a foreign world, but the hues in which this world is
painted and the emotional reactions it elicits vary widely under the
influence of forces often removed from the initial will or knowledge
of the newcomers.
                                —PORTES AND RUMBAUT (1990a, p . 179)

## THE RACE OF LATINOS

Latinos can be white, black, American Indian (or indigenous), Asian, *mestizo* (mixture of Indo-American and Spanish or other European groups), or
mulatto (mix of African and Indo-American with European groups), or any
racial combination of these. There is no such thing as a distinct Latino or
Hispanic race, in spite of census and other forms that list Hispanic as a race
category. One can be a Latino Asian, a Latino white, or a Latinegra. U.S.
census figures in 1990 show that 52% of 22 million Latinos said they were
white, 3.4% said they were black, and 42% said they were "other," the only
third choice. A large number of those who checked white were *mestizos* or
mulattos (brown-skinned people).

Mexicans belong to a variety of races. A relatively small number are
distant descendants of the Spanish conquerors or other Europeans
(French, German) and preserve light skin color. The majority are *mestizos*
in different combinations of indigenous groups with Europeans. A small
minority of Afro-Caribbeans, living in Veracruz in the south of Mexico, are

descendants of African slaves brought to Mexico before slavery was abolished there in 1829. The significant variation in race and skin color among Latinos worldwide may be less acknowledged in the United States because of the influence of American Indian ancestry (Mayas, Aztecs) among Mexican immigrants—others are prone to classify the whole group as one race with "definite" dark skin color and Indian physical features.

Puerto Ricans are also a racially mixed group. Their ancestry is Taino Indian, Afro-Caribbean, and Spanish. Puerto Rican immigrants suffer remarkable discrimination and prejudice in the United States, an effect of longstanding white racism against black people. Consequently they are the poorest among Latinos.

Cuba's population has a rich mix of mestizos and mulattos of Afro-Caribbean, Spanish, and other European and American Indian heritage. In contrast to poor Mexican and Puerto Rican immigrants who immigrated in search of work, Cuba's political and ideological exiles of the 1960s were white, educated, and wealthy. They encountered welcoming arms, emotional approval, and federal subsidies rather than prejudice and racial contempt. The 135,000 refugees that came from Cuba in the early 1980s had a much larger proportion of Afro-Cubans and working class or poor immigrants, and they encountered a much colder and more hostile reception upon arrival in the United States.

## RACE AS A SOCIAL CONSTRUCTION

Racial groups have been historically linked with positive and negative social constructions. The distinguishing features of any racial category are socially defined (Baca-Zinn, 1995). In most societies, the social hierarchy favors those with light skin while excluding and devaluing those with dark skin. In their countries of origin, Latin Americans of dark skin color may also suffer ingrained but unacknowledged racism.

From the time of the Spanish colonization of Mexico, social status and economic class were clearly tied to racial purity, and lighter skin bore greater privilege. After centuries of intermarriage this dichotomy still exists, although there is greater gradation between the white and very dark skinned. This racial hierarchy, part of the established and unchallenged social order, perpetuates the status quo and implicitly condones discrimination.

Puerto Rico and Cuba, like most Caribbean islands, share a significant population of dark-skinned people who, over generations, have mixed with whites and together have generated a wide range of racial characteristics and color. Puerto Ricans have been labeled as the "rainbow people." Dark skin may be considered less attractive than fair skin, but it carries with it no implications of genetic, intellectual, or work inferiority (Ramos-McKay, Comas-Díaz, & Rivera, 1988).

Some writers (Shorris, 1992; González de Alba, 1994) have tied the historical origins of racial prejudice in Latin America to the inferior status assigned to colonized Indians by arrogant white colonizers, the Spaniards. The marks of colonization and the deprecating gaze of "the other" have not disappeared in these countries and is often re-created in the anti-immigrant sentiments of many American whites.

Linking the dynamics of the colonizer and the colonized, the oppressor and the oppressed, to the internalization of negative self-evaluations, these writers have speculated about the passivity and resignation of the Mexican Indian, and about the lack of aggressiveness and fatalism of the Puerto Rican. They offer an analysis, albeit stereotypical, of these traits based on centuries of oppression, first by the Spanish and later by Americans.

Similarly, Fortes de Leff and Espejel (1995) suggest that underlying racial issues reflect and re-create the relationship between the Spanish conquerors and the conquered Indians. In a fascinating paper, the authors note that from the time of the conquest of Latin America, to be white (or *güero*) has implied the power and privilege of a higher social class. To be dark (or *indio*) has signified the conquered, dominated, and intellectually inferior (*tonto*). These constructions may well survive in the dynamics of the modern-day Mexican family.

Further, therapy itself can represent a form of conquest—the family may feel pushed toward a new way of living and relating that conforms to the values of a more powerful therapist. But while therapeutic change can represent a threat to a family's way of life, it can also be framed as an opportunity for positive transformation or gain. The introduction of "conquest" myths in the therapeutic conversation can unlock frozen systems by generating intense affect and bringing together family subsystems previously split by real or imagined color differences. As with many *mestizos*, for example, a hybridization of Indian and Spanish heritage, of dark and light skin, mends conflicts based on distorted and harmful social constructions.

## RACISM AND MIGRATION

Racism, discrimination, and prejudice are very much a part of the cultural history and social experience of Latinos in the United States. The classification of "Hispanic" as a race has its roots in political and racist motivations. Until 1954 Latinos were considered "Caucasian" or "white" in America. That year they became a "colored minority" along with African Americans and Asians. This label was used by racist schools as a way to circumvent the

1954 desegregation order by arguing that such schools already enrolled people of color: the "Hispanics." Over time Latino activists used this classification to gain some measure of political advantage, whether to obtain federal funding for community agencies or to secure political representation in local government.

Migration vastly exacerbates the sting of discrimination and racism. It is strikingly different to be poor and dark-skinned in one's homeland, where one shares national origins and a sense of entitlement to an ancestral land and a community, than to be poor and dark in a foreign land, a minority isolated from heritage and loved ones, with no entitlement whatsoever. Migration shifts one's place in society from the center to the periphery, and the psychological consequences are vast.

For immigrants, encounters with discrimination fluctuate with historical trends toward inclusion or exclusion. These in turn generate either ethnic affirmation or ethnic shame, a wish to assimilate to the dominant culture or a desire to isolate from it. In *Mexican Voices, American Dreams* (Davis, 1990), a book based on oral histories of immigrants, Mary Margaret Navar begins her story:

> "My older brothers are named José Adalberto, Rafael Francisco, and Luis Seferino, Spanish names as ancient as you can come up with. But I was born in the assimilation years [the 1950s] so the name Mary Margaret, or as my aunts, the matriarchs, call me, Maria Margarita. Because of the heavy, heavy racism of the assimilation years, they [the parents] decided I would learn only English." (p. 334)

There is much in a name. A therapist may assume that by saying a name, say Rafael, Dolores, Concepción, or Carlos with the correct Spanish pronunciation she conveys respect and knowledge of the language or culture and therefore expects to be received somewhat more favorably. But she may be mistaken. Even if a clinic intake record shows a Spanish name, the person or the family may have adopted the English version and pronunciation in an attempt to assimilate. A choice to deny one's given name or language, so deep a part of the self, may stem from experiences of racism or discrimination related to society's current attitude toward exclusion or inclusion. And attitudes toward immigrants are rarely hard to detect.

> Growing up in a Jewish enclave of Buenos Aires, I often heard complaints about discrimination and insults toward Jews. I had grown to dread and be ready for the moment I might be called a "dirty Jew." Yet that did not prepare me for the put-downs Latinos endure in the United States. I spent two days in Miami Beach in 1963, and while there, I went to a drugstore to get some aspirin. I walked in and had yet to ask, "Where can I . . . ?" when I was abruptly ordered to the back of

the store by a male clerk. I looked and saw a large sign: "Spanish spoken here." Then I said, "But I speak English . . . " to which he swung his arm impatiently and exclaimed, "Just go there . . . " in no uncertain terms.

It was unseasonably cold in Miami that day so I went to a hosiery store for some stockings. I began browsing through the bronze, brownish colors as I always do, to match my olive skin and dark hair and eyes. Suddenly a sales lady intervened: "Honey, no offense but your complexion is dark, not too dark . . . , but you know what I mean, you have to be careful, watch what you wear, you don't want it to look . . . you know what I mean, why don't you get a light hose, you'll look so much better. . . . " Although her intentions were good, she summarily dismantled any hope I had of total acceptance in the United States. I knew I was short, small, and the owner of a Spanish accent, and now I could tell those elements darkened my skin. I learned about the emotional power and insidious rejection of racism. It taught me, too, how a seemingly sensitive assumption about lack of language proficiency on the basis of physical appearance or accent can in fact be experienced as humiliation.

Mary Margaret reflects about the discrimination suffered by immigrants: "I also know other Mexican Americans who are very intimidated by the whole thing, scared. All they know is that some people may be prejudiced against them. So the only sense of cultural heritage they have is a sense of something dark hanging over their heads" (Davis, 1990, p. 344).

The label of racial inferiority applied to Latinos in the United States may be connected to a poor person's dress, Spanish accent or surname, slightly darker skin color, or immigrant status. The significant connection between social status and race is evident in a 1989 National Opinion Research Center study in which Mexicans, Puerto Ricans, and Gypsies were ranked 35th through 37th of 37 racial and ethnic categories ranked by social standing (*New York Times,* January 8, 1992, p. 34).

## RESIDENTIAL SEGREGATION AND SOCIAL MALADIES

In Latin American countries, social interaction between rich and poor and between light- and dark-skinned people is a daily occurrence. Segregation occurs through the class structure but does not equate with the remarkable, race-based separation of residential neighborhoods seen in the United States.

In their richly documented book, *American Apartheid,* Douglas S. Massey and Nancy A. Denton (1993) demonstrate the persistent significance of race over ethnicity by considering patterns of housing segregation among Caribbean Hispanics. This group shared many similarities with Puerto Ricans and Cubans of all races: they entered the United States under similar immigration conditions and had the same cultural background, the same class composition, and similar family characteristics. What differentiates them is race. Housing segregation indices for Latinos in three racial groups (white, mixed-race, and black) indicate that the average level of segregation increases steadily when one moves from white Hispanics, with an index of 52, to mixed-race Hispanics, with an index of 72, to black Hispanics, with an index of 80, which is comparable to that observed for African Americans. Massey and Denton conclude that when it comes to housing and residential patterns, race, not ethnicity, is the dominant organizing principle. By concentrating poverty, residential segregation also concentrates social maladies, most notably drug abuse, domestic violence, gang activities, and crime.

Racial characteristics ultimately lead Puerto Rican and Cuban blacks to suffer more socially induced behavioral and emotional problems than lighter-skinned Latinos. Black Puerto Ricans are more frequently diagnosed with mental illness than white Puerto Ricans (Rabkin & Struening, 1976). Further, racial discrimination and income are closely related. White Puerto Rican families that come from urban cities in Puerto Rico and have marketable skills are likely to successfully establish themselves in the United States and have children who advance in school and work. But for the rest, darker skin, racism, and poverty become hopelessly intertwined. One-third of 2.5 million Puerto Ricans in the United States are very poor, and of all the Latino men in jail in New York, the majority are Puerto Rican (Novas, 1994).

In contrast, Mexicans tend to live in neighborhoods with larger proportions of whites. These neighborhoods remain commercially viable and maintain some social order through residents' surveillance of public places and collective, community action.

Learning about a family's neighborhood and housing is critical to understanding its entire ecological niche. Starting with the client's address, the therapist can expand her lens to understand the resources of the ethnic neighborhood and the role of racial discrimination and poverty in the lives, and problems, of individuals and families.

## RACISM AMONG LATINOS

A Latino's experience of racism in the United States is further complicated by the existence of within-group segregation—a hierarchy of racism exists among Cubans, Mexicans, and Puerto Ricans. Enduring their American context of discrimination in the workplace, in housing, and in political representation, the three Latino immigrant groups project their experiences of racism and hurl national and ethnic stereotypes at each other. The assumption that Latinos would relate better and be able to create a more intimate connection with each other than with members of other cultures may be true at the level of language and for certain values and traditions. But race affects intragroup relationships, too. Exploration of cross-group racism may be needed in the clinical arena.

A 17-year-old Mexican American girl, Lupe, in her junior year of high school developed bouts of crying and a persistent refusal to talk and to attend school. Her parents were concerned that Lupe might be hiding a pregnancy, but found it difficult to discuss this possibility openly. After many interrogations, Lupe finally said she wanted to be transferred to another school but would not explain why. Only in the privacy of an individual interview did Lupe "confess" that she was infatuated with a Latino boy in her school and feared her family would disown her forever if she continued the relationship.

When the therapist suggested alternative ways that would allow her to remain in the same school and test out the reality of her feelings, Lupe related another story. Teresa, her older sister, had fallen in love with Roger, a Puerto Rican youth. When her father discovered a token of love that the young man had given to Teresa, he broke her lip with a slap and told her in no uncertain terms that she had tarnished her family's name. The father objected to Roger's "inferior race" and threatened that he would be the first "to warn" other respectable, interested young men about her past. Teresa had been paradoxically condemned to be "only worthy" of the Puerto Rican boy, and she was no longer allowed to date.

Lupe's refuge into total silence could be interpreted as the response of a person familiar with a double-bind situation in which she was damned if she defied parental authority or damned if she obeyed it.

Earl Shorris (1992) makes a useful distinction between racism—discrimination at the dominant culture level, based on xenophobia—and *racismo*—discrimination from inside the same cultural group. The latter may stem from a need to establish subgroup hierarchies for a variety of psychological reasons, including internalized racism, self-rejection, or the need to project onto others denigrated parts of the self. In this context, Shorris offers his observations about a hierarchy of racism based on myths about the prestige of national origin and race among the three Latino groups. He says Cubans in Miami act as the most conceited and are perceived by other Latinos as arrogant and as identifying more with Europe than with Latin America. They appear to flaunt their white skin and economic progress and may use it to denigrate other Latinos in a racist way. Mexicans are racially prejudiced against dark Puerto Ricans and many other darker-skinned Latinos. Puerto Ricans are critical of blacks in the United States.

In Shorris's view, no one suffers *racismo* as much as Mexicans and Mexican Americans. As in Mexico, discrimination is based on Indian heritage. In the United States, discrimination by other Latinos is fueled by the Mexican's frequently nondocumented status and willingness to take any job, no matter how low the pay or how unfair the working conditions. Perhaps this is one reason Mexicans cling most fiercely to their national identity. In fact, Mexican immigrants themselves may focus a more vitriolic attack against particular members of their own group than against darker-skinned Caribbean Latinos. A notable target is a *pocho*—a Mexican American who has "traded" his language and culture to adapt and take better advantage of life in the United States. A *pocho* is regarded by his compatriots as a traitor, a cultural pariah (Villareal, 1970).

## Double Labels, Doubly Scorned

The movie *Selena*, starring Jennifer López and directed by Gregory Nava (1997), recounts the story of the Mexican American Tejano singer whose life was tragically cut short. Her father, Abraham Quintanilla, poignantly laments about the specific challenges that Mexican Americans face as a group. He states: "It is very difficult, very difficult to be Mexican American" and goes on to explain that the hyphenated designation means something different for them than for other minority groups. For Mexican Americans, it signifies a painful, no-win situation—they are at once despised foreigners who speak poor, accented English in a land that belonged to their ancestors, and they are unwelcome visitors south of the border who speak poor, broken Spanish. Abraham tells his children that to face this double rejection they need to be better than Mexican and even better than American, a daunting task. And that was Selena's highest, near-impossible dream: to be a crossover artist, loved by Mexican and by Anglo-American audiences.

The Chicano movement of the late 1960s and early 1970s was initiated by the English-speaking children and grandchildren of Mexican immigrants and was precipitated by the dilemma of bearing a double label. It was, in part, a reaction to being dubbed "too Mexican" by Anglo-Americans and "too American" by Mexicans. These young Mexican Americans started to use the terms Chicano and Chicana as an affirmation of pride and identity and to state: "We are not Mexicans, or Americans. We're a combination—a special group with our own history and culture." The desire to legitimize their mixed cultural identity has won some recognition in the creation of Chicano Studies programs at universities, particularly on the West Coast.

Therapists may encounter identity conflicts between Mexican or Mexican American parents and their Chicano children. It is important to realize that these are not picky labels. The terms carry serious implications for political and personal definitions (Martínez, 1997), which need to be explored for each person. It's possible that a parent's criticism of a child's Chicano identification may stem from negative racial stereotypes associ-

ated with the Chicano label as compared to the Mexican American label
(Fairchild and Cozens, 1981). Parents may be trying to protect their children from further discrimination. Therapeutic conversations about these
issues can uncover common pain and personal desires to rescue ethnic dignity. Along the way, therapy builds generational bridges.

A similar need to resist assimilation underlies the criticism by Latinos
of compatriots who have moved away from the inner city. They are sometimes viewed by Puerto Ricans in New York as having joined the world of
the *blanquitos* (a diminutive word scornfully used for the white race), the
Anglo-American world of the dominant middle class. This parting between
"them" and "us" has implications for therapy—distrust of Anglo-American
therapists may be likely, but even Latino therapists may be viewed with suspicion, having "defected" from the Latino world to go to the Anglo-American side. Later in this chapter we discuss what therapists can do to diminish
the family's distrust and their fear of discrimination.

## Skin Color, Family Esteem, and Self-Hate

It is not uncommon for Latino family members to differ in skin color, the
result of a complex mix of Indian, African, and Spanish blood. Color and
race identification are toxic issues in the mainstream culture, and they
penetrate individual and family life even more intimately than economics
and politics. They become tied to family acceptance and self-image.

> You should know, my son, that you are very, very dark. Now that you are going
> to move (from Guadalajara) and come to live here in Mexico City and that
> you soon will have a girlfriend, you must find one who is very, very white so
> that in case you get married you will have white children.
> Advice given to Luis González de Alba (1994, p. 28)

> First of all, I was brought up with the notion that it was much better to be
> white. It was much better. Just, you are a better person if you are white. I didn't
> feel sorry for myself but I longed to be white. I just felt they were better peo-
> ple. They couldn't possibly do anything wrong. This was from education but
> also from my family. I remember saying to my uncle about getting into
> Berkeley on a minority status. He said, "When they asked you what you were,
> you didn't say you were Mexican, did you? Oh, my God, how could you be
> so stupid!"
> María Aguirre, Pediatrician, Redlands, California (in Davis, 1990, p. 395)

The advice given to the Mexican writer Luis González de Alba in the
first quote did not surprise him. He grew up in Mexico with the Spanish
nickname *el prieto*, or *el moreno*, or *el negrito*, all meaning "darky" in English.
He also grew up hearing the lavish, enthusiastic praise given to his brothers' light-colored eyes. He was a witness to the family's joy at the birth of a
blond, blue-eyed cousin (*la güerita*), who was followed by 14 equally white

siblings (*güeritos*), "all the better," he sardonically comments, for the "glory of the race."

In summing up these and many similar experiences, González de Alba calls the family "the school of esthetic values—the scales of whiteness—and the painful center of racism." For those like him who are "the (dark) fly in the soup," the family also becomes a fountain of anxiety (*zozobra*), resentment, self-hate, and self-rejection. In his opinion, "The family *constructs* in small scale what the country incorporates in large scale. The *mestiza* (mixed IndoHispanic) family with children of all the colors, but with an unmistakable preference for the light-skinned ones, is the representation of the Spanish contempt for the Indians." But humiliation inflicted by the family, González de Alba claims, is "more subtle ('the color of that shirt does not become you . . . '), but also more painful because they come from those whom we love."

The directionality of causes proposed by González de Alba is questionable. The family can't "construct" a scale of whiteness and proceed to enculturate all of its members on the practices of racial discrimination. More likely, the family, like the individual, internalizes and reflects inward society's racism. In the classic autobiographical novel *Down These Mean Streets*, Piri Thomas (1967) vividly portrays the impact of differences in color between himself, his siblings, and each of his parents, and the destructive interactions that follow when these color differences lead to widely divergent opportunities for work and social life.

The second quote, from María Aguirre, suggests that her uncle, in urging her to hide her ethnic identity, wants to protect his niece from the racist disqualification she will suffer in the educational system. The heart-wrenching social and psychological consequences of prejudice for the individual's identity and self-esteem are always devastating, but a family like González de Alba's that practices internalized discrimination is different than one that recognizes racism as an external injustice, as does María Aguirre's uncle.

Clearly race is one construction in which "material heavy with meaning" (Seltzer & Seltzer, 1983) can emerge. Racial pride in families, for example, is often based on denial or distortion, revealing the socially constructed nature of such perceptions. Fortes de Leff and Espejel (1995) relate a surprising case of an elite family that described its members as *güeros de ojo azul* (whites with blue eyes). The parents were very distressed over their daughter's choice of a dark-skinned fiancé from a lower social class. When Fortes de Leff and Espejel met the family face to face, they were astonished to find not a single blue-eyed, light-skinned family member. In such cases, it is as though the fear of racial mix and shift from one socioeconomic or cultural way of life is intricately tied up in a family's internal dynamics, even if differences in skin color are more imagined and symbolic than real. Such meanings extend to the value parents ascribe to their children. Fortes de Leff and Espejel observed that many parents take pride in and overvalue having light-skinned children. The presence of dark-skinned children can precipitate shame and conflict. Later in life, children or parents may present with symptoms of depression or with subsystem alliances based on skin color.

## Family Racism as a Cultural Mask

On occasion, racial tensions manifested inside the family serve as mechanisms of psychological distancing and may be part of the presenting clinical picture. When the person being blamed in a family is dark-skinned or a member of a foreign or minority subgroup, one might assume that marital or family interactions replicate larger ethnic or racial prejudice. A closer (and necessary) examination might reveal that other problematic processes are at work between people who are intimately and painfully connected. Racism may be providing a cultural mask or deflector from these other problems.

Under situations of acute stress or loss, such as an impending divorce, an affair, illness, or death, intermarried couples in conflict may use ethnic explanations to blame the other, prove a point, obtain support, and vent anger, even though those ethnic characteristics were not problematic when the couple was getting along (Falicov, 1995a).

Therapists can detect the defensive use of a "cultural mask" by looking for distortions in a couple's cultural explanation of its problems and by noting the degree of emotional intensity connected to these attributions. The question "Why is culture an issue now?" is essential for understanding such cases. The answer often reveals severe, underlying stress, perhaps the impending loss of a spouse through divorce or death.

A couple that was contemplating divorce consulted me as a last resort. Previous marital therapy had not resulted in any change. Susan, a blonde American who traced her ancestors back 300 years, spoke in a very derisive manner about her Cuban husband of 18 years, Luis, a successful engineer whose father was Afro-Cuban. She blamed many of his objectionable features on his ethnic origin and minority status. She said that he had an "inferiority complex" and was "very insecure," "insensitive and undemonstrative," "incapable of love," "selfish," and "uncaring."

Upon examination, these statements and their attribution to ethnicity were flawed. First, the traits did not really have any identifiable ethnic roots. Second, during their nearly 20 years of marriage, the two had endured tensions due to cultural and language differences, but these had been seen as surmountable. If anything, the wife had joined the husband's culture—she had learned a little Spanish and gained considerable knowledge of Cuban history. There had been many attempts at integrating cultures. They had given each of their children two names: one Spanish, the other English. Although Luis was visibly disturbed by his wife's references to his ethnic background, he behaved like a gentleman and never returned in kind the cultural insults. In fact, he tacitly supported his wife's rendition of their problems as primarily ethnic based.

I did not question the validity of Susan's ethnic stereotypes or mention the couple's previous adaptations to cultural differences because I sensed something else was happening. To explore matters further, the spouses were interviewed separately. When alone, Luis said his marital dissatisfaction had been long-standing. Recently he had abruptly taken the initiative to move out of the house. He was living in an apartment with a younger Mexican woman, with whom he had fallen in love. His wife knew this but had refused to take it seriously and had taken every opportunity to invite him to move back home.

In the context of this marital crisis, the use of ethnic stereotyping could be understood from various perspectives. By selecting to blame her husband's Latin culture for his behavior, Susan protected herself from recognizing the possibility that he no longer loved her and also allowed herself to indirectly criticize her husband's choice of new partner, who was Mexican. The adjectives Susan used to describe Luis's character could be heard as metaphors for the feelings his behavior evoked in her: He was "insensitive" (toward her), "uncaring" (toward her), and "inconsiderate" (of her feelings toward him). Luis had been emotionally estranged from her for some time. Perhaps his wife's use of ethnic stereotypes could have stirred additional emotions, at last provoking a powerful reaction on the husband's part.

To confront the wife—perhaps by examining which of Luis's traits were truly Hispanic or how these traits clashed or fit with her own cultural preferences—would have been therapeutically incorrect. Rather, it was important to discuss the protective function of blame, which helped her avoid dealing with the impending loss of her husband. Consideration for the couple's adolescent boys and the balanced picture of father that would benefit them in the future became a therapeutic avenue to help Susan search for her strengths and a measure of equanimity.

The notion that differences are maximized and prejudice increases in the face of stress has been the subject of classic social psychology experiments (Kretch & Crutchfield, 1948; Simpson & Yinger, 1958). In the face of a situation that is hard to understand or accept, prejudices can be adopted to "explain" the crisis and bring meaning where confusion and ambiguity abound. They are a search for a reason, or even an alibi, a way out for oneself or the other person. In this light, comments about race or culture can be heard as metaphors for other relationship issues, such as separation or loss, and should be given clinical consideration (Friedman, 1982).

## THE SUBTLE PREJUDICE OF PROFESSIONALS

Racism in the therapy encounter can be insidious and unexpected. Whether it occurs covertly or overtly, within family relationships or therapeutic ones, the ramifications are great indeed. Latino mental health professionals are not immune to internalized racism that is manifested in subtle messages. Martínez (1994) relates a case in which a white foster mother was not allowing her two Mexican foster children to speak Spanish. The foster mother also spoke about the biological Mexican mother, who was in therapy with the children, in a condescending and disparaging way. She implied that the mother, being Mexican, was backward, an incompetent parent, and did not care about education. A Latino supervising case manager, filling in for a trusted Latino caseworker, supported the foster mother's beliefs and credited her value on learning as especially helpful to the children. At every family session the children were becoming increasingly more reluctant toward and rejecting of their biological mother and did not want to speak with her in Spanish.

The fact that the supervising case manager was a Latino lent tremendous power to his opinions. Social service agencies are usually at a loss when trying to understand people of a different culture or language. A professional who speaks the language and understands the culture has tremendous impact because he is viewed as an expert on both Latino and Anglo-American cultures. Aware of this power, Latino therapists must examine their own family and institutional experiences with racism, their prejudices toward other ethnic groups, and their internalized racism toward their own cultural group. Regardless of their ethnicity, if therapists feel removed from or consciously prejudiced against an ethnic group, they should be cautious about counseling these clients and refer them.

When professionals get caught in a process of ethnic stereotyping they may use their power in ways that perpetuate injustices. Sometimes professionals may subtly criticize or discriminate against clients who don't fit an expected cultural stereotype. Such covert behavior impinges on the client's individuality. The problem of unacknowledged professional prejudice is illustrated in the following case of a lawyer and his Mexican female client, who was being divorced by her Anglo-American husband. The case study begins with a history of the couple's stormy relationship.

Consuelo Jones (née Acosta), a Mexican woman from Rosarito, Baja California, came to see me in great distress over an impending divorce from her Anglo-American husband, Tom Jones. Before the separation, the couple lived in San Diego with their three children, 7-year-old Jessica, 5-year-old Jimmy, and 18-month-old Scotty. The couple had originally met at a street music fair. They both struggled with the other's language, but no other cultural incompatibilities surfaced during their courtship. Eight years later, Tom initiated the divorce and a fierce custody battle was brewing.

It is not surprising that Tom was so attracted to Consuelo initially. She was a stunningly beautiful woman, with light brown skin, black hair, dark brown eyes, and a vivacious and ambitious disposition. She had wanted to have children but had also wanted to better herself by learning English. Tom supported all of this for awhile, but he also began to criticize Consuelo, intensifying the verbal attacks during her second pregnancy. Tom found her too loud, too disorganized, and too unrealistic in her ambitions. He frequently confided, in English, with a male friend and Consuelo sometimes detected that he was speaking critically about her. Once Scotty was born, Tom began to object to the children being babysat by Consuelo's mother, sisters, and aunts in Rosarito, even when they came to San Diego.

Although Tom had at one time enjoyed Consuelo's family very much and had favorably contrasted their warmth to the relative emotional distance of his own family, now he hated them. He found her family intrusive and felt they were a negative influence, spoiling the children with sweets, toys, and permissiveness. He felt they would make the children become lazy, *mañana* types and "dumb" Mexicans as he believed they had raised Consuelo to be. Slowly Tom began to cultivate relationships with his own family members, who had always felt Tom had married beneath himself.

During their marriage Tom had occasionally become abusive toward Consuelo, locking her in the bathroom so she would learn how to behave and not throw temper tantrums. During one fight he wanted to force her to move out, go to work, and give him child support so he could stay home and raise the children. He attempted to prevent her from attending sports and other school activities for their oldest child, and wanted to celebrate the children's birthdays without her. By the time I became involved, Tom was pursuing sole legal custody and implying, through indirect statements and partial anecdotes, that Consuelo was mentally or emotionally unstable. To be fair, my knowledge of this case comes from Consuelo's account, her lawyer's description, and the legal records which contained many letters of various allegations and attempts at resolution by both parties.

Consuelo was referred to me by her attorney, a white Anglo-American, a seasoned middle-aged man, who was looking for a Spanish-speaking therapist for his client. After I met with her once, Consuelo told me that her lawyer wanted to talk with me. When we spoke, he was very explicit. He wanted my help in getting Consuelo to be more compliant and less reactive to Tom's provocations, and to quickly settle the case out of court. He hoped Consuelo would understand me better because of our common language. He was surprised that she was so assertive and eager to negotiate everything rather than settle quickly. She was, he said, "too pushy for her own good." The lawyer wanted me to help Consuelo get past her anger and behave more rationally. He told her that the solution to her problem was "in her hands," if only she would change her attitude.

Unlike Tom's lawyer, Consuelo's lawyer may have had her best interest in mind, but he was also operating with several biases—in addition to labeling Consuelo "too emotional," he deemed her lacking in the submissive quality he expected from a Latina, an ethnic stereotype he assumed was a fixed trait. If Consuelo could become more submissive, the lawyer could secure her agreement with his proposals, which turned out to be pretty similar to those of Tom's lawyers, and the divorce would quickly become a "done deal." The faster the case closed, the more likely he would be paid for his time. In fact, the lawyer feared that Consuelo would never be able to pay his bill if the fight became protracted. From their earliest meetings he had predicted that because Consuelo was Mexican she would not have enough money to pay him. The lawyer had thus insured his compensation by bartering for goods with Consuelo's parents who, defying the lawyer's stereotype of hand-to-mouth subsistence, had a lucrative business in Mexico.

Equally disturbing was my realization that, just as Consuelo's concerns were being ignored, the lawyer was dismissing my concerns and expecting me to follow his instructions. He told me, another Latina, what to do in therapy and he had little interest in or patience for my point of view—I was not supposed to have a mind of my own. I told the lawyer of my concerns about Tom's violent temper, the vengeful tone of his accusations, and his wish to exclude Consuelo completely from her children's lives. I felt that his belligerent and litigious tone indicated the beginning of a long future of many trips to court. I suggested that a psychological evaluation of both parents' competence might be helpful. It could clarify each parent's contribution and perhaps challenge or support certain customary arrangements. The lawyer disagreed, fearing that such an exploration would ignite the other team further. He believed Tom and his Anglo-American, middle-aged lawyer, who was "pro ex-husband" in divorce cases, were very strong. He clearly was more impressed by the team of Anglo-American men than by the Latina women.

No doubt similar disqualifications could have occurred between a male lawyer and a white, English-speaking woman who was just as reactive and overwhelmed as Consuelo. The difference is that an English-speaking client would have her language with which to express herself, her voice would have been heard with somewhat more respect and less racial and ethnic prejudice, she may have had a network of friends that had gone through divorces and legal battles and lent their savvy to her case. The jeopardy of gender is compounded by the jeopardy of color, language, and cultural ignorance.

Consuelo and her family engaged a new attorney—one of three I recommended (two Latino and one Anglo-American). I favored a Latina lawyer who could listen to Consuelo in Spanish and understand the complex blend of gender and ethnic issues involved, and who believed that decisions about what is fair cannot be made on the basis of a priori assumptions about cultural styles or monetary interests. Consuelo went for interviews and quickly settled on a lawyer who was a white South American woman. She spoke perfect Spanish and excellent English, and her name didn't sound Spanish—a definite advantage against the prejudice that may have befallen her too. The new lawyer was a brave woman who obtained a less complacent and more fair settlement for Consuelo and her children, and one that allowed for the multiple relationships the children had developed with their mother's extended family.

While I believe professional territories and boundaries need to be respected, the relationship between each client and other larger professional systems crucial to the client's welfare in which decisions are made needs to be part of the therapeutic conversation (Imber-Black, 1986; Korin, 1994). With disempowered clients, vulnerabilities to be treated as "the other" are greater than with mainstream clients. Therapists must help them think aloud about the nature of those interactions and the consequences that could stem from them. This critical examination is part of an empowering process, a necessary rebalancing of social relationships.

## Talking about Race and Racism in Therapy

In spite of its enormous weight, the issue of race is often beyond awareness or is kept quiet or hidden for Latinos. This makes race and racism a very difficult topic to bring into the therapeutic conversation. In their pioneering book *Counseling the Culturally Different* (1990), Derald Wing Sue and David Sue challenged the prevalent "myth of color blindness" for therapists and discussed how a history of oppression, discrimination, and racism (and classism, I would add) has affected the way minorities perceive psychotherapy, which is basically a white, middle-class activity.

Many of the barriers identified by Sue and Sue (1990) that impede a strong therapeutic alliance with African American clients also apply to Latinos. Suspicion, apprehension, verbal constriction, indirect communication, distractions, and above all, passivity and inconsistency of commitment to the therapy process may all be present. While passivity and superficial compliance may confuse the therapist into believing that an alliance is being forged, the client may simply be carefully observing the therapist.

Kenneth Hardy and Tracey Laszloffy (1994) maintain that therapists must always validate the importance of race for the client. Race should not be underestimated as an organizing principle in their lives and in therapy. Since clients rarely communicate in a direct fashion about race, therapists need to learn to identify "racial metaphors." For Latinos, racial references may be tied to skin color but also to other physical characteristics such as stature or height. Being a *chaparrito/a* (shorty or of small build) is considered problematic in a society such as the United States, where height is considered desirable. Or clients may comment about their own accents or limited knowledge of English in alluding to their fear of discrimination.

Latinos, like all other minorities, are cognizant of the racial prejudices of the dominant culture. They will be alert, sensitive, and prepared to encounter prejudice among white professionals. They may also detect "microaggressions" (Hardy & Laszloffy, 1994; Pierce, 1970; Pinderhughes, 1989)—those small acts, often outside the awareness of both people of color and whites, that degrade, put down, or express indirect aggression against racial minorities.

## The Question of Matching

Given that racism and discrimination are ubiquitous experiences for many Latinos, and that most helping professionals belong to a dominant culture that harbors myriad prejudices, one might wonder if the gap between the two could be sufficiently bridged for effective therapy to occur. Or is ethnic/racial matching a more viable alternative? The truth is that opportunities and vulnerabilities lie in both "mismatched" therapist-client combinations and in those in which client and therapist share race and ethnicity.

Clearly not being Latino should not disqualify a clinician from working with Latino families. Many non-Latino therapists are sympathetic and respectful of Latinos. This client-therapist match, however, calls for certain precautions. Non-Latino clinicians concerned about their lack of experience with Latinos may be excessively "curious" or may overcompensate by spending a lot of time inquiring about cultural details at the expense of focusing on other issues of greater concern to the client. This problem is what Comas-Díaz and Jacobsen (1991) have aptly dubbed the "clinical anthropologist syndrome."

The non-Latino clinician may also be very eager to label as cultural, and therefore nondysfunctional, issues that are problematic but appear superficially as culturally consonant. Martínez (1994) describes this as "cultural interpretation gone awry" or "joining the family's denial system." This is an important warning. Don Jackson (1965) also alluded to family members' invoking "our culture" not as a sociological norm but as an interpersonal tactic or homeostatic device to control each other's behavior. Braulio Montalvo and Manuel Gutiérrez (1983) and Edwin Friedman (1982) caution that therapists may, in an effort to respect cultural differences, inadvertently collude with a family's "cultural camouflage" between members themselves or between the family and various institutions. Families may flash their "cultural masks" or otherwise hide their problems behind the guise of their culture.

Shyness, self-sacrifice, overdependence, domestic violence, child abuse, alcoholism, or religiosity may be minimized in the name of such Latino cultural code themes as *familismo, respeto,* honor, machismo, or Catholicism, when in fact any of these may have reached unhelpful excesses or become manifest in dysfunctional ways. In a case in New York, for example, a judge with "the best of intentions" sent a 6-year-old Latino child to her death by returning her to an abusive parent, dismissing the parent's behavior on the basis of cultural differences in child-rearing techniques.

Language is, of course, a serious barrier if therapist and client don't share a thorough knowledge of the other's tongue. The use of translators with first-generation immigrants is less necessary with Latinos than with other immigrants—it's often possible to find Spanish-speaking therapists to refer to or collaborate with if the clients don't speak English. When translators are used, it's important to be aware of the potential for subtle, unwitting distortions of meaning.

A common language, together with similar experiences and values, increases empathy for the immigrant's situation and facilitates easy rapport between the Latino therapist and the Latino client. However, this match isn't immune to pitfalls either. The most disturbing of these are the emotional fluctuations between idealized and denigrated views the therapist and the client may have of each other.

At the idealized extreme, immigrants, in particular, are vulnerable to regarding a therapist who is of the same ethnicity and race, but who is bilingual and holds a higher position, as a fairly omnipotent figure (Grinberg & Grinberg, 1989). It seems likely that therapists project an image of having competence and control over life in a way that immigrants of limited economic means do not experience. The status gap may stir confusing feelings on both sides. Countertransference in the Latino therapist may also include a wish to maintain positive views of the client. This vulnerability to take an idealized view is similar to that described for non-Latino therapists who miss problematic behavior in the name of cultural sensitivity. The same vulnerabilities can tempt Latino therapists to rescue Latino clients from discriminatory, oppressive situations, and in so doing, unwittingly disempower them or rob them of their sense of personal agency.

On the other hand, at the denigrated extreme, Latino clients may view Latino therapists through the lenses of *racismo* (Shorris, 1992)—the internalized autoracism or self-hate that oppressed groups often project by rejecting, distrusting, or invalidating the competence level of their own cultural group. Therapists themselves may not be totally exempt from a similar vulnerability toward internalized racial/ethnic prejudice and the projection of negative evaluations on clients of their same culture.

Montalvo and Gutiérrez (1990) accurately remind clinicians that alertness to preconceptions, a generic tool in all therapy, is of critical importance in working with minority families. This caution applies to all preconceptions but particularily to emotionally charged views implicit in idealization or demystifcation.

Cultural and racial differences and similarities between clients and therapists can be judiciously brought out as a subject for conversation and exploration, the onus being on the therapist's ability to be sensitive about these difficult subjects. My personal opinion is that therapists need to share their own ideological position with clients when issues of culture are discussed. This helps create a collaborative dialogue and conjoint reflection that enhances the therapeutic encounter.

## ON TRUSTING PROFESSIONALS

The development of trust in a setting that may harbor hidden or overt prejudice for minorities presents a particular challenge for therapists who are members of the dominant culture. Certainly therapists are defined as people who are capable of intuitive empathic understanding—someone who can imagine what it must be like to have lived and be living the experiences of the other. C. Wright Mills (1959) coined the term "sociological imagination" to describe the ability to connect a person's biography with the sociocultural and sociohistorical circumstances of his or her life. But how does this look in practice?

Earlier I discussed the importance of the development of *confianza* (trust) in interpersonal relationships. This trust is created not through an efficient task orientation that follows procedures or provides prompt services, but rather through the gradual development of a relationship based on *personalismo*. For therapists, this means an ability to be respectful of the client's dignity by communicating kindness, fairness, and simple courtesies and personal interest rather than by "doing" anything in particular.

Experiences of discrimination and feelings of inferiority and foreignness lead many Latinos into institutional dealings with a deep sense of *desconfianza* (mistrust). Even middle-class, educated Latinos may be wary of subtle racial or ethnic discrimination, or fear being misunderstood, or show caution for the nearly inevitable indoctrination into American ways when they interact with agents of the larger society, including therapists.

Therapists can help to mitigate this natural distrust in a number of ways. First, they need to face and examine their own positive and negative stereotypes about Latinos, because these will inevitably be transmitted. Bilingualism, biculturalism, and empathy are helpful, but not necessary, in developing trust with Latino clients. Second, therapists can practice a number of attitudes and approaches that build trust: they should be open and honest about the clinical setting and the goals of therapy and repeatedly offer to answer any questions family members may have, even if they never take up the offer. Further, it's important to be pleasant, sociable, nonconfrontational, and show genuine interest. The interview should be a pleasant, enjoyable experience, helped along by some small disclosure from the therapist, such as "I am a parent, too," or "I have experiences as an immigrant." I am convinced it is impossible to build *confianza* in a hurried or impatient way, or through a therapist's reputation alone. In the end, conviviality may not take more than five extra minutes of each hour, but once *confianza* is in place, it is stable and greatly speeds up future work.

Lloyd Rogler, Osvaldo Barreras, and Rosemary Cooney (1981) provide some useful insights into dealing with distrust. In easing the minds of their Puerto Rican participants, these researchers employed Spanish-speaking Latino interviewers, who offered home visits and gave their phone numbers so the families could call with any questions about the study. Trust-building, they noticed, was further helped by close attention to generational differences. For the older generation, they followed a more formal address, using the pronoun *usted* (*señor, señora, Don*, or *Doña*). These forms connote respect, maintain appropriate distance, and convey to elders that they are worthy and honorable persons. Interviewers also avoided anglicisms that might create feelings of alienation in non-English-speaking people. Accepting hospitality and other offerings was also encouraged because a rejection would have diminished the generous intent. Showing interest in *vuestra manera de ser* (your way of being) further helped interviewers demonstrate that they wanted to understand each family's meanings about their culture. This invitation may evoke intense feelings of *añorar* (nostalgia) about the past and the home country. Empathic listening fosters trust and rapport.

With the younger generations of couples, the interviewers used the informal form of address, *tú* (you), which indicates a more fluid, less structured relationship between speakers. Much of the informal talk referred to cultural changes in the life cycle of the interviewees—the effects of women's drive toward equality, child-rearing issues, or contemporary Latino culture in the United States. English was spoken more often with this group, as was an alternation between English and Spanish, with some hybrid "Spanglish" words thrown in.

More fundamental for trust-building practices than the external amenities that create conviviality are the internal attitudes of the therapist, revealed through the types of explorations, statements, and conclusions she makes. If the therapist conveys a belief in the "deficit model" that focuses only on specific details of the family's psychosocial problems, not much headway will be made in creating a working relationship. The family's despair may only increase, or they may feel the therapist has good intentions but has little to offer beyond sympathy. A therapist can empower the family by commenting on its "relational resilience" as a functional unit (Walsh, in press)—a group that demonstrates survival and coping skills, ethnic and network resources, situational triumphs, and affectional capacities in spite of racial and economic discrimination. These messages can offer a family a more solid, hopeful base as they gain trust in the therapist's capacity to appreciate and help them.

## The Therapy Office as Cultural Context

Because culture is both material and ideational, therapists can send powerful cultural messages not only at the ideational level, but also at the material level. In fact, entering the therapy office is the first time and space for this cultural encounter.

> Years ago, while browsing in a bin of old lacy napkins and handkerchiefs in an antique shop in Wisconsin, I came across an embroidered piece of thick natural cloth depicting a map of the United States. Within each state's embroidered outline some characteristic attribute of that state was shown, such as yellow corn in Iowa, red clay pottery in New Mexico, or brown quarter horses in Montana. It reminded me of a canvas map of Argentina I once had. I cherished this map of Argentina because it allowed me to walk my land (which was different than my parents' land) with my hands and my mind, much before my feet could take me anywhere far from home.
>
> Because the United States is my children's country (and perhaps because I needed to learn the geography of my new home), I bought this homemade United States map and framed it in natural wood. Over the years it traveled from one of my three daughters' bedrooms to the next until it no longer fit any of their tastes in decor, and finally it ended up in the family room. I have often chuckled about the fact that many visitors have delighted in its quaintness and have chosen to spend quite a bit of time examining it, over other more impressive art in the house. The eager onlookers usually zero in on the states they are from, or those they have lived in.

The presence of objects, as cultural signifiers, such as that old map, conveys powerful emotional and ideational messages. A culturally sensitive therapist can help clients feel less alien by creating a therapy environment that is more diverse and somewhat international. Symbols can create a sense of familiarity for the clients and increase their trust and confidence about the therapist's friendliness and sensitivity. Many studies attribute Latinos' underutilization of mental health services to doubts about the possibility of being understood, or of finding culturally consonant solutions to their problems. A physical environment that reflects the national groups, and the communities it serves, may facilitate engagement in treatment (Inclán & Ferrán, 1990).

Maps of Mexico and Central and South America may help locate towns of origin and places along the route of migration. In addition, a map of the United States may help children and parents talk about where they have been, where they are, and even where they are going, using a sort of "geographic genogram." Even the presence of a globe helps convey movement, location, and diversity. Games, magazines, and books in Spanish are wonderful tools for engaging parents, children, and even adolescents in conversation about language, customs, and memories, and may even encourage storytelling about the extended family or the parents' past experiences (Martínez & Valdéz, 1992). Dolls of different skin colors and racial features, cooking utensils from various cultures, and other identifiable objects and symbols are useful in making the family therapy context consonant with the minority client's experience of living in a multicultural environment. Clearly if one takes the view that we share cultural borderlands, then creating a physical environment that reflects this belief will convey immediately a sign of acceptance and respect.

In conclusion, focusing on the dimensions of a client's ecological context opens up conversations about the psychological impact of feeling like a marginalized minority, whether because of race, poverty, or immigrant status. These conversations help to discover possible associations between the presenting problem and powerlessness or lack of entitlement, or the therapist may discover the opposite—that the family is proud of their fierce zest for life in the face of adversity. It is imperative that therapists examine their own subtle prejudices about Latinos and strive to create an atmosphere of genuine mutual trust. We offer suggestions that help build trust, but clinicians may exercise their own humanity and creativity in this respect. Failing to acknowledge the hard social realities of ecological contexts and Latinos' own coping resources can lead to confusing the effects of social marginalization with ethnic value preferences. In the next chapter I focus on two particular contexts in which Latino children and adults may experience this marginalization: the classroom and the workplace.

# 7

# The Challenge of
# School and Work

## IMMIGRANT CHILDREN AND SCHOOL ACHIEVEMENT

Perhaps more than any other institution, the school of the majority culture is the arena in which many of the problems of young Latinos are played out. School is often where problems begin, or simply intensify. Further, educational attainment for all Latino groups except Cubans is significantly lower than for other ethnic populations, including American Indians and African Americans. U.S. Census Bureau statistics show that 79% of all Latinos have not completed high school. Among Cubans, 63% of children born here or who arrived at a young age complete high school as compared to 55% of Puerto Ricans and 44% of Mexicans, all below the rate of 80% for non-Hispanics. Only 9% of all Latinos go on to complete a college education (Pathey-Chávez, 1993; Suárez-Orozco, 1993; Trueba, 1989; Trueba, Rodríguez, & Cintrón, 1993; Vigil, 1988).

Poverty among Latinos is the main correlate of limited educational achievement (Chapa & Valencia, 1993). In addition to the well-known psychosocial stresses of poverty—parents who are stressed by unemployment or underemployment and lack of education, bleak or dangerous neighborhood life, and overcrowded housing—Latino children also experience the deleterious effects on academic success of linguistic and cultural marginality, generational conflicts, and the impact of racial and ethnic discrimination (Rumbaut & Cornelius, 1995; Delgado-Gaitán, 1988).

The literature on factors involved in Latino school performance is extensive, particularly as it relates to desegregation and bilingual education. In this chapter, however, the discussion is limited to two school problems that are likely to be encountered by clinicians: academic underachievement and school dropout. In discussing theories that attempt to explain these problems, I move away from deficit models and focus on protective factors that are conducive to school achievement. Programatic approaches that promote academic success and empower children and parents are included.

Of the two theories that address school problems in Latino groups, one relates to the primary, cultural discontinuity of values between home and school. The other focuses on the ecological, child-school rifts that are secondary to discrimination and a youngster's minority status (Bernal, Saenz, & Knight, 1995).[1] Let's examine these two theories briefly.

## Cultural Disparity or Home-School Mismatch?

Incompatibilities between home and school in primary languages, cognitive and relational styles, and values may cause confusion and conflict for Latino children who live with two sets of cultural codes. Parents must deal with these cultural clashes whenever their interactions with children involve school issues. Teachers also experience dissonance when they struggle to understand Latino students and their parents. Family interdependence may prepare young children to expect help from adults, perhaps in tying shoes or taking off coats, while teachers may see this as a sign of dependency or a lack of self-reliance. Or the young child may show deference and respect to authorities by lowering his eyes, while teachers expect directness and openness. This behavior may be perceived as being shy or "sneaky" rather than respectful (Escovar & Lazarus, 1982).

In a study of low-income Puerto Rican mothers and their children in a Headstart program, Ortiz-Colón (1985) found that mothers preferred children to be obedient and conforming while their Anglo-American teachers preferred behavior that was assertive, verbal, self-directed, and independent, and of course, they both thought these choices of behavior were connected to future success. Later I will discuss how ideas about proper demeanor and self-maximization permeate child socialization and parenting styles (see Chapter 9).

Immigrant parents from many countries seem to favor external conformity over autonomous behaviors. They may regard motivation and social skill as important, if not more important, than problem solving and verbal ability in defining what constitutes an intelligent child (Okagaki & Sternberg, 1993). In a study of the child-rearing values of Puerto Rican mothers, González-Ramos, Zayas, and Cohen (1993) found that mothers stressed family closeness, respect for parental authority, and religious beliefs as the driving elements in their parenting. Indeed, qualities that stress responsibility for others and affectional ties have been found in successful children from ethnically diverse backgrounds (Werner, 1990).

Zayas (1994) suggests that the common, deficit-oriented view of Hispanic parents as authoritarian fails to take into account the survival strategies these parents developed in response to their environments. Democratic parenting may not be sufficient to protect and deter children from the negative pull of urban dangers and temptations, such as drugs, violence, and racism. Zayas cites studies in progress that show parents who have limited support become more controlling and firm when faced with ecological stress, while those who have adequate social support can turn toward more "autonomous teaching" approaches. Once again, a family's ecological context must be examined before assessing the relative influence of cultural styles and present external circumstances.

In general terms, it seems the American educational system uses primarily competitive motives to promote and reward academic achievement, while the Latino family emphasizes cooperation, affiliation, and proper manners. It would be a mistake, however, to conclude that Latino children are passive, cooperative, and compliant in all contexts. They may be fiercely competitive in a soccer game where the rules of the game require it. Further, while ethnic socialization may account for some of the differences Latino children and their teachers encounter together, migration clearly has its own effect. In an extensive review of the literature, Aranowitz (1984) suggests that shyness, nervousness, and quietness in the classroom may stem from a sense of unfamiliarity and many of the fears that accompany migration.

The theory of primary cultural discrepancies helps orient therapists to explore possible misunderstandings between the family and the school, and to be aware that underachieving children may be experiencing confusion and dissonance in language and cultural codes. Attendance at parochial rather than public schools seems to decrease this dissonance somewhat, perhaps because of small class sizes and a shared history of Catholicism. A number of other, powerful elements related to minority status also play a significant role in a Latino child's experience at school, as I discuss in the next section.

## Secondary Ecological Discontinuity

The theory of secondary ecological discontinuity stresses the influence of low income, prejudice, and discrimination on minority children's school resistance and failure. The most ardent proponent of this view is John Ogbu (1987). He maintains that when poor and dark-skinned minorities first establish contact with white-dominant groups, only primary differences in their cultures emerge. But as children become more familiar with American culture through the school years, secondary cultural differences develop. These represent reactions, response styles, and attempts by minority children to adapt to the treatment they receive from the dominant group. Such adaptations may include more aggressive or more withdrawn communication styles, stronger ethnic alliances, and rejection or distrust of the cultural values of the dominant group. Most importantly, minority children may come to believe that their chances of educational and economic success will never compare to those of their white classmates. According to Ogbu, these youngsters then develop behavioral styles that involve at least two features detrimental to academic success: cultural inversion and oppositional social identity.

Cultural inversion is the tendency of minority groups to see behaviors, meanings, and symbols of the dominant group as undesirable for themselves. The result is a framework of opposition—peers exert pressure on each other to avoid acting in accordance with dominant group values, such as working for good grades. The new, oppositional identity promotes behaviors that lead to school failure and ultimately to dropping out.

Different factors predict dropout among Latino groups (Vélez, 1989). For students of Mexican descent, cutting classes, suspensions, heavy dating, being older, and being female increases one's odds of dropping out. Among Cubans, suspensions were the primary predictor of quitting school, while for Puerto Ricans, being female, older, and confrontational were significant factors. Cubans were the least likely to drop out, correlating with a larger number of two-parent households, higher socioeconomic level, and relatively recent migration. Although less so than for Cubans, recent immigration from Mexico and Puerto Rico is a protective factor for dropout. Exposure to American society tends to hurt, not help, the prospects of immigrant children. Grades, school attendance, and motivation tend to slip the longer immigrant children are in the United States.

Other empirical evidence supports the theory of reactive discontinuity over that of primary cultural mismatch. Particularly interesting are the findings of a recent study of 13- to 18-year-olds. Anthropologist Marcelo Suárez-Orozco and psychologist Carola Suárez-Orozco (1995) investigated how concerns and attitudes regarding school achievement and family orientation differ among Mexican youth living in Mexico, Mexican immigrant youth (born in Mexico), Mexican American youth (born in the United States of Mexican parents), and non-Latino white students in southern California. Studying all of these groups allowed for cultural comparisons between uprooted minorities and those who have the advantage of family and school stability in their home countries, uninfluenced by the dislocating experiences of migration and culture change.

A surprising finding was that achievement motivation was more frequently self-initiated among Mexican youth born in Mexico than among non-Latino white students. This finding contradicts the stereotypical belief that the cultural "background" of Latinos, which stresses fatalism, present orientation, low aspirations, and noncompetitiveness may largely account for school failure in the U.S. system, a system that upholds quite different cultural values. In the Súarez-Orozcos' study, the Mexican students' narratives spoke of a cultural background that stresses self-initiated achievement and truly values hard work as the road to success. These strivings coexist with familism, interdependence, and obtaining help from others more than in non-Latino groups (see also Delgado-Gaitán & Trueba, 1991; Trueba et al., 1993).

The study concludes that limited achievement by Latinos in the United States cannot be attributed to cultural differences. Rather, we should look at the negative shift that occurs after children and their families become part of a discriminated minority—one that suffers economic deprivation, school alienation, and internal and external pressures to join the work force.

These findings clearly point to the importance of looking beyond the individual child to identify and intervene when school problems loom. Efforts should always be made to elucidate the actual school situation, including interaction with teachers and peers. Emphasis on the school setting per se does not mean disregarding the contribution of parents. As for children everywhere, parental attitudes have a strong impact on Latino children's school performance. As we will see, efforts to empower both parents and children to deal with the school are critical avenues of change.

## IMMIGRANT PARENTS AND THE SCHOOLS

The dream of Latino immigrant parents is to educate their children and thus provide a way out of poverty. Yet, besieged by overwork or by underemployment, and by insufficient knowledge of the culture and language, parents may rely on and even overburden their children with the multiple responsibilities of translating, cleaning house, and babysitting. Further, many immigrant parents feel lost and intimidated by the school system. They may be unsure of the best ways to support and encourage their children in this unfamiliar environment. Youngsters may be left feeling profoundly alone, unprotected, and incompetent. Latino parents frequently report being misunderstood, misinterpreted, or not listened to by school personnel. Similarly, school staff report frustration and inability to communicate problems or expectations to Latino parents.

Immigrant parents may feel inadequate when dealing with the school, and justifiably fear prejudice. They are aware that larger systems and institutions are often carriers of unexamined negative attitudes toward ethnic minorities, women, and the poor (Imber-Black, 1986). In addition to their genuine lack of understanding of language and institutional procedures, anxieties about detection of undocumented status and subsequent threat of deportation also contribute to the guardedness observed by well-meaning but frustrated teachers and principals. These fears may be passed on to the children, who are already coping with their own shame and doubt.

For Latino parents, education and schools stir emotional meanings that are deeper than in those who have never experienced life as an immigrant.

The year we moved to San Diego, my two oldest children were 6 and 10 and had been attending a very good school in Chicago. To show our appreciation and to bid everybody good-bye before the move, we went to the "end of the year" ceremonies. At one point during this event I began to cry softly, and pretty soon could not control an inconsolable sobbing. My husband didn't know what to do to comfort me—I couldn't readily explain to him what it was about this particular setting that stirred me so profoundly. That memory and some of the sadness have returned at times, usually around some school event involving my children.

School has always had a lot of emotional significance for me. As the first child of unschooled immigrants, entering school in Argentina was to enter a realm of profound loneliness, fear, and shyness. Until (as a new immigrant to the United Sates myself) my first child entered school in the United States, I never understood or forgave my parents for never visiting my elementary school, never meeting any of my teachers, and not attending my high school graduation. As a parent of children in an American school, I experienced total culture shock and began to feel empathy with my own parents' immigrant predicament. The classrooms, arrangements of tables and chairs, the blackboards, the sounds of the silence and of the noise were completely different from what I remembered them to be as a child in my own country. I felt intimidated by the teachers and principals, ashamed of my accent, and in a state of vulnerable regression—truly outrageous feelings considering that I had gone to graduate school in the United States.

Over time I have come to believe that many immigrants do not feel entitled, let alone welcome, to make use of the institutions of a country that is not their own. It is as though you are always a guest in a place to which you have not been invited, and therefore you can never go farther than the entrance threshold and remain coyly standing up—the way I was when I entered school alone for the first time in my own country, fighting hard to hold back my tears. As time went on, growing up in Argentina, being brave in a new world my parents had not experienced paid off. School became a site of autonomy and mastery, of hope and even elation, a second home. But it also took me to an internal place of no return, very far away from my parents. The fear that a physical and philosophical separation might happen some day could also have been part of their resistance to know about and support my schooling.

I have come to accept that, for me, contact with American schools will always be tinged with the inevitable unease of the foreigner in a national setting or the trepidation of the working-class interloper in a middle-class world. The threshold of the two worlds, the old language and the new knowledge, the envisioned excursions from one social class to another are right there, almost palpable at the school. Those symbolic meanings give me clues to the conflicts, tensions, and considerable suffering of Latinos in school. I use these feelings and experiences in my work with children and adolescents, their families, and their teachers. As part of exploring their own cultural genograms, young therapists can profit from sorting out their own school experiences, feelings, and attitudes. This awareness can help them develop sympathy with all family members and particularly with parents who often appear passive or disinterested in their children's schools.

For all its trials and tribulations, school is the place where Latino children *and* parents learn about American society. Increasingly, programs are being developed in which parents participate either with other parents or with their own children in sharing problems and finding community support.

## PROGRAMS FOR PARENTS AND CHILDREN

Many avenues are opening to help parents and children raise levels of school achievement, prevent dropout, and encourage a sense of belonging in the school, the community, and the future.

## School Consultation

The practice of having therapist, teacher (and sometimes other school personnel), and parent meet for an assessment or conjoint problem solving[2] is a very useful method of intervention with Latino parents who speak English fairly well, but it can be an overwhelming experience for immigrant parents. The latter can profit from a one-to-one interview with a teacher and a translator or an interpreter.

Cognizant of the fundamental role played by parental support, a number of programs around the country involve Latino parents with their children in the school setting. These range from group therapy-like approaches to mentoring efforts, including the following:

### Folktale or Cuento Therapy

Latino parents readily cooperate with special interventions that can enhance their children's chances of school success. An after-school program that taps cultural consonance and ethnic respect and provides excellent results in enhancing school performance is offered by *cuento* therapy. Starting with the notion that a culture's folktales use metaphors to concretize abstract ethical concepts such as obedience, honesty, or filial love while transmitting a cultural heritage, Giuseppe Constantino, Robert Malgady, and Lloyd Rogler (1986) devised this unique treatment modality. *Cuento* therapy is a form of narrative "modeling" in which *cuentos* (folktales) from indigenous Puerto Rican folklore are adapted for use with children and adolescents to present models of adaptive behavior in multiethnic, urban inner-city situations.

In one study, children from kindergarten to third grade presented anxiety symptoms, conduct problems (aggressiveness, disruptiveness, inability to delay gratification), poor social judgment, and low self-esteem. The typical *cuento* session took place in a school classroom from 3:00 P.M. to 4:30 P.M. Two therapists and five mothers sat with their children in a circle. After the mothers read the stories bilingually, the therapists conducted a group discussion of the character's feelings and behavior and the moral of the story. A third step involved the mother-child dyad dramatizing the story and resolving the conflict presented. Videotapes of the role-playing exercise were reviewed and therapists led a discussion of the group members' experiences, focusing on which solutions they found to be effective for similar conflicts. The results of 20 sessions of the *cuento* therapy were dramatically more effective in reducing symptoms, promoting growth, and increasing IQ measurements than the control group which participated in traditional play/activity sessions conducted by a therapist and a schoolteacher (see Constantino & Rivera, 1994).

In a second study designed for adolescents, Malgady et al. (1990) developed *cuento* therapy using biographical stories of prominent Puerto Rican athletes, artists, and politicians who have overcome poverty and prejudice. These stories provide "heroic" adult role models that can help bridge the identity, bicultural, and intergenerational conflicts confronted by Puerto Rican adolescents. Mothers did not participate because the adolescents felt inhibited by their presence. Group members read the biographies and therapists led the discussion. The biographies embodied themes of cultural conflict, such as expression of ethnic pride in the face of discrimination, and the structured group discussion compared each group member's experience with the model's biography. The discussion was followed by imitative role playing that explored adaptive behaviors. The main positive findings were decreased anxiety symptoms and increased ethnic identity and self-esteem, all of which enhanced a sense of empowerment and increased personal agency.

## Parent Education Programs

Latino parents play a crucial role in their child's education, even before age 3. A number of programs are aimed at helping them understand and utilize this important position. A combined goal is to increase the parent's sense of personal efficacy, positive interactions with the child, and use of community resources (Powell, Zarubrana, & Silva-Palacios, 1990; Powell, 1995a).

Many programs are culturally based—they take into account the child-rearing techniques and personal qualities Latino parents want to inculcate in their children—rather than constructed on a framework of acculturation. Furthermore, the ecology of poverty, with its developmental risks and limited access to resources, guides formats that encourage parents' input and supports their initiatives in their neighborhoods and schools. For descriptions of settings, activities, and the psychological benefits of such programs the reader may want to consult Duany and Pittman (1990), Rodríguez (1994), and Shapiro (1995).

Until recently, most parent education programs and discussion groups have been oriented toward Latina mothers with an almost all-female staff. New educational projects are being oriented toward Latino fathers and male staff. Although based on a small sample of 28 Latino fathers, research conducted by Douglas R. Powell (1995b) provides a good starting point for collaborative programs that accommodate the characteristics of local communities. In this particular sample, fathers expressed a preference for meetings that included mothers and fathers (as well as extended family members); liked a combination of parent discussion groups and home visits; preferred groups in which they were already familiar with some of the participants; favored program staff who were professionals knowledgeable in child rearing; and preferred information given in verbal dialogue rather than materials for reading. These patterns, consistent with the results of a sample of immigrant Mexican mothers, reveal a cultural ideology of familism and community, and of respect for professional expertise in a context of personalism. The possible content areas chosen by these parents were child rearing and the relationship between family and environment. With regard to the latter, most of the concerns centered on the consequences of poverty, language, and minority status.

The preventive potential and therapeutic value of programs that are attuned to the family's ecological niche can be invaluable in providing emotional support, psychoeducational input, and adaptational empowerment.

## Community Empowerment

The work of Concha Delgado-Gaitán and Henry T. Trueba (1991) focuses on immigrant families learning community empowerment and democratic participation both at home and in school. These authors make a very important theoretical contribution by developing an ethnography of the empowerment stages parents undergo as they interact with schools. They contend that by learning to form community organizations that have direct input in the schooling of their children, these parents not only help the self-esteem and performance of the children, they also emerge from a sense of social isolation and helplessness and become more aware of their common rights and responsibilities.

## Mentoring Programs

Many large cities have after-school mentoring programs. The children come from public elementary and junior high school settings with large Latino populations. The staff is comprised of volunteer, bilingual adults who provide educational enrichment by pursuing with students interests in history, museums, art, music, or other cultural and sports activities. The mentors are role models of successful Latinos and provide an informational bridge for Latino parents who often lack the resources to guide their children toward higher education and to cross the institutional barriers.

Therapists working with Latino families of school-age children need to be familiar with information and resources about local community support and educational and mentoring programs, either as the primary or adjunctive form of help for parents and children.

## WORK IN A NEW WORLD

Latinos are hard workers—they left their countries with a hopeful determination to better their family's socioeconomic status. Their commitment to work differs from the middle-class Anglo-American belief in self-improvement, getting ahead, and achieving personal recognition and individual success. Latinos immerse themselves in hard work because they firmly believe they have to sacrifice themselves for the survival and well-being of their children and other loved ones. This is the sustaining motive behind the endurance and tolerance (*aguantar*) of heavy work schedules, holding two or more jobs, working overtime, moonlighting, accepting low wages, and withstanding grueling, exploitative working conditions.

Only Cuban men represent sizable numbers in management and professional jobs, while Mexicans and Puerto Ricans are more likely to be employed as operators or laborers. Labor force participation of Latino women has increased sharply in the past 20 years. Women in the three groups are more likely than men to be employed in technical, sales, and administrative support positions to almost the same degree as the non-Latino population, though a large number are also involved in service occupations. Unemployment rates are 4% higher among Latinos than non-Latinos (Chapa & Valencia, 1993; Ortiz, 1995).

Median household income is lower for all Hispanic groups than for non-Hispanic households. Median incomes for Cubans are the highest while those of Mexicans and Puerto Ricans are the lowest—almost half that of non-Hispanic families. Puerto Rican workers have median incomes comparable to other Hispanic groups. The greater poverty of Puerto Rican households derives from their greater likelihood of being single-parent homes.

## Respect and Dignity at Work: *Buen Trato, Mal Trato*

A very significant source of work stress for Latinos is their relationship with employers and other workers. Latinos describe their interactions with bosses in terms of *buen trato* (respectful treatment) or *mal trato* (disrespectful or demeaning treatment, lack of consideration, or exploitation). *Buen trato* reflects *respeto,* but more than anything it accords *dignidad* (dignity) to an employee. There is nothing more meaningful to a Latino than to be treated with dignity, because it grants worth and respect, regardless of position or status achieved in the social or economic hierarchy. *Mal trato* leads to depression, either through internalized feelings of worthlessness or internalized anger. These feelings rarely find expression—complaints will likely result in losing a job that was difficult to get in the first place.

*Buen trato* offers other benefits. When *buen trato* has been established, employers become the trusted advisors that can be sought for solutions to problems, financial loans, suggestions for resources such as schools for children, second jobs, or additional work, legal help, translation of documents, and health or dental care. This type of relationship is most marked between household employees, both live-in and day workers.

Employers can become part of a helpful network in a class system, or they can be an additional, and powerful, source of constant stress. The relationship between employers and household employees is a complex one involving psychological and familial processes that may be played out in therapy in a variety of ways. Working women who suffer *mal trato* often present at mental health clinics with depression. I often encourage them to become more verbal and ask their employers for time off to return to their countries to see their children, or to help them find out about English classes in the neighborhood, or to facilitate getting a second opinion from a family physician or gynecologist.

In other words, an employer can officiate as social intermediary for relatively new immigrants or even for those who have been here longer but lack access to information. The therapist can encourage immigrants to voice their human needs and their limits and to ask for help rather than to continue to serve and self-sacrifice silently. Although this represents a different type of negotiation than for Anglo-Americans, who may be more concerned about maintaining clear boundaries and privacy, I have witnessed successful systems of mutual help, particularly among women, across class and ethnicity.

## The Connection between Work and *Machismo*

Theories about Latino men's dominant attitudes toward women and children have stressed traditional ethnic beliefs about what is proper behavior for men. Some authors have questioned this ethnic-based explanation (Baca-Zinn, 1982) and regard *machismo* as a response to structural or socioeconomic class and work limitations. Even though I have observed many economically powerful Mexican men bent on maintaining a patriarchal system of financial dependency and behavior control in their families, male dominance may take on a different meaning when society excludes minority men from fair rewards and economic advancement. Under these circumstances, the family may be the only arena in which a father and husband can maintain a compensatory sense of pride in his stereotypical manhood.

Both men and women are prey to these stereotypes. Women too expect men to be capable providers and may look down on the man who fails at this task. Latinas raised in upper socioeconomic settings may come to expect all the material comfort, hired services, and security of status that wealth provides. This wealth is often dispensed by a domineering but generous father. Their disappointment in a husband who cannot fulfill this expectation can be devastating to the love connection. In therapy I have encountered considerable resistance on the part of women to the suggestion of exercising "cultural resistance" to this induction into a social definition of men as dispensers of money, comfortable homes, vacations, or expensive jewelry. Appeals to *pobre pero honesto* (poor but honest) do not seem to sway the learned expectation even in contexts in which remaining rich may entail devious maneuvering on the man's part.

The social and economic inequality theory of machismo is of particular relevance to working class Mexican and Puerto Rican men. If an immigrant father's promise of offering protection and a better future never materializes, he becomes not only internally demoralized but he also loses his prestige and his influence with his wife and adolescent children. In our discussion of family structure (Chapter 9), we note that the more a Latino man perceives these losses the more forcefully he may attempt to assert his authority with his wife and children. The adolescent children may side with mother and become increasingly scornful and distant from father. Powerless, the father may fall back on the empty gestures of a "paper tiger" with nothing but a cultural stereotype to hold up his dignity.

## Working Women: Benefits and Costs

Today many Latino households have dual incomes. This transformation in gender roles appears to be more economic in origin than ideological. In a comparative ethnographic study, Kelly and García (1989) contrasted the experiences of Cuban women in Miami and Mexican women in Los Angeles. They found Mexican immigrant women to be in a process of "proletarization" because their labor has become essential and would most likely continue to be required for family survival. Cuban women, however, had left the labor force as soon as short-term goals of improving the family's living standards were achieved. These decisions probably reflect a preference by both women and men for a traditional gender division of labor, when it is financially viable.

Research shows that Latino families have always been able to adapt to socieconomic conditions via the wife's incorporation in the labor force (A. R. Del Castillo, 1996). But the employment of Latinas is often a sign of economic marginality, a necessity that may cause considerable conflict for both partners. A husband in my office reproached his wife for her "failing to fulfill her wifely duties" (a euphemism for having sex) to which she responded much more directly: "If you fulfilled your husbandly duties of supporting this family, things would be different. . . . " Each one of them earned under $10,000 a year, but the husband worked two shifts. The wife's reproach did not mean, however, that she failed to derive considerable agency and power through her work. Clearly a subscription to rigid sex roles can be at cross purposes to financial survival for many Latino couples, and a serious source of stress as a result (Vásquez & González, 1981).

The wife may be gaining independence precisely when the husband is struggling to find stable employment and is feeling his deficiencies more keenly. The husband may feel he is losing his function as protector and provider, his only cultural reward. He may increase his social drinking and become psychologically or physically abusive with his family. The home becomes the only place where a man who is in a subservient occupation, unemployed, or underemployed can express the aggressive masculinity he has been socialized to exert but unable to.

For the wife, work may be a place to gain experience, competence, and confidence. One result may be a change in her tolerance and expectations of marriage. While her income and need to work lowers her husband's status, it may increase her own contempt, especially if she comes home from work and still has to carry out all the traditional homemaking and childcare tasks. These are common sources of marital tension and may lead to the woman's disinterest in sex. Some of these cases include violence that escalates as a husband tries to reassert his dominance.

Parallels between the gender role conflicts of Latinos and other groups are many, and therapists may be tempted to generalize from assumptions based on the difficulties white women experience in striving for egalitarian rather than patriarchal arrangements. However, Vásquez and González (1981) suggest that feminist issues among Latinos have some important differences from those of Anglo-American women. While seeking equal access to work and pay, Latinas continue to embrace commitment to family, community, and ethnic group, and seek respect for the roles traditionally performed by women. This prioritizing of the family has been called "political familism" by Chicanos, in the sense that the Chicano family has been a mechanism of cultural resistance that afforded protection, security, and comfort in the face of oppression (Baca-Zinn, 1975). Latina clients may be reluctant to remain in therapy if they detect the therapist supports a feminist ideology. They may not share any goal that, directly or indirectly, devalues traditional feminine roles or emphasizes a focus on self. A multicultural perspective needs to become more central to the development of feminist-oriented therapy theory and practice (Brown, 1995).

## Adult Work and Children's Work

A parent's problems at work often intersect with a child's difficulties at school. Children may worry a great deal about the perils of parental unemployment, discouragement, or financial woes. They may feel disloyal or guilty about succeeding in school when a parent is failing at work. They may consider dropping out or may express anger at their parent for not trying hard enough or for failing as a role model. Several of these issues were present in the following case:

> Javier Reyes Balán, a 16-year-old boy, was referred by his school for persistent truancy. Nine years ago, his mother, father, and four younger siblings (two boys and two girls) moved from Michoacán, Mexico, to San Diego, California, to better their economic situation. Javier was bilingual and served as the family interpreter in their dealings with outside institutions. He preferred to speak English and was clearly more savvy about American values and ways than his parents.
>
> Mr. Reyes began the session by complaining bitterly about Javier's unruly behavior, lack of cooperation with his mother, and lack of respect toward his parents. Mrs. Reyes appeared to agree with her husband's view about Javier, although she protested that she didn't need much help around the house. (This triangular interaction occurs frequently in Latino families. It's probably patriarcally based in that mother may not ask much for herself, and father orders the children to help their mother rather than helping her himself.)
>
> Whenever the father demanded greater obedience from Javier, the teenager became more rebellious and threatened to leave home to find a job. Because Javier was highly acculturated, he clearly had more power in the outside world than did his parents. And, influenced by the autonomy he observed in his American peers, it seemed difficult for Javier to assume a compliant attitude. The father, feeling defeated in his attempts to control his son, would turn to the mother and blame her for not raising the boy properly, for being too "soft," and for not demanding enough of him. This situation escalated into a marital conflict of mutual accusations.

An inquiry about Mr. Reyes's occupation revealed that he had hoped to start his own small business as a car mechanic after moving from Mexico. He had not succeeded and was supporting the family precariously with occasional small jobs. He was proud of his competence and honesty as an automobile mechanic (visibly emotionally moved, he displayed a very old, tattered letter of recommendation from a client in Mexico). But now he refused to work in a company under an Anglo-American foreman who would subject him to *mal trato*. In his view, "they [Americans] don't respect us Mexicans, and when you turn around they exploit you." The father's position in the family appeared to be debilitated by his unemployment, yet it was difficult to discuss this subject without undermining him further. In addition, his arguments against oppression were a double-edged sword—he felt empowered by his determination not to be exploited by Americans, but without work he was sliding toward impotence and helplessness.

I decided to express my admiration for the father's sacrifice and integrity. He had come to the United States where he expected racial discrimination and had remained honest in the auto business where there is so much dishonesty. He also had maintained his pride in the face of scorn for his Mexican identity, in spite of the financial difficulties it had occasioned him. I wondered if his family appreciated all of these qualities and efforts, which should only deserve *buen trato*. Mr. Reyes was moved to tears and said he did not know. The son intervened, saying that his father was very stubborn and that if he was not going to work, he should let him find a job to help the family. Mother remarked that she also wanted to look for a job, but her husband would not allow it because their two young children were too small. This interaction gave me the opportunity to reframe the son's defiance as showing care, concern, and a wish to sacrifice his own future and education for the family. Perhaps he had tried to grow up too fast and had tried to be practical in a rather American way, but the values of loyalty and family solidarity in contrast to "selfishness" (the Anglo-American values of individualism) had been successfully inculcated by his parents.

Reframing their viewpoints in a positive way was a necessary first step in bridging the values of parents and child, and in narrowing the cultural gulf between father and son. It also seemed important to decrease the son's power by encouraging his right to autonomy in certain areas, while supporting his parents' authority in others. In this case, as in many others, it was worthwhile to acknowledge that teenagers often have greater power through mastery of the language and social protocols of the new culture. Yet it was also important to "shrink" the adolescent to size when his power led to distortions. In Javier's case, his desire for a job was validated by respectful questions that asked what kind of job he liked and what kind of job he would be able to get, which uncovered the fact that his job opportunities were almost nil. I wondered aloud if he should use his last year of high school to better prepare himself for the job market.

The father was asked if he felt prepared to reassure his son and his wife that he would do whatever was necessary (including taking on work he was not proud of) to improve the financial situation. He began to emerge from his depression and inertia to ensure the welfare of the family, without abandoning his dignity. Because the parents could not really help Javier, the school counselor's cooperation was enlisted in dealing with the teen's plans for the future. I continued to work with the parents alone and focused on removing roadblocks to the father's employment. I saw Javier alone, too, and worked on his goal of completing high school.

Whenever school problems are present, therapists should thoroughly explore parental difficulties with work and economic survival. As with almost all problems that present in a therapist's office, understanding and intervening requires a careful investigation of the family's ecological context. Particularly for minority families, if we fail to consider relevant migration experiences, idiosyncratic and ethnic family styles, life-cycle issues, and contextual factors such as racism and discrimination, we seriously limit our ability to connect with and help Latino families.

As we explore with curiosity the family's unique experience of life in America, we are apt to discover solutions that are meaningful, attainable, and culturally congruent. Oftentimes these solutions will involve a return to the religious and spiritual beliefs and practices that are an integral part of many Latinos' lives. In Chapter 8 I explore some of the traditional, indigenous, and mainstream religious meanings and coping styles that alter how Latino clients view health and illness.

## NOTES

1. These theories fall into the same two broad categories that I proposed in the introduction to this book: the study of cultural differences and social power differentials as two ways of understanding the mental health stresses of minority groups.

2. In a classic article written in 1976, Harry Aponte describes the school-family consultation in rich technical and clinical detail.

# 8

## Belief Systems: Religion and Health

And so *la Virgen* [de Guadalupe] is called upon to cure ills north and south for loved ones or for anyone else who suffers. This gathering in L.A. [to celebrate the day of the Virgin of Guadalupe] might not be as monumental as the festival in Mexico City. But there is an intensity here that matches or maybe even surpasses the devotion back home. Perhaps it is the yearning to remain rooted in a rootless time where one's address can't be changed by twists of the economy or the border patrol.

—MARTÍNEZ (in Castillo, 1996, p. 111)

Latinos share with other people universal and personal beliefs and cultural meaning systems, all deeply embedded in their original ecologies. In this chapter I address two interconnected, key sets of belief systems that are especially relevant to psychotherapy with Latinos. These are the constellations of beliefs about health and illness, and religion and spirituality. In spite of increasing professional interest in and inquiries into traditional theories of illness and healing practices, we know little about the degree to which Latinos adhere to systems of folk medicine and beliefs in magic or bewitchment.

Most of the pertinent literature portrays Latinos as maintaining a dual system of beliefs and practices concerning physical and mental problems—mainstream medical and psychotherapy approaches and traditional folk-oriented approaches share the stage. Rather than viewing them as unconventional alternatives, we consider the folk approaches as having their own wisdom and effectiveness, and as playing a complimentary part alongside conventional methods. During developmental transitions, for example, immigrant families turn more intensely to the comfort and continuity of past traditions, such as prayer and folk medicines. The tendency of people to find meaning in life changes by revisiting cultural beliefs and rituals has been called "ideological ethnicity" (Harwood, 1981). This draw toward one's primary ethnicity can be used as a therapeutic resource to help families discover practices that enhance continuity and belonging, and propel the life cycle forward while reaffirming past ties.

Even for Latinos who are normally doubtful of traditional folk practices, there may be a tendency to fall into the "psychological ruts" of their ancestors' core beliefs when times are especially uncertain and stressful, what McKay and Fanning (1991) refer to as "mental grooving." Once a therapeutic alliance is firmly established, clinicians may be able to explore this realm of beliefs and examine how clients view the potential use of those avenues as supportive resources. We should hear each client's own ideas or aspect of cultural beliefs and help them discover their own best use of cultural practices.

## FOLK HEALTH: ILLNESS BELIEFS

The word "belief" is used to denote the constellation of assumptions, meanings, explanations, and attitudes that underlies the way people view various aspects of human experience at any given time. The health beliefs of Latinos can be grouped in several categories: belief in traditional folk illnesses; belief in hot/cold theories of illness; and belief in the supernatural, magic, and bewitchment (or witchcraft).

### Traditional Folk Illnesses

A "folk illness" refers to the layperson's conception of a physical or emotional problem. These problems are identified with nonmedical labels that summarize observed clusters of symptoms, and they derive from knowledge that is passed on informally from generation to generation. Older people in a community are the repositories of this knowledge and life experience. Although more prevalent in rural settings, urban dwellers may also identify and refer to these illness explanations occasionally.

Folk syndromes are sufficiently different from the conventional diagnostic classifications that the fourth edition of the *Diagnostic and Statistical Manual of Mental Disorders* (DSM-IV; American Psychiatric Association, 1994) includes in its appendix a glossary of culture-bound syndromes, several of which are relevant specifically to Latinos. The descriptions help clinicians make a differential diagnosis between folk syndromes and conventional categories of illness such as anxiety or depression. The recognition of culture-bound syndromes also legitimizes the therapist's exploration of folk illnesses and corresponding folk approaches for cures.

Harwood (1981) reviewed a number of taxonomies for Mexican American traditional folk concepts and noted that the majority are collected under *males naturales* (natural illnesses), while a smaller number fall in the category of *mal puesto* (witchcraft). The most common natural illnesses are *mal de ojo* (evil eye), *susto* or *espanto* (fright), and *empacho* (indigestion). Two other natural syndromes are very important for understanding Latinos: *nervios* and *ataques de nervios*. Underlying folk illnesses are beliefs in the power of strong emotions—one's own or another's envy, anger, fear, and frustration—to influence bodily health.

*Susto* or *espanto* (fright) is a syndrome that can affect people of either sex and of all ages. A parent may bring a child to a clinic after a fall from a bicycle saying that the child seems to have lost his appetite or the gleam in his eye; a woman may say that her nerves are out of control after she was frightened by her husband's threats to kill her when he was drunk; or a young man who witnessed a friend die of an asthma attack now appears blunted in his affect. The common element in these cases is the underlying explanation of *susto* or *espanto*—all three people were deeply frightened by the experience they witnessed. This explains their symptoms of restlessness, listlessness, diarrhea, vomiting, weight loss, or lack of motivation (Tseng & McDermott, 1981). *Susto* can be thought of as an acute reaction to trauma. Sometimes *susto* is used to justify a passive sick role or to manipulate and control social interactions, perhaps in situations where few socially legitimate avenues exist for avoiding overload of psychological stress.

*Mal de ojo* (evil eye) is a concept widely found in Mediterranean cultures. It embodies the belief that social relations contain inherent dangers to the equilibrium of the individual. A person with *vista fuerte* (strong vision) can exert inordinate attention on another person. His or her covert glances produce a stronger power over a weaker person, robbing the latter of their ability to act on their own accord. The victim of *mal de ojo* may experience severe headache, uncontrollable weeping, fretfulness, insomnia, and fever. *Mal de ojo* is thought to more commonly attack women and children because they are believed to be weaker beings. Professionals should be cautious in accepting the psychological and superstitious explanations of this folk diagnosis because they may obscure the detection of organic pathology, such as severe influenza.

*Empacho* refers to a type of indigestion or gastrointestinal infection that afflicts children and adults and is thought to be caused by a complex interaction between physiological and social factors. Stomach pains are thought to be a symptom of intestinal blockage and fever that causes thirst and abdominal swelling. It is believed that the afflicted person has been forced to eat against his will, either by allowing another to override his personal autonomy or by excessive politeness in accepting food when not hungry.

Beliefs in natural folk illnesses exist throughout Latin America. They are unrelated to religious beliefs, and even to social class, though they are more prevalent among poorer and less educated Latinos who have limited access to conventional medical diagnosis and treatment.

Curiously, as a child in a Jewish immigrant family in Argentina, I was taken several times to a folk healer to be cured of *empacho*. These trips were charged with a blend of trepidation and a giggling excitement—I anticipated the mysterious neighborhood, the dark, cavernous house, and the candlelit room where my bare back and belly were rubbed with gray ashes that were not to be washed off for several days. The skin around my spinal cord was lifted and pinched, a procedure that is the standard treatment for *empacho*.

In retrospect, one could appreciated the cultural hybridizaton of immigrants who may find in the "new" folk illness treatments elements of their own peasant mythologies.

*Nervios* (nerves) refers to a general state of distress connected to life's trials and tribulations, but it also describes a specific syndrome that includes "brain aches" or headaches, sleep difficulties, trembling, tingling, and *mareos*, a form of dizziness, or simple anxiety and nervousness. A person may be said to *sufre de los nervios* (suffer from nerves) or *está enfermo de los nervios* (be ill from nerves).

*Ataque de nervios* has been dubbed "the Puerto Rican syndrome," incorrectly so, as it also appears in other national groups. A common feature of *ataque de nervios* is a sense of being out of control. The symptoms may include dissociative experiences, hyperkinesis, seizure-like or fainting episodes, mutism, hyperventilation, crying spells, or shouting. The victim may experience amnesia of what happened during the ataque (Fernández-Marina, 1961). *Ataques* appear to be more common among women in lower socioeconomic levels. Some *ataques* are socially acceptable responses to certain situations, such as when one has witnessed or received news of a shocking family event, or has faced a dangerous situation. An *ataque* may be interpreted as a call for help or a way out of an impossible social situation.

Fifteen-year-old Verónica moved with her parents and two siblings from Mexico City to San Diego, California, less than 2 years ago. Her parents were worried that Verónica had developed *ataques de nervios* over the past 6 months. Not wanting to embarrass Verónica, her parents had difficulty providing details of the episodes in which the girl had epileptic-like trembling, rolling of her eyes, and sometimes foaming at the mouth. During these episodes, she appeared unable to move—she felt like "dead weight" and resisted her family's intervention by screaming. These attacks could last up to half an hour and then stop on their own, but Verónica would often be morose for several hours afterward. Medical evaluation failed to uncover any organic issues.

Verónica had been a model student in Mexico, and in spite of the new language and cultural stress, she continued to be at the top of her class in the United States. With fierce determination she told me, "*Yo quiero ser alguien*" (I want to be somebody). By "becoming somebody," Verónica hoped to justify the extreme hardships her hard-working parents had endured to bring their children to the United States and to rent a small apartment in a middle-class neighborhood so the children could attend a good public school. But Verónica also hoped to increase her own odds for a better economic future and avoid the stresses that led her parents to quarrel ferociously about money.

This concern with achievement motivation, "trying to become somebody," coupled with a wish to help her family and to alleviate ongoing parental hardships have been described for first-generation Latinos as a form of intense guilt and "compensatory achievement" (Suárez-Orozco & Suárez-Orozco, 1994).

An even greater stress came through Verónica's involvement in a love triangle that involved competition with Ligia, her 15-year-old cousin, for 19-year-old Raúl. Although the young man had pursued Verónica with declarations of love, just when Verónica began to respond to his interest, Ligia succeeded in enticing Raúl with her sexual provocations. When Verónica confronted Raúl about Ligia, he confessed to having gone out one night to dance with her, followed by kissing and heavy petting. Verónica was very anxious and mildly depressed over the threat of losing two meaningful relationships—her lifelong closeness with her cousin Ligia, who was like a sister to her, and the newfound romance with dashing, experienced Raúl.

Life stresses such as school, work, family pressures, love torments, and attempts to maintain interpersonal harmony by suppressing anger may all contribute to *ataques de nervios*. In Verónica's case, information about one particular episode shows how anticipatory anxiety followed by situational frustration may trigger an *ataque de nervios*.

On that particular day, Verónica could not avoid attending a weekend youth retreat organized by her Catholic church. She had not wanted to go and would have preferred to be with Raúl instead. She wanted his support and affection, particularly as she struggled to maintain a semblance of harmony with her cousin Ligia, as both her mother and her aunt (Ligia's mother) expected. Verónica also suspected the retreat discussions would address sexual activities among youth, a topic that stirred a great deal of conflict for her. The moment she entered the building where the retreat was being held, she began to feel suffocated, she "hated the way the corridors were dark and lit with ugly and infrequent lights," and felt dizzy, nauseated, and uncomfortable. She asked the counselors to let her return home. In spite of her vehemence, her request was repeatedly denied, a situation that frustrated her greatly. She then asked to be excused to go the bathroom where she sat in a shower stall and had an *ataque*.

In going over the event, Verónica seemed conscious and even mischievously amused by the possibility that sometimes the embarrassing *ataques* saved her from an unwanted situation that she could not refuse directly. Later I discussed with the family the many ways in which Verónica created or responded to a demand for perfection in school and in family relationships. This motivated the parents to relieve Verónica of some of their expectations that she be a super "good girl."

Because we had a good therapeutic alliance, I was able to ask the parents if they knew of any folk cures for *ataques de nervios*. They giggled, thinking I might be humoring them. I explained what I knew of the syndrome and the studies that show many Mexican people often try mainstream *and* folk systems of health care. The mother said she had been thinking of sending Verónica to Mexico to be with her grandmother for a summer vacation. At the time, I thought the mother meant it would be good for Verónica to get away from the stresses in San Diego. I reflected to myself on the timing of her response and on the considerable economic hardship and risks of sending Verónica, undocumented, back over the border. I wondered if the mother thought it would be easier to find a good folk healer in Mexico.

At any rate, Verónica went to Mexico and returned free of her symptoms. Her parents were getting along pretty well, and Verónica's relationship with Raúl had not only survived the crisis with Ligia, but seemed stronger for it. Though these two changes probably took a considerable burden from Verónica's shoulders, there may have been some special magic done by the folk healer, of which I will never know.

## Hot/Cold Theories of Illness

Anthropological literature points to a previous blend or syncretism of native Latin American medical theories of disease and 16th-century Spanish medical knowledge and concepts of illness. One important element in this syncretism involves ideas about magical and emotional causation of illness. Native ideas revolve around the concept of "soul loss" occasioned by fright or by spirit intrusion, and these phenomena are ultimately attributed to shame, anger, or envy.

A Spanish component relates to certain beliefs in the pathology of Hippocratic bodily humors, as expressed in the hot/cold theory of illness (Currier, 1966; Harwood, 1981). According to this theory, the healthy body is in an equilibrium of hot and cold that produces optimal warmth. Disequilibrium occurs after excessive internal or external exposure to hot or cold. Natural elements, foods, temperaments, and emotional experiences may underlie this disequilibrium. Even mechanical situations are seen as contributing to illness; for example, ironing clothes with hands cold from washing clothes is thought to cause arthritis. The imbalance needs to be counteracted or neutralized with the opposite—cold remedies and topical applications work for excessive heat and hot remedies for excessive cold. At the psychological level, strong emotional experiences such as fright are thought to cause heat that should be treated with cooling herbal teas or soothing cold compresses. (For a table Puerto Rican hot/cold classifications of illnesses, medicines, and foods, see Harwood, 1981, pp. 424–425.)

Mexicans and Puerto Ricans vary greatly in their subscription to the hot/cold theory of illness. The belief and practice appears to diminish with increased levels of acculturation to Western theories of health and illness (Castro, Furth, & Karlow, 1984). It is interesting, however, that although hot/cold theories may be decreasing in prevalence, the underlying idea of balance or homeostasis is still viable and can be part of a therapeutic conversation about striving for mental balance and personal harmony by counteracting or neutralizing excesses and imbalances.

## Beliefs in Disorders of the Supernatural

### Magic and Bewitchment

*Mal puesto* or *brujería* (bewitchment) provide explanations for prolonged disorders that cannot be accounted for by natural and hot/cold illnesses or for which treatments for natural illnesses have not worked. In spite of a declining belief in witchcraft, serious disruptions in social relations are sometimes thought to be followed by various forms of bewitchment. Among these disruptions are unrequited love, quarrels and breakups among lovers, and conflicts among close family members. Following these incidents, it is believed that one of the parties may have hired the services of a sorcerer (*brujo* or *bruja*) to bewitch or place a hex on the other party. *Mal puesto* is used as an explanation for infertility and various forms of mental illness or "insanity" including schizophrenia. Chronic and treatment-resistant illnesses are thus more likely to be diagnosed as the result of *brujería* or (witchcraft).

Here again we see elements of cultural syncretism. In pre-Hispanic Mexico, natural elements were invested with god-like, supernatural qualities and magical powers. These gods (of the sun, the rain, and so on) needed to be revered, sometimes through ritual sacrifice, for the order of the cosmos and earth to be maintained. Magic was thought to benefit human beings in individual health and group survival. But it also had its dark side—it could be used to harm enemies through poisoning, drought, plagues, fatal illnesses, or other forms of harm. This became known as "black magic" performed by "black witches," while benevolent magic was consequently dubbed "white magic." "White witches" were called upon to cure illnesses or to resolve life problems, while "black witches" were contacted to help one retaliate by placing hexes or bewitching.

The Spanish conquest brought a different religion, Roman Catholicism, with its own beliefs and magical practices. The cult of the saints had its own stories of miracles and its own physical sacrifices and punishments to gain favors or concessions. The devil was believed to be the cause of all malignant forces and witches were thought to have made a pact with the devil.

## White and Black Witches

Both world views and conceptions of magic, the indigenous and the European, operated separately at first, but over time a blending of concepts developed. Today, white and black witches are still consulted for a wide variety of problems. White magic is called upon to ward off dangers, alleviate illnesses, locate work, bring success in a new enterprise, provide luck in romance, or recuperate from a lost love. Black witches are consulted when one wishes to harm an enemy, defeat a rival, or revenge another evil hex. Specific rituals are part of the armamentarium of *brujos*. For a comprehensive book on the subject, consult Scheffler (1983). The doors to this surrealistic underworld of magic and witchcraft opened for me in 1994 and gave me a glimpse into these fascinating mysteries.

At that time I was living in Mexico City. A 23-year-old woman, Adelina, helped me with housework. Her family and home were in Puebla, in the mountains about an hour and a half away from the city. Her mother and sisters had jobs in town and on weekends both her parents and some of her sisters would come to fetch her. Two of my daughters had become friendly with Adelina and we all liked her very much. One day, Adelina rather abruptly burst into tears and told me she had to have an operation because she had cancer of "the female parts." I was immediately worried about whether she was getting good medical care and if the diagnosis was accurate. When her mother came, I tried to talk with her about these issues but found her unreceptive and angry towards Adelina. Mother and daughter spoke among themselves in an Indian dialect and from what I could gather, the mother believed Adelina had done something wrong for which she was being punished.

A few days later, Adelina returned with some family members to pick up her belongings. After she left, I went to her room and while cleaning her bathroom, came across a brown clay pot carefully tucked behind the toilet. I lifted it and found inside two large dark candle figurines, one shaped in the form of a man, the other a woman. Inside the pot were three small plastic bags containing different colored powders, a box of matches, and a little bag of metal straight pins. I had no idea what to make of this and so consulted with four Mexican friends who were having dinner at my home that night.

At first there was much laughter and commotion. The most common guess was that Adelina was performing some sort of ritual with those objects and that in the haste of the move, she had forgotten the hidden container. The youngest of my dinner guests was a little worried that Adelina, out of envy, may have wanted to harm or scare my daughters in some way by leaving the clay pot. No one wanted to take it seriously but, nonetheless, everyone agreed that it would not hurt to be cautious and take some preventive steps—to ward off evil spirits, we put a large glass of pure water in a prominent spot, and I was told to change it frequently and keep it pure for several days. My friends left at midnight.

At around 1:30 A.M., one of my guests called me, saying that he and his wife had been discussing Adelina's container and they thought it best that I buy several types of white flowers and place them in every room of the house as a *limpia*, a form of cleansing ritual for my home. White flowers are my favorite, so I told them it would be a pleasant outing to go to the flower market the following morning.

I was attempting to ignore a subtle hint of fear in my psyche when early the next day, another thoughtful dinner guest called. She knew I was going to the market and suggested I visit a natural herb and remedy stand. She thought the owner might have helpful hints about counteracting any negative energy left by the clay pot. While these precautions seemed exaggerated and unnecessary, I wrapped the container in plastic and took it with me to the market. The owner of the shop looked at it suspiciously and sold me a large plastic bottle with a bluish liquid that smelled like ammonia. She said I should stand first at the entrance to my house and then at the threshold of each room, in each instance sprinkling the liquid in front of and behind me to exorcise any bad omen that may have entered my dwelling. She also advised me not to bring the clay pot back into my house but to burn it with kerosene, perhaps inside a trash can.

I walked away pondering this last directive, which sounded rather daunting, when I heard a kind voice behind me. It was a healthy, roundish Indian woman with long beautiful braids and the signature apron that identified her as a houseworker in a wealthy home. She had heard the advice given to me at the herbal shop and she didn't trust the wisdom of the shopkeeper. She was on her way to a *señora* who was very knowledgeable and would help allay my concerns about the meaning of the strange clay pot. She encouraged me to take the next bus with her, reassuring me that I had nothing to fear.

By this time I must have been in some sort of trance that made me much more suggestible and less cautious than usual. Before I knew it, I had embarked on an odyssey to the outskirts of the city. We arrived at a poor neighborhood without paved streets or sidewalks, potable water, or even telephones lines. After a long walk from the bus, we arrived at a modest home with a garage. Attached to the garage was a small, narrow room with a protruding roof under which there were two benches. Two women were waiting on the benches for their turn. My companion greeted them and invited me to sit down.

After a while the three women began talking. First they discussed the amount of time it would take for each one to be seen and the chores that were awaiting them at home. All of them were due home after a morning of work or errands and were expected around 3 P.M. for the main meal. They complained that if they did not cook, the family would go without eating. Cautiously they began to share why they were coming to see the *señora*. One wished her husband to stop drinking because he was a good man but became abusive when he drank. The other wanted her husband and oldest daughter to be less lazy, and to go to work or help around the house rather than sleep and loaf around the two-channel TV all day. They felt *la señora* gave them good advice to have faith and not doubt themselves, but also to be less involved and overbearing. My companion was more reserved but finally hinted that she had health problems, mostly high blood pressure, which was difficult to control medically. She admitted to often being full of anger toward her husband and had repeatedly threatened to throw him out if he did not stop hitting her. She had come to realize by coming to *la señora* that she was hurting herself by being so frustrated, making empty threats and never getting any results. By responding less intensely and urgently, and trusting the answers that would come in time, she had managed to decrease her high blood pressure and was even getting more help from her family. She saw *la señora* regularly to report her progress and receive support and encouragement.

When my turn finally came, I walked into a small narrow room with tables covered with burning candles, small altars, crucifixes, and religious stamps of the saints and of the Virgin of Guadalupe. In between tables there stood a middle-aged woman of medium build with short white hair and a plain white cotton dress. She had a radiant face and a kind, welcoming expression. As I explained the reason for my visit, she took the plastic bag with the clay pot from me and examined it and its contents. She explained that Adelina must have been experimenting with a plan to harm a rival. Her guess was that perhaps she was in love with a man who was committed to another woman, as suggested by the two candles in the shape of a couple. The different powders were symbols of various evils that Adelina hoped would befall the couple in order to separate them. The red powder was pepper and was intended to make them have a nasty quarrel. The black powder was to poison the relationship symbolically with doubt and suspicion. This white witch then looked squarely into my face and told me that I had nothing personal to fear, that I had the face of a gentle, kind person who would never harm anyone and therefore should not fear the harm of others. Only people who have the wish to harm others, she said, experience fear because they see their wish in others, an idea that seemed to me akin to the concept of projective identification, a psychoanalytic mechanism. She then added, "That poor Adelina, she must have been suffering a lot to want to inflict pain. . . . "

The white witch proceeded to tie a knot in the plastic bag and, taking it aside, she announced very clearly that these things were not mine, they did not belong to me, and they had not been intended for me. I should let her dispose of them in an appropriate manner and without any participation on my part. She wrote on a small piece of paper three ingredients that I could get at an herbal pharmacy downtown if I would feel better having my house smell fresher. A great relief overtook me. I was enormously grateful. I thanked her and asked her how much I owed her for her help. She responded that I owed her nothing but that she would accept a small donation for her altar. I later learned that white witches customarily do not charge a fee.

Outside, my companion was waiting for me, perhaps she was practicing not rushing to satisfy her husband's needs. She then walked me to the bus stop. When I put some money in her palm for her help, she gently refused it, saying that it was part of her good deeds to help others and that no money was expected. I sensed that I might offend her if I insisted so I just thanked her profusely.

A few weeks later Adelina called me to ask me if I would write her a letter of recommendation for a new job. I invited her to come over. When she arrived, I told her that I was concerned about her and interested in what may be happening in her life. To my surprise she confirmed the white witch's theory. She had been seeing a married man in her home town. At the time she began dating him, she thought he was single, but later found out he had a wife and child. He promised Adelina he would leave them to be with her but he never did. Then, laughing nervously, Adelina told me she had been using her salary to get the advice of a black witch on how to win him over. (She didn't mention the clay pot, but I learned later that it was indeed a tool of black witchcraft.) To make things worse, when Adelina's parents found out about her relationship with the married man they became furious with her, particularly because she had lost her virginity. The operation they wanted her to have for "cancer of the female parts" was a hymen repair, an operation commonly advertised in telephone directories throughout Mexico.

I left this situation with a tremendous appreciation for the white witch's skills. Her customers felt better and had developed new ways of thinking and behaving. Through her wisdom about human relationships she had become the equivalent of a local psychotherapist. In my case, she had managed to positively connote every person involved, had reassured me, and had created a boundary and a closure to the event that was surprisingly smooth. Further, she constructed a compassionate narrative that made Adelina's behavior intelligible and human.

## FOLK, RELIGIOUS, AND MAGICAL HEALING

The world of white and black witches exists but it is secret and not readily accessible in conversation. More acceptable and more public is the world of natural healers who use herbs and massages but may also prescribe tasks and even talk to spirits.

*Curanderismo* is the indigenous method of cure for many natural folk illnesses such as *susto, empacho,* or *mal de ojo,* but *curanderos* (folk healers) may also be consulted for impotence, depression, or alcoholism, even by those who do not profess to believe in folk illnesses or cures. *Curanderos* are a heterogeneous group distinguished by specialties in particular disorders or by particular healing powers. Women healers or *curanderas* are sometimes called *señoras.* They use a range of treatments: herbal remedies, inhalation, sweating, massage,[1] incantations, and a variety of ritual cleansing treatments. Among the latter are stylized manipulations of raw eggs and palm leaves (Gafner & Duckett, 1992).

*Curanderos, brujos,* and *espiritistas* frequently perform *limpias.* These are important and widely used cleansing rituals that require branches of various plants, eggs, perfumed waters, religious images, dissected animals, and candles specific to each problem. Rituals take place next to their *altares* (altars), which are decorated with ritual objects, candles, incense, and images of saints, the devil occasionally, or of supernatural beings.

Sometimes *curanderos* specialize in certain "Western" medical problems such as menstrual cramps or prolapsed uterus, and may have anatomical charts or other objects found in modern medical offices. Yet *curanderos* do not see themselves in competition with medical providers, particularly with regard to serious health problems. They are willing to refer clients for medical care and even to use the services themselves. The clients too see value in using a dual system of health care, alternatively or conducted together (Applewhite, 1995). Reluctance to accept conventional treatment may signify a family's concern that mainstream medicine may interfere with alternative approaches, such as prayer. In other situations, the family may not comply with drug treatment for reasons that are embedded in their ecological setting. The parents of 9-year-old Raimundo, who had been diagnosed with hyperactivity (ADD) and given a prescription for Ritalin, were reluctant about the medication because they feared it would begin a drug addiction and a life in the streets, as they saw daily in other youngsters in their *barrio.*

Innovative public mental health programs for Latinos such as the one offered by San Francisco General Hospital and the University of California at San Francisco provide conventional medical approaches and complementary options for intervention by creating provider networks and community partnerships that accept *curanderos, sobadores, yerberos,* and other folk healers (Navarro & Carrillo, 1997). A balanced, nonidealized, and informative account of an interview with a *curandero* in California, as narrated by a physician and a nurse, can be found in Mull and Mull (1983).

These studies indicate that *curanderos* are skillful at creating a warm and intimate atmosphere and pay tribute to values on family connectedness by including relatives and asking them to take an active role in decision making about treatment. They are reassuring and paternalistic, exuding confidence in their ability to diagnose and cure the illness, factors which may contribute to success or satisfaction through suggestibility.

Although *curanderos* do not ask or answer many questions, they do allow for ventilation of fears and hostilities on the client's part. For example, it is believed that *susto,* if left untreated for some period of time, can lead to "soul loss," a belief that generates even more fear. The cure is a ritualized recapture of the soul and its fast reentry into the body. But close observation of a *curandero*'s healing shows that much more than a ritual is involved. Tseng and McDermott (1981) report that a client with *susto* developed a transference-like attachment to the *curandero.* She expressed a lot of her fears to him and received plenty of reassurance both in words and medicine. In addition, she was distracted from her symptoms by a series of tasks that provided her social contact, increased her self-worth, and gave purpose to her days. The tasks of recapturing her soul, preparing medicines, and conducting relevant ceremonies brought the network of relatives and community together in support of the client. Again, one can reflect on the convergence of therapeutic elements in the *curandero*'s practices and conventional psychotherapy and psychopharmacology.

*Yerberos* (herbalists) are especially knowledgeable of home remedies and the use of hundreds of wild and domestic plants to treat body and mind. *Yerberos* are an important and widely used health resource in Mexican communities. Unlike *curanderos,* they do not use traditional rituals.

*Espiritismo* (spiritualism) refers to an invisible world of good and evil spirits who can attach themselves to human beings and thus influence behavior (Delgado, 1978; García-Prieto, 1996; Steiner, 1974). Everyone has spirits of protection, the number of which can be increased by performing good deeds or decreased by doing evil (Wittoker, 1970). Beliefs in spiritualism are embedded deep in history—among some Puerto Ricans, for example, a belief in spirits has been traced to the Taino Indians, who felt that everything in nature had a spirit. Today the enduring spiritual presence of a loved one after death is common among Puerto Ricans, although it may vary among family members according to acculturative influences (García-Prieto, 1996; Shapiro, 1994).

Some interpretations of spiritualism come from a social justice perspective. Fanon (1967) suggests that colonized people live in tension, containing anger that may be released destructively or displaced into magic and spiritual systems. When political action is not possible and self-determination is limited, placing oneself under the protection of benevolent and powerful spirits may help counteract fear, powerlessness, and lack of agency (Comaz-Díaz, 1995; Lechner, 1992). In this context, spiritualism is thought to act as an adaptive stress-reducing mechanism among Puerto Ricans in the United States (Pérez & Andrés, 1977).

Many Puerto Ricans and some Cubans, particularly those who come from the eastern region of the island, rely on *espiritistas* ( spiritualists or mediums) who can communicate with the spirits and have the power of healing. In the book *Families of the Slums* (1967), Minuchin, Montalvo, Guerney, Rosman, and Schumer describe how these indigenous agents "speak" the inner language, a kind of "spiritualese" reserved to describe psychological distress. This distress is often seen as originating from supernatural sources rather than one's own inner life. The locus of control is external, and motivation for change may come in the form of a visit by God, hearing a voice from beyond, or seeing a ghost who summons a person to return home or to stop drinking. In a cultural consonant vein, these compelling spiritual experiences may be invoked to bring on necessary change without requiring clients to openly acknowledge responsibility or remorse, or give in to family pressure.

In that same book a situation is described in which a couple couched the wife's infidelity in terms of possession by the spirit of a prostitute. With the problem framed this way, the spouses were freed of responsibility and joined together in going to an *espiritista*. The spiritualist, working within a cultural framework that endorsed externalization, accepted the couple's explanation. He assigned them a "task" to bring the estranged husband and wife together cooperatively—they were to take a long trip to dispose of a chicken leg stuck with a nail in order to exorcise the spirit of the prostitute. The authors comment that a middle-class psychotherapist would have directed the couple to reinternalize and personalize their problem. While this frame would be much more congruent with the therapist's own cultural set, it could have rendered the problem unsolvable for the couple. Ways to bridge mainstream therapy and *espiritismo* are offered in an enlightening clinical article by Comas-Díaz (1981).

*Santería* is a religion prevalent among Cubans, some Puerto Ricans, and other Caribbeans, and appears to be widely practiced among Cuban Americans in South Florida (Martínez & Wetli, 1982). It combines deities of the Yoruban or Orichas (Africans from South Nigeria) with Catholic saints (Sandoval, 1977). In Cuba this religion is known as *lucumi* and in Brazil as *macumba*.

No specific religion predominates in Cuba now but there has been a significant increase in religiosity, perhaps as a spiritual refuge from recent economic hardship. Cubans are adept at blending beliefs and practices, and they do not insist on theological consistency. It is not uncommon for a person to believe in the Catholicism of Spain, the African cults combined with Haitian voodoo, and in European spiritism with a touch of American Protestantism. Variations on these blends are many—one individual may rely mostly on Catholic practicees that offer peace and hope after death, while another may regularly turn to a *santero* for help, depending perhaps on their particular ecological niche.

*Santeros* are very practical and will try to resolve concrete problems here on earth as well as predicting through divination the immediate future. *Santeros* are priests or priestesses who function as healers, diviners, and directors of rituals. They treat *bilingo* (hexes and spirit possession). A *santero*'s "diagnosis" of possession and a client's experience and report of the same may complicate differential diagnosis for psychotherapy practitioners, who may think the client is psychotic (Alonso & Jeffrey, 1988). Some *santeros* operate *botánicas*, stores where special herbs, potions, candles, and other ritual objects may be purchased (Bernal & Gutiérrez, 1988; Boswell & Curtis, 1984; Comas-Díaz, 1989). In the United States, *botánicas* can be found in Miami, Los Angeles, San Francisco, New York, and other cities with large ethnic neighborhoods. The most comprehensive treaty on *santería, espitirismo,* and *botánica* accessible to all audiences is *Santería: The Religion* by a long-time expert on the topic, Migene González-Wippler (1996). For herbal aspects of *santería* see Brandon (1991).

It may be apparent by now that health for many Latinos involves a complex interaction of physical, psychological, social, and spiritual factors. It is difficult to distinguish discrete causation between psychological and somatic disorders and between naturalistic and spiritual or magical elements. Often these elements combine and influence each other, and include the significant role played by Roman Catholicism.

## RELIGIOUS BELIEFS

Roman Catholicism is the predominant religion of Latinos. As I discuss in other chapters, Catholicism influences the meanings assigned to life cycle transitions and the many values that affect marital and family life. Catholicism provides a common denominator of beliefs and values for many Latinos. Differences in specific content and blends of native religions vary considerably from country to country, group to group.

Religions other than Catholicism are increasingly present in Latino communities, partly because of exposure to new faiths in the United States. Further, a large number of missionaries proselytize to individuals and communities in Latin American countries. These include various branches of Protestantism, Pentecostalism, Jehovah's Witnesses, and numerous evangelical and fundamentalist faiths. A number of Latinos are Jewish.

In this section I am concerned with the Catholic beliefs that shape interpretations and attitudes toward physical and mental illness. These are primarily Christian beliefs in God as a supreme being, in life after death, and in the existence of a soul. Beliefs about heaven and hell, sin, guilt, and shame also play a role in meaning making and in attributions of responsibility.

Catholicism also encompasses some magical thinking, belief in miracles, propitiatory rituals, promises (*promesas*), and prayers. While small altars to saints are everywhere in the streets of Latin America, immigrants create home altars with flowers, crucifixes, bottles of holy water, and saints depicted in plastic statuettes or postcards. These practices are not gratuitous—they bring emphasis to the Latino's value on enduring suffering and denying self in exchange for needed favors.

Devotional offerings, daily prayers, masses at home, vows of penance, and even pilgrimages to shrines may be offered to special saints in return for their intercession and commendation. Numerous prayers are offered to the Virgin of Guadalupe, the patron saint of Mexico who is also revered in Puerto Rico and other parts of Latin America. This deity offers enormous psychological protection and unity among people. Her portrait, a most powerful icon, hangs in living rooms and dangles over automobile dashboards and from key chains from Mexico to East Los Angeles and to many cities in Texas and New Mexico. She is a perfect fusion of indigenous Aztec and Catholic European elements, the only brown-skinned virgin who validates the promise of Catholicism for indigenous people. In fact, the Virgin of Guadalupe has many Indian names. The most common is Tonantzín, and the legend of her miraculous appearance on Mexican soil in 1531 to a poor priest, Juan Diego, is lovingly retold by children and adults alike. A most interesting book edited by the Chicana writer Ana Castillo titled *Goddess of the Americas: Writings on the Virgin of Guadalupe* (1996) demonstrates the multiplicity of meanings and symbols and the profound love bestowed upon this Virgin by gang youth, feminists, social justice activists, and writers concerned with identity construction.

Religious beliefs and practices are receiving increased attention by health professionals. Allen Bergin (1991) has urged an examination of the usefulness of religion and spiritual practices in enhancing mental health and compared the impact of religion to psychotherapy. Larry Dossey (1993) examined the efficacy of prayer in producing physical changes in his review of a large number of medical studies. He concludes that the ritual of prayer may trigger emotions that seem to lead to healing changes by affecting the immune and cardiovascular systems. The essential ingredient is belief or faith in the process of prayer rather than particular religious content. For an excellent book that conceptualizes the impact and multidimensionality of beliefs in the process of physical illness and healing, see Wright, Watson, and Bell (1996). In spite of the widespread importance of religious beliefs and practices for Latinos, very little has been written about the interaction of religion and psychotherapy for this population.

It seems clear, however, that churches and church life provide support and a sense of community. They are an important part of a client's ecological niche and often are a great resource for families in therapy. Immigrants sometimes attend church in the United States because it provides a place of belonging, a way to meet other immigrants, and a socializing and educational setting for their children and themselves. A priest, pastor, or rabbi may become a key figure in times of stress. Sending children to parochial schools and getting involved with church activities and needs can provide an avenue for self-expression and status for men and women who have little opportunity for stimulation or acknowledgment through their jobs or life situations.

Adherence to church doctrine, regular church attendance, and the roles played by priests and organized religion vary in the three Latino groups. Mexicans are a devout group to which churchgoing and observance of religious holidays and rituals is considered vital. For older Mexicans, the church provides spiritual support in the form of hope or by helping individuals face pain and accept suffering. Religious leaders may be important auxiliaries to the treatment process. Therapists should ask if the client finds spiritual solace or any form of support through church attendance. For many Puerto Ricans, the church is a place for communions, weddings, or funerals. Church is not considered necessary, however, to reach God or the supernatural. Puerto Ricans have a special relationship with saints, whom they believe can be personal emissaries to God (García-Prieto, 1996). Cubans partake of Catholic values and rituals but perhaps with less vigor. Exposure to other Protestant and Afro-Caribbean religions has led to the incorporation of other beliefs and rituals for a considerable number of Cuban Americans.

## The Marriage of Religion and Folklore

The wedding of religion and folklore among many Latino groups is particularly apparent during such transitions as death and bereavement. Mexicans, for example, do not ignore or avoid the subject of death as is common among most Anglo-American traditions. The "Day of the Dead" is an annual public fiesta in which folklore, religious litanies, sugar candy skulls, and tissue paper skeletons poke fun at death. Jokes and sayings about astute maneuverings that confuse and defeat death are common and may represent a counterphobic approach to death.[2] Octavio Paz (1961) eloquently describes the Mexican attitude toward death: "The word death is not pronounced in New York, in Paris, in London, because it burns the lips. The Mexican, in contrast, is familiar with death, jokes about it, caresses it, sleeps with it, celebrates it; it is one of his favorite toys and his most steadfast love. True, there is perhaps as much fear in his attitude as in that of others, but at least death is not hidden away: he looks at it face to face, with impatience, disdain, or irony. As in a popular folk song, 'If they are going to kill me tomorrow, let them kill me right away'" (p. 49).

The Day of the Dead includes a ritual of grieving that takes place each year for 4 years after the death of a family member. The family erects a portable altar at home with a photograph of the dead person, some favorite objects surrounded by *zimpazuchis* (deep yellow and purple flowers—the only ones that can be used for this ritual), and the deceased's favorite foods. After a day's vigil at their open home, the family transports the altar with its hanging objects, foods, and covers of beautifully embroidered clothes to the cemetery. Family and friends light tall candles and sit around the grave chanting and swaying. Close family members, particularly women and children, sleep next to the grave until the following morning, *para acompañar a nuestros pobrecitos muertos* (keep company to our poor dead ones). This ritual offers emotional release, and some household variant could be used as a natural therapeutic resource if the ritual has been meaningful to the particular family, although it would be hard to fathom an American cemetery as a place to spend the night with one's deceased relatives.

Less lavishly, Puerto Ricans and Cubans also celebrate the Day of the Dead. Their funerals, processions, and street caravans to accompany the dead are very expressive, especially for a child's funeral (Santiago, 1994). Gasping for breath, heart palpitations, or *piquetes* (chest pains) in the deeply bereaved are accepted as natural expressions of grief—emotional states are not conceived as separate from bodily reactions in most Latino cultures. For Anglo-Americans who adhere to a mind-body dichotomy, these reactions may be pejoratively construed as "somatizations."

Hallucinations of the deceased, including "visitations" of spirits and ghosts, may occur for several years following a loved one's death, especially among Puerto Ricans who practice *santería* and Cubans who engage in *macombe* (an Afro-Caribbean religion). Shapiro (1994) provides an excellent example of bereavement therapy for a Puerto Rican client who felt the ghost of her dead mother lingering. Thus, as many Latino cultures offer a blending of religion, spiritualism, and folklore, therapy may blend these elements into mainstream modalities to fashion more meaningful and culturally congruent treatment.

# LOCUS OF CONTROL AND STYLES OF COPING WITH ADVERSITY

The belief systems of most Latinos share a "trait" that is critical for therapists to understand—when illness or trouble strikes, the cause may be attributed to sources outside or beyond the victim's influence or control. It is
not unusual to attribute physical or emotional problems to external trauma
with its ensuing internal reactions and interpersonal tensions. Many Latinos will automatically add *si Dios quiere* (God willing) or *Dios mediante* when
speaking of their plans for the near or distant future. These statements
transmit a recognition that their lives are not under their control. The Chicana writer Sandra Cisneros (1995) sees the relatively infrequent use of this
linguistic expression among Anglo-Americans as evidence that they must
feel "in audacious control of their own destiny." For many Latinos, fate,
destiny, or God is in charge—*el destino, o Dios, así lo ha querido* (destiny, or
God, has willed it).

## Fatalism

The notion that little in life is under one's direct control is described in social science as an external locus of control—a world view that is often as-
cribed more frequently to minority groups. But as Sue and Sue (1990)
point out, it is important to distinguish various meanings of externality,
particularly when working with culturally diverse clients. These authors
note that "high externality may be due to (a) chance-luck, (b) cultural dictates that are viewed as benevolent, and (c) a political force (racism and
discrimination) that represents malevolent but realistic obstacles" (p. 143).
*Fatalismo*, a cognitive orientation or belief system (Comaz-Díaz, 1989; Garza
& Ames, 1972; Rotter, 1966), may resemble some of these aspects of externality. While many studies have attributed fatalism to the Mexican culture,
others have found it less a characteristic of ethnicity than a function of social class. The latter theories postulate that fatalism is more prevalent in
lower socioeconomic classes because poor people learn through recurrent
experiences that powerful others and unpredictable forces control their
lives (Sue & Sue, 1990). The assumption is that limited opportunities to get
ahead and change life circumstances result in feelings of helplessness, a
sense of failure, and of futility about pursuing an active orientation.

According to some authors, this fatalistic outlook increases psychological distress (Ross, Mirowsky, & Cockerham, 1983). *Fatalismo* from this perspective contributes to a deficit view. In my opinion, it is important for
therapists to distinguish between a "deficit-oriented" theory of *fatalismo* and
a "resource-oriented" one. The ecology of lower socioeconomic status can
indeed disempower individuals and limit their hopeful outlook, a situation
that requires the use of empowering therapeutic approaches. On the other

hand, selective coping by trying to accept losses that are beyond one's control (aging, an incurable disease, or an unexpected death) may be a strong resource based on a different philosophical or spiritual orientation than American instrumentalism. Holding a both/and frame in conversation with Latinos about how they conceptualize control over problems and solutions is probably the most respectful approach.

At first glance it appears that belief in an external locus of control would "fit" with externalizations used by narrative therapists such as Michael White (1989), who purposely separates a client's symptoms from the client himself as an avenue to stimulate personal agency or choice. In fact, Wright et al. (1996) suggest that externalization techniques in which the illness, rather than the victim, is accused are similar to those employed by witch doctors. On closer examination, however, externalizing conversations are often based on talking about a problem as if it could eventually be defeated or escaped, and so conversations about struggle, conflict, and control prevail. This type of language use is very different from a world view that encourages acceptance, resignation, and coexistence by making peace with an externally induced problem, as in the following case of Mrs. Moreno Carrillo. A distinction is made by Tomm, Suzuki, and Suzuki (1990) between an outer externalization, in which the problem is placed outside of the person and therefore can be confronted and struggled against, and an inner externalization, in which the problem will remain inside the individual and must be accepted, though perhaps not allowed to take over one's life. This differentiation can be helpful if we consider that an outer externalization appeals to instrumentalism, or the capacity to control and prevail. On the other hand, cultural inclinations to see problems as the result of fate or luck reveal several internal coping mechanisms—*aguantar, controlarse, no pensar,* and *sobreponerse*—that may be supported or reinforced by inner circumscriptions or externalizations that are more syntonic with the Latino world view than the usual "true" externalization.

## Controlarse (Control of Self)

While many Latinos hold that individuals are not usually thought to be responsible for bringing about their own problems, various degrees of self-control are possible. According to Cohen (1980) and Castro et al. (1984) *controlarse* (control of the self) is a dynamic theme of Latinos, a central cognitive and behavioral mechanism for mastering the challenges of life by controlling one's moods and emotions, particularly anger, anxiety, and depression. The concept of *controlarse* includes the following ideas: *aguantarse* (endurance), or the ability to withstand stress in times of adversity; *no pensar* (don't think of the problem), or avoidance of focusing on disturbing thoughts and feelings (see Chapter 4 for a discussion regarding mothers who migrate alone and who often use this coping mechanism to manage the sadness of leaving children behind); *resignarse* (resignation), or the passive acceptance of one's fate; and *sobreponerse* (to overcome), a more active cognitive coping that allows for working through or overcoming adversity. The following case illustrates a rather typical manner of coping with severe mental illness—the family draws together and keeps the illness within its realm.

Jerónimo Moreno Carrillo, a 32-year-old Mexican American juvenile court counselor, had come to therapy off and on for several years with his Mexican American girlfriend, Azucena. The focus was Jerónimo's apparent inability to make a commitment to the relationship. It had taken a long time for him to separate emotionally from his family and solidify a romantic relationship. After Jerónimo and Azucena finally married, I saw them occasionally. At some point, Jerónimo asked me if I would have a consultation with his family of origin. He wanted to see if anything could be done to ameliorate a volatile home situation that involved 8 of his 16 siblings who were living with his parents. The whole family was fighting daily with the second-to-youngest daughter, Mónica, a 27-year-old woman who had displayed aggressive behavior and paranoid ideation for many years. Recently the quarrels had escalated into physical altercations. Mónica was provocative, often saying terribly hurtful or insulting things to the others and refusing to cooperate with household chores or to comply with any requests. Everyone felt intimidated by her and didn't dare suggest the need for psychiatric care because she had always violently refused to hear it.

I agreed to see the family and asked that everyone who lived in the household come. Mónica was invited and was told that the purpose of the meeting was to discuss current family relationships. The day of the scheduled session, the mother, Mrs. Moreno Carrillo, six of the siblings who lived at home, and Jerónimo, who lived separately, came to my office. The father and the youngest daughter had to work and Mónica had refused to come but was reported to have been very restless and inquisitive all day. The siblings' descriptions of Mónica's behavior coincided with what Jerónimo had reported: their lives were constantly disrupted by Mónica's behavior. Recently most of them had become so angry with her that they either avoided her or shunned her. What was surprising was Mrs. Carrillo's reluctance to be involved in the session. Poised and beautifully groomed, she impressed me with her quiet strength. I felt admiration for what seemed to me a totally impossible task—raising 16 children closely spaced in age, without household or family help, all on her husband's meager salary. As we sat down she turned to Jerónimo dryly and said, "It was your idea to come here, why don't *you* say what you had in mind?"

As the family story unfolded, it turned out that Mónica was not the only one who had a history of mental problems. The mother had plunged into a depression shortly after having the last son, now 23. A

31-year-old sister had mental problems and was never able to maintain a job. She had been diagnosed as schizophrenic about 8 years ago and only got better when she began to take antipsychotic medication. Jerónimo himself had recurrent and unexplainable bouts of depression.

Mónica had been a very challenging, unruly child from the beginning, leading the family to believe she was born this way. She was very bright and talented in many areas, but was unable to focus consistently or develop any potential skills. From her adolescence onward, she had suffered recurrent delusions of being followed, of being loved at a distance, of being deceived by others, and even of being in danger of being poisoned or infected. In recent years Mónica attributed sexual fantasies to family members. She thought her mother was having an affair with the priest who led their bible study class because he had remembered her mother's first name. According to Mónica, her sister was trying to seduce the neighbor because she went to close a window while wearing a nightgown.

As we went over the families attempted solutions to Mónica's problems, Mrs. Moreno Carrillo would shake her head and show distrust that any of these problem-solving ideas would have any effect. Thinking that she should oppose the illness more, I suggested, though kindly, that she sounded diffident, perhaps even defeated by the problem. "Defeated, Oh no!", she said, "but I do not struggle" (*no le hago la lucha*). Indeed, Mrs. Moreno Carrillo had tried very little in terms of consulting physicians, psychiatrists, or teachers. She had not told neighbors or even the family physician in Tijuana about their problems with Mónica. Several years ago, when Mónica was sent home from a convent that she had joined, her mother accepted it without inquiry, let alone protest.

Mrs. Moreno had two explanations for her silence and apparent inaction. One was that her own mother had told her to "never murk up the waters from the river, because you may have to drink from those same waters later." In other words, privacy and decorum with outsiders is protective, because speaking about problems may hurt one's reputation and deprive one of help in the future. Mrs. Moreno also knew that Mónica's problems were intractable—she had always asked God to give her the strength to accept and save her energies *para sobreponerse* (to overcome adversity) for the sake of the other children.

In my mind I entertained many possible scenarios about Mrs. Moreno Carrillo's coping style and the world view behind it. On the negative side I wondered if there could be a touch of insulation and suspicion about the world in the mother's refusal to reach out. Or could it be that Mónica's delusions were a metaphor for a theme of sexual repression and excessive modesty in the family's Catholicism, a misguided attempt to balance for the family a developmental issue that appeared to be somewhat skewed? On the positive side there was the possibility that the mother's decision to accept rather than to struggle was similar to the acceptance and resignation I had seen in Ricki's great-aunt (see Preface) when she realized that the boy would not survive heart surgery.

From our Westernized vantage point of optimism and even hubris about endless possibilities for change, we equate quiet acceptance with a type of resignation or fatalism. In fact, acceptance of a severe illness about which we know little and control even less might just simply be sensible, humble realism.

What would be an appropriate intervention for this family? I experienced a real dilemma. If I could be reasonably certain that pursuing individual therapy, family therapy, or psychotropic medication would be of help with Mónica's hostility and delusional disorder, I could express my opinion and go against any cultural coping mechanisms that might stand in the way of relief. But I was far from confident myself that Western approaches had much to offer. I opted for a both/and approach, what Cade and Cornwell (1985) call a "split opinion interaction"—I praised the mother for her resilience and endurance in bearing a very heavy cross. I reflected that perhaps her acceptance of fate was the wisest choice given the nature of Mónica's problem. After all, the methods that health care professionals could offer would be experimental, with a combination of approaches that work in some cases but not in others. On the other hand, I wondered aloud about the recent escalation of aggression and whether it would continue if nothing was tried at all.

The siblings became curious about this latter statement and asked me to elaborate. I wondered if Mónica had increased her attacks because she had felt increasingly more isolated by the silence and rejection of each of the siblings. After all, anger is a form of contact that may be preferable to abject loneliness and frustration with one's limitations. I suggested that attention to her emotional and social isolation might provide a more beneficial connection than their usual attempts to be objective and correct her delusions.

The siblings were mobilized—they started to discuss in very animated terms how to implement these ideas among themselves. Mrs. Moreno Carrillo seemed calm and unimpressed. On the way out she thanked me and kissed me. She told me that she appreciated my efforts, but that what she trusted was to pray and go to confession. Perhaps in concession, she said she would add two or three prayers to her usual number so that things would not get worse. Clearly, she was telling me that her power and her comfort lay in prayer because the events themselves were beyond her control.

A week after the session I received two thank-you cards and payment beyond what I had requested from Jerónimo and another sibling. The notes thanked me for providing a place to talk about their distress and perhaps find some constructive things to try. This led me to believe that perhaps sibling therapy could be useful even without Mrs. Moreno Carillo's participation.

The attitude of the mother in this case provides a good example of what has been described as an external locus of control, in this case, with regard to mental illness—emotional and psychological problems and solutions are seen as the result of luck, fate, or powers beyond the control of the individual. Sometimes mental illness is perceived as God's test, other times, it is simply God's will.

## Somatization: The Mind-Body Connection

Another form of coping related to locus of control lies in somatization, those medically unexplained physical symptoms that commonly denote emotional distress. Somatization is observed more frequently among women and older individuals, and also among individuals from developing nations and those with lower education and income. Depression is correlated with somatization (Barsky & Klerman, 1983). Recent studies that attempt to disentangle the effects of social class from ethnicity and from migration have concluded that a higher level of unexplained somatic symptoms is present across social classes, gender, and age groups in Puerto Rico (Angel & Guarnaccia, 1989; Canino et al., 1992; Escobar & Canino, 1989). This finding has not been made conclusively for other groups, with the exception of older Mexican women, who also show an elevated number of functional somatic complaints.

To explain the tendency to somatize rather than "psychologize," Canino et al. (1992) argue that Anglo-Americans may be more likely to postulate a mind-body Cartesian dichotomy than other cultural groups, which are more likely to integrate mind-body experiences and express them somatically. Complementary hypotheses focus on ambivalent judgments toward mental illness that may make it more socially acceptabie to express psychological distress through physical complaints. Also, among the poor, health care is more readily available for medical than for psychological complaints. These reasons may also explain why somatization has frequently been found to characterize the behavior of immigrants and refugees. The connection between posttraumatic stress disorder and somatization also remains largely unexplored (Castillo, Waitzkin, Ramirez, & Escobar, 1995).

Physical complaints for which medical causes cannot be found may have a number of symbolic meanings or emotional explanations. These meanings can be readily accessed by asking Latino clients if they have any guesses or attributions about the emotional reasons for their symptoms. Beliefs are enduring aspects of people's collective and personal cultures. Understanding and respecting clients' beliefs and traditional theories and syndromes about health, illness, and healing enhance the successful engagement and unfolding of psychotherapy. Similarly, accepting the complimentary nature of folk healing resources in the community, such as *curanderos, yerberos, santeros, espiritistas,* and *sobadores,* can lead to open discussion and even fruitful collaboration as opposed to the parallel, guarded use of these services by the client.

Mainstream religious practices such as regular church attendance, praying, and confession are important sources of comfort, solace, and moral guidance for Latinos and may coexist with other practices based on indigenous magical beliefs. A therapist can access these meaning systems using an experimental, creative searching approach. Further, a consideration of cultural preferences in coping styles that stress quiet acceptance and internal endurance opens the way to questioning instrumental theories of therapeutic change, especially with clients who may already have their own cultural strengths. In the end, what helps is to envision a holistic mind-body connection that allows for emotions to manifest in bodily expressions, and for problems to reside in the mysteries of relational sin and revenge, thus entering the poetic realm of human drama. Harry Aponte (1994) describes this process with clarity and caring:

> When it comes to our work, however, spirituality is an arena where we need our clients. It will require that we see ourselves not as proprietary experts on the subject, but as companions on a journey, *their* journey. We do not own the expertise about the spirit. As therapists, we are not the new priesthood. We all have our own personal philosophical, social, and spiritual perspectives. We have varying degrees of commitment to our values. We have, in effect, our respective "religions." However, the poor come to us sometimes clothed only with their ethnicity, culture, and spirituality. It is not for us to dress them with our apparel. (p. 246)

In the next section we move on to another domain of MECA—Latino family bonds. Perhaps in few other areas are therapists as at risk for applying stereotypes of the Latino family or for misconstruing a family's distinctive meanings around relationships. The hazard of applying pathological labels of "enmeshment" or, conversely, idealizing a family's remarkable closeness is very real indeed. Thus it is with particular caution that we explore this dimension of life and recall that even these definitions are constantly changing.

## NOTES

1. Massage therapists are often called *sobadoras*.
2. Psychoanalysts have thought of this custom as counterphobic, yet it is also possible to think of it as an existential attempt to banter with a difficult but inevitable companion.

---

# PART IV

# Latino Family Bonds

---

Imagine for a moment what it must be like to have a very large number of people to relate to on a daily basis. The range and diversity of attachments and relational possibilities soars when an individual has not only the closeness of his own nuclear family, but a continuous bond with two large extended families. Growing up in the company of all of the descendants on mother's side and all those on father's side, the Latino adult's extended family expands once again when he marries and adds his mate's two families of origin to this burgeoning group of relatives.

From a general systems viewpoint, open and stable systems of such size and complexity offer more diverse alternatives for outcomes and solutions than small systems. Indeed, large family size augments the options and resources available to many Latino families, whether they organize as nuclear bigenerational, single- or two-parent arrangements, or even trigenerational units, and whether they live under one roof, in the same neighborhood, or within a few miles' drive of each other.

Despite the occasional complications and conflicts of life in a large group, and the imposed fragmentations caused by migration, most Latino immigrants share a preference for traditional family arrangements that support lifelong, parent-child cohesion and respect for parental authority. Limited economic resources and Roman Catholicism further support and reinforce large families of four, five, or more children, with extended family involvement through life (Bean & Tienda, 1987). The presence of extended networks in the United States and back in the native land facilitate the continuation of traditional and ethnic values, and provide bridges for leaving and returning periodically. The absence of such networks robs families of child care and other vital supports. A study of Mexican American families at different levels of acculturation (Rueschenberg & Buriel, 1989) found that the longer families had been in this country, the more they were able to adapt to "external system variables," such as developing stronger achievement and competitive orientations, or an understanding of politics or sports. Yet the "internal system variables," such as family connectedness, interpersonal controls, and communication styles that fall under the domain of "family organization" endure in various manifestations of Latino life.

Living within such a large family network clearly has consequences for social and psychological well-being and differs dramatically from life in a small, nuclear family. Yet most family therapy theory is based on the nuclear family model, and most Anglo-American thinking emphasizes individual autonomy, personal authority, and such nonblood relationships as husband and wife. A first critical point for therapists to know is that, while Latino families may organize in a variety of ways, their meaning systems and interactional patterns flow from a collective rather than an individual ideology and usually focus on blood relationships (e.g., mother and son). These differential styles and meanings influence connectedness and separateness, gender and generation hierarchies, and communication styles and emotional expression among family members and with outsiders. In Chapter 9 I explore these issues and the many strengths, constraints, and dilemmas of living in a collectivistic setting.

The world of couples comprises its own remarkable beliefs and behaviors within a veritable galaxy of children and parents, aunts and uncles, grandparents and godparents. Nowhere are cultural stereotypes of Latinos more obvious or more problematic than in definitions of what it is to be a man or a woman. And nowhere is the political discourse as heated as in conversations about the impact of these definitions on intimate human relationships. Faced with rapidly changing gender roles, decisions about incorporating dominant views, and attachments to traditional gender mystiques, Latino couples are entangled in a complicated web of hope, ambivalence, and contradictions.

In Chapter 10 I consider the meanings—traditional and evolving—that many Latino couples give to marriage. I also examine the dilemmas and opportunities behind two marital ideologies that would appear to compete: the intergenerational view and that of the nuclear and relatively isolated family. The myth and reality of such gender mystiques as *machismo* and *marianismo* are considered for the role they play in the problems and solutions of couples. While increasingly complex dynamics are at work in both marital and family life, I attempt in this section to illuminate some of the ubiquitous cultural themes that influence the domain of family bonds.

# 9

# Family Organization: The Safety Net of Close and Extended Kin

I do not belong to the culture of 911 (there is always a relative I can depend on to rescue me).

—A LATINA CLIENT (1996)

## CONCEPTS OF CONNECTEDNESS

The basic social unit of Latino culture is the extended family. *La gran familia* comprises three or four generations of relatives and includes horizontal relationships between adult siblings, cousins, and myriad others who place considerable value on their day-to-day, or at least weekly, interactions.

The sheer size of the household changes the texture of family life. There is a buzzy, noisy, chatty atmosphere in small spaces. Many people are part of a family's daily life, and a grandparent, an uncle, an aunt, or a godparent can always be counted on to change a diaper, keep an eye on a toddler, or monitor an adolescent's high jinks in the neighborhood. Overwhelmed parents get a much needed break and their children find some individual attention as this relative or that lends a hand.

What accounts for this connectedness among such large kinship groups? Scholars and researchers use such concepts as *familismo* and the "familial self" to describe the cultural meaning systems that are the ingredients of a richly connected family.

### Familismo

*Familismo* encompasses meanings about inclusiveness and participation in large family networks. In many Latino extended families, visits are frequent and helpful exchanges commonplace. Rather than move away from extended family, as Anglo-American adults often do, Latinos migrate toward them (Mindel, 1980). And unlike the dominant culture, boundaries around the Latino nuclear family are flexible, expanding to include grandparents, uncles, aunts, or cousins with natural ease (Alvirez, Bean, & Williams, 1981; Keefe, 1984; Ramírez & Arce, 1981; Vega, 1990). Children who are orphaned or whose parents are divorced may be included in the household of relatives, along with adults who have remained single, become widowed, or divorced. Both vertical and lateral kinship ties, up to third and fourth cousins, are often close.

*Familismo* also suggests collectivism or interdependence. Many family functions, such as caretaking and control of children, financial responsibility, companionship, emotional support, and problem solving are shared. The emphasis is on collective rather than individual ownership or obligation, affiliation and cooperation rather than confrontation and competition.

## The Role of Family Rituals

Nowhere is *familismo* better reflected, and reinforced, than in family rituals—a key component of Latino family life. Latino rituals are extended family celebrations that proclaim and reaffirm unity and connection. They may mark special events or occasions, but they also have a place in daily life (see Chapters 8 and 9 regarding life cycle rituals).

Larissa Adler Lomnitz and Marisol Pérez-Lizaur (1986), a Chilean anthropologist and a Mexican anthropologist who live and work in Mexico City, comment that to be part of a Mexican family is to participate in a complex system of symbolic actions that amount to a way of life. Not one week goes by without one or both extended families requesting the presence of all nuclear family members for some type of gathering. The most common ritual for many families is *la comida semanal* (the weekly meal) at each of the two grandparents' households, which usually takes place on weekends. This weekly custom includes all the unmarried or married offspring with spouses, children, and drop-in relatives of all ages. Visitors of any of the regular members may also be present.

Middle- and upper-class families from Mexico, Puerto Rico, and Cuba often continue some form of these gatherings in the United States, in part because they have the space and economic means. But most immigrant families are poor and have shrunken extended networks. Still, informal rituals may persist or emerge—a weekly stroll through a city park, a family picnic in a public space, or a get-together for no other reason than to watch TV.

As a great believer in the weekly shared meal and its importance for family connection and identity, I often ask immigrant clients if they might create a modified version of *la comida semanal,* perhaps eating together after church on Sunday or going for an ice cream after the children's soccer game. A weekly family meal may involve parents and adolescent children in cooking and cleaning, and this ritual in turn may renew the tradition of inviting significant others, if only to share a pizza and eat group style. Whatever their form, these gatherings symbolize *familismo*—solidarity, family pride, loyalty, and a sense of belonging and obligation to one's blood ties.

## The Familial Self

An Anglo-American therapist raised with values of autonomy and independence may wonder how the individual functions in such a collective world. A partial explanation lies in the concept of *personalismo* (Levine & Padilla, 1980), which denotes a high level of emotional resonance and personal involvement with family encounters. The term "familial self" may also explain how Latino individuals participate in life among many.

Psychoanalyst Alan Roland (1988; 1994), in observing Japanese and Indian people, coined the term familial self to describe a sense of self that includes one's close relationships as part of who one is. This self-family construction is useful in understanding Latinos' dedication to children, parents, family unity, and family honor. Money, objects, home, and other possessions are shared easily, perhaps because a familial self is tied to a different conception about individual rights and property. The familial self is balanced by an inner reserve of unshared feelings, which Roland calls a "private self," behind which all kinds of secret feelings and fantasies are kept. This inner separateness may explain in part how Latinos can individuate from their parents' nurturance and controls, while maintaining considerable emotional closeness and mutual dependency for a lifetime. The brilliant Mexican writer Octavio Paz has offered over the years his interpretations about the Mexican national character, particularly in his book *The Labyrinth of Solitude* (1964). Many of his ideas about Mexicans' ideations and communications coincide with the construction of a private self, shielded and evasive.[1]

## Closeness Pathologized

*Familismo* and the familial self extend our understanding of the Latinos' preference for close connections with family. They also serve as important comparisons to mainstream Anglo-American ideas about family life, and as such, help therapists avoid applying diagnostic labels (such as enmeshment) that do not fit. Indeed, what constitutes "excessive" connectedness in one culture may have entirely different meanings in another.

Tamara, my 27-year-old-daughter, is going to graduate school in San Diego and lives at home with me. The money she earns covers only her university fees and minor expenses. She gets free room and board at home. We get along very well, and each of us has total autonomy to travel, socialize, work, and shop at her own discretion. Yet we also share many meals, events of the day, news or gossip, and entertaining at home. Like many Latinas, we think a shared daily life is a rich life and have no resentment toward the small curtailments of freedom, the collective economics, or the emotional dependency. Her somewhat bewildered American classmates question Tamara frequently about this arrangement. They find it odd. They worry that she is not meeting all the challenges of growing up, as defined by the Anglo-American cultural narrative about "leaving home."

While Anglo-American therapists are at risk for pathologizing normative Latino closeness, they may also incorrectly label the behaviors that characterize such close family connections. For example, gender socialization motivates women to be supportive of their children and their husbands and to "sacrifice" themselves in silent ways that may be alien to Anglo-American culture. In mainstream American psychotherapy, this can look very much like codependence.

Jaime Inclán and Manuel Hernández (1993), two Puerto Rican psychologists who work at the Roberto Clemente Family Guidance Center in New York, wrote an interesting and useful cultural critique of codependence, the construct so widely used as the basis for self-help and treatment approaches to chemical dependency. Inclán and Hernández argue that the concept of codependence is embedded in Anglo-American values of separation/individuation and individualism. Clearly the notion of codependence needs critical review before application to Latinos because the changes these "codependent" clients are expected to make amount to a total rejection of *familismo*. Familismo stresses the duties of family members to help one another always, but even more so in the face of serious problems such as alcohol or drug addiction.

Poverty and family honor also play a role in intensifying *familismo*, because they promote even stronger family ties as a survival safety net. Further, family honor dictates shielding family conflict, shame, or deviation from external scrutiny. Misunderstanding of these Latino values can result in labeling *familismo* as pathological codependency or enmeshment, particularly in families that have been in this country for more than one generation.

In multicultural work, then, therapists need to examine their own personal and professional values and philosophies about family structure and connectedness, while exploring the specific meanings of closeness and attachments for each family.

## THE CAST OF CHARACTERS, ROLES, AND HIERARCHIES

Understanding the unique brand of connectedness of many large Latino family networks helps us "read" and compare maps of family organization. But just as crucial to this familial drama is a knowledge of the players and their specific roles and relationships. In this section I explore cultural meanings about nonkin "family members," godparents, the unquestioned authority of parents, the devotion between mother and son, and the life-long bond among siblings.

## Kith and Kin

As a therapist working with Latinos, you may be fascinated by the gradual appearance of new characters in the family drama of your clients. The nuclear family models most therapists use are too narrow for application to many Latinos, so we must think beyond their confines. It's important to ask if other people live with the family you're seeing in treatment. For new immigrants and poor and working-class Latinos, it is not uncommon to have seven or eight people sharing a room, with three or four people sleeping in one double bed. The family will likely reveal the important "others" as the barriers of institutional mistrust melt away.

I recently encountered a family consisting of mother, father, and three children who, after a few sessions, began talking about "the other family." In their rented apartment they were housing another family of four who had recently arrived from a town near their own native home in Oaxaca, Mexico. The "new" family was paying to rent one of the two bedrooms. Both families shared one bathroom and kitchen. Although it helped pay the rent, the arrangement was creating serious tensions and jealousies rather than the anticipated help and child care, and may have aggravated marital problems and fighting between the children.

Another family from Ensenada, Baja California, Mexico, consisted of a mother, three grown daughters, and a wealthy father who apparently lived with them on and off and paid for their therapy. But this was the father's "on-the-side" family, his *casa chica.* He had another legal family of wife and five grown children, his *casa grande.* He was very reluctant to participate in the therapy because he was going with his legal, first family to therapy somewhere else and his therapist had prohibited him from seeing his second family while he was solving problems with the first. The other therapist had quickly promoted an acculturative stance and wanted the father to conform to monogamy with his "first" family, not considering the possible disservice to his "second" family.

Raised and trained in Anglo-American culture, clinicians may back off in these situations and feel somewhat inhibited, to the detriment of the therapeutic process. It is best to ask questions politely and give each family member an opportunity to voice their feelings and opinions: "Is this type of family composition common in your culture? Among your family and friends? How does it work? Does it cause any problems?"

Another family consisted of a single, professional Puerto Rican mother who had raised her two teenage daughters "alone" since they were babies. Then I learned that Lupita, maid, cook, babysitter, and jill-of-all-trades, had lived with the three of them and slept with the girls for the past 10 years. Lupita had just now brought back from Mexico her 12-year-old son to join this "family." When Lupita came at my request for an information session, not only did she know much more about the girls than the mother, but she also turned out to be the best cotherapist I ever had, and the mother's most sensitive coach.

Maids have both a silent presence and a great impact in the lives of children and adults in Latino families, and they should be considered part of the extended family network.[2] They are present not only in middle- and upper-class families, but also in many working-class families. Maids allow mothers to work outside the home for profit, perhaps experiencing less stress around child care issues than their Anglo-American counterparts. The emotional attachment between these helpers and children, and occasionally between the adults, is often very significant.

Nelly was an illiterate, indigent 18-year-old Argentinian Indian who came from the north down to Buenos Aires to work for my family when I was a baby because my mother had become pregnant again. She quietly vanished from my life 19 years later, just prior to my wedding, when she was "no longer required" in my parents' household. Although she never told me, I always suspected she had wanted to leave much earlier, but must have known that I so very much needed her warm and comforting presence in my life. That she could not continue to be part of the family when she ceased to be *una empleada* (an employee), represents another excrutiating social injustice toward "service" people. I later learned that she had a baby girl and had named her Celia Beatriz, my first name and my sister's first name.

The involvement of extended family and nonfamily helpers or friends with the nuclear family should always be explored. To what degree are these other players part of the problem, or part of the solution? Would therapy with the nuclear family benefit by participation from others? A simple question such as, "Does anybody else live with you? Or "Who helps you with the children when you're working?" begins this exploration.

For example, unmarried Latino men and women whose parents have died may be more likely to live with married siblings than on their own. The presence of a maternal or paternal aunt is so commonly seen among my client families that I have come to label it *la tía* (the aunt). The therapist usually discovers the importance of *la tía* serendipitously, similarly to "the other family" pattern mentioned previously. In some cases, the aunt serves useful affective and instrumental functions while subsystem boundaries are maintained. In other cases, depending on her age and role interactions within the family, the aunt may form a cross-generational coalition with a parent or child, or may attempt to act as an intermediary between the two, sometimes benefiting growth but other times blocking it, as in the following example.

Charito Pérez, an unmarried, 33-year-old woman moved in with her brother, his wife, and their children. She quickly formed a coalition with María, her 14-year-old niece, against María's father, Mr. Pérez. María claimed that her Aunt Charito understood young people much better than her father, especially in areas of fashion, curfew, and friends. There was some truth to this, in that the aunt had recently arrived from Cuba with "more advanced" ideas than Mr. Pérez, who had migrated 20 years before and held to traditional ways, especially with regard to his expectations of women. The aunt's role as mediator was a resource at times, but her protective stance sometimes prevented Mr. and Mrs. Pérez from reaching agreements directly with their daughter. In addition, this coalition also inflamed the covert conflict between Charito and Mr. Pérez, who exerted his control as older brother rather sternly.

In these situations, the therapist needs to be careful not to conceptualize automatically the presence of the unmarried "stranger" in the family as a problem. Nor should the therapist believe that a triangle always reflects underlying marital conflict. Sometimes sibling therapy among the adults is helpful in addressing old ledgers and loyalties from the family of origin.

Relationships with same-sex peers, whether relatives or friends, are so important for Latinos that it's not unusual for them to be implicated in the presenting problem of an individual or family. Occasionally these relationships are a source of support, but often they are conflictual in themselves and comprise a stressor that affects the individual client, and in turn, his or her family. Whether working with individuals, couples, or other groupings, therapists are challenged to expand their unit of observation beyond the nuclear family, while keeping in mind that problems often reverberate as part of *familismo* rather than pathology.

## The Value of Godparents

In Anglo-American culture, godparents typically play an honorary role in family life. In Latino culture, godparents may be vital participants with significant status in families. The Latino custom of *compadrazgo* establishes two sets of extended family relationships: one between *padrinos y ahijados* (godparents and their godchildren); the other between the parents and the godparents who become *compadres* and *comadres* (coparents). Many Mexicans and Mexican Americans live in the same towns as their *compadres* and use their help in a variety of ways (Keefe, Padilla, & Carlos, 1978). Godparents are equivalent to an additional set of parents who have acquired formal kinship through a religious ceremony. They may act as guardians or sponsors of the godchild and care for him or her in emergencies, and they may be chosen from among members of the extended family or from outside. Godparents perform different roles and functions at various life cycle transitions and rituals, such as baptisms, communions, weddings, and funerals.

In many instances, migration separates the family from the godparents. But near or far, godparents can have auxiliary functions as advocates for the child, adolescent, or even for the parent. They can provide temporary relief for a sick or stressed parent or become an intermediary between parents and children. They can be especially valuable resources when therapy is addressing life cycle impasses. In the case of an out of control adolescent, a godmother provided a "demilitarized zone" so the parents and adolescent could begin to deal with their conflicts. Given their relative formality and emotional distance, godparents are often more effective with unruly adolescents than the biological parents and even the grandparents who sometimes are too partial to the child. Although godparents are seldom mentioned by Latino families in therapy, therapists might find a valuable resource if they take the initiative to ask about any *compadres* and *comadres*.

## The Unquestioned Authority of Parents

Despite the presence of godparents, aunts, uncles, maids, and other players in the life of a Latino family, parents clearly have top billing. While parents certainly care for and enjoy their children, affectional closeness and cohesion does not necessarily mean permeable boundaries, or even a great deal of self-disclosure, because too much closeness could threaten another strong organizing value: parental authority. Rules organized around age are the most important determinants of authority, with older men and women granted the greatest leadership and influence.

Latino parents command the *respeto* (respect) of children. While the Spanish word *respeto* translates as the English "respect," the internalized meaning of the word is quite different. For Anglo-Americans it reflects a fairly "detached, self-assured egalitarianism." For Mexicans, *respeto* means a relationship involving a "highly emotionalized dependence and dutifulness within a fairly authoritarian framework" (Diáz-Guerrero, 1975). For example, a 40-year-old Mexican woman recently told me she considered it a sin to be disrespectful of one's parents needs for contact, involvement, and financial support the way her American boyfriend was with his parents.

In general, the status of parents is high and that of children low, although there are spoiled Latino children too, particularly in the upper classes. Complementary, vertical transactions between parents and children are stressed, while symmetrical, horizontal transactions are discouraged or tolerated only in jest.[3] The unquestioned authority of parents persists throughout life, only slightly attenuated for adult children (Clark & Mendelson, 1975). Compare this situation with the Anglo-American concept of "personal authority" (Williamson, 1981), which underlines autonomy from parental approval as the hallmark of optimal adult development.

## The Status and Sacrifice of Mothers

Certain cultural prescriptions pertaining to gender also bolster parental status. The idealized role of the mother has been equated with self-denial and abnegation. When her patience is exhausted, a mother may become upset, nervous, or quietly suffer, but she is not expected to take time off or demand collective cooperation. A therapist may fail to convince a Latina mother that she needs time for herself and relief from her children. She may not share the Anglo-American mother's resentment at being "other-invested" rather than "self-invested," a value that underlies the individualistic nature of most dominant therapeutic goals.

The role of mother comprises a "mixed blessing." Latina mothers may experience considerable anxiety in relation to their children's safety and an excessive sense of responsibility. Mexican and Puerto Rican mothers may feel especially anxious about the dangers of the street and the vulnerability of their children to Los Angeles or New York gangs and believe this danger may increase in proportion to the child's separation from his mother's lap.

On the positive side, the social position of "mother" carries considerable status and commands respect. A 52-year-old Mexican woman who is married to an Iranian man was totally devoted to mothering and homemaking. She considered these roles as the highest calling for an individual, because "it passes on the essence of family to the next generation." Furthermore, she felt that the household atmosphere she created played a very decisive role in enticing a great fellow to marry her daughter. "When he saw," she said, "my clean house and the fresh, warm food I prepare, he was smitten with my daughter."

In payment for their sacrifice and dedication, mothers are the subject of much devotion, especially apparent in the lavish Mother's Day celebrations of Mexico. Indeed, mothers enjoy a lifelong reverence by their children, and especially by their sons.

## The Mother-Son Bond

Nowhere is parent-child closeness and devotion greater than in the relationship between mother and an oldest, or an only, or a favorite son. This bond is mutually supportive. The mother may have a strong influence even over a grown adult son, and he in turn may always worship and side with his mother. A number of hypotheses about this powerful attachment go beyond mere emotional connectedness and enter the realm of family politics (A. R. Del Castillo, 1996). Some writers speak of the emotional isolation of the mother from her husband, and the subsequent formation of a supportive subfamily unit of mother and children that excludes the husband. Still others regard mother's instilling a fierce loyalty and devotion in her son as a way of undermining the authority of the patriarch and gaining ascendancy over him (Lamphere, 1974).

In the earlier discussion of connectedness, I addressed the danger of pathologizing *familismo* as enmeshment or codependency. At the other extreme lies the danger of romanticizing Latino family connectedness, including mother-son bonds that may be maladaptive. Clinicians who endeavor to be culturally respectful may be at risk for disregarding a number of fairly extreme, possibly universal, human problems that may appear as "closeness" but actually transcend cultural stylistic preferences. These problems are evident in repetitive, rigid behaviors, and in imbalances of interpersonal influence that lead to developmental impasses and undifferentiation instead of growth. Such was the case of Frank González Torres Jr.'s family. This family of three illustrates parent-child connectedness gone awry, even though it has a culturally consonant flavor.

Frank Jr. was 9 years old when he was referred to therapy for night terrors and multiple fears. His mother, Mrs. Eudora González Torres, was a heavy-set and very properly attired 45-year-old woman who looked much older. She was born and raised in Mexico and lived with her parents before she got married in her mid-30s. She had wanted to go to nursing school but her mother did not let her for fear she might get sexually involved with somebody. Frank's father, meanwhile, had come from a very poor and chaotic family. He had left his family in his early teens and had fended for himself on the streets, ultimately becoming very suspicious and distant from almost everybody. When Eudora met Frank Sr. he was a single, very heavy, slow-mannered man a few years older than herself. Frank Sr. was ready to get married then, but Eudora felt she had to wait until her ill mother died before she could leave home. After her mother died, Frank Sr. and Eudora got married and migrated to the United States.

Their initial marital adjustment was smooth until Frank Jr. was born. In their words "the apple of the discord" was planted. Instantly mother and son became an inseparable unit. They slept in the same bed, displacing Mr. González Torres to the living room sofa. Disagreements about handling the boy mounted. Eudora protected the son and called the father a brutal and uncaring ugly monster. My impressions were to the contrary—the father's thoughts about his son's needs made more sense to me than did those of his wife.

The family first attempted to get help for Frank Jr. in kindergarten when he developed extreme separation anxiety. Prior to the boy entering first grade, mother and son suffered a conjoint psychotic break and were hospitalized and heavily sedated. The psychiatrists felt that the mother-son symbiosis was a hopeless situation, sending the boy to Mexico to live with relatives. Although Mrs. González Torres said the separation was "like death to me," she complied with the plan.

After some time, Eudora recovered, Frank Sr. returned to the matrimonial bed, and the marital discord subsided. But very soon after, the relatives in Mexico reported that Frank Jr. was having nightmares again. Immediately the mother went to fetch the boy. Like a powerful magnet mother and son embraced each other again and locked the father out in mind and body. Soon Frank Jr. developed terrors about everyone and everything. He could not go anywhere alone, not even to the bathroom.

I supported and engaged the father in therapy because he offered a hope for movement in a rigidly closed system. But when Frank Sr. began to respond, Eudora wanted him out of the session. Creating an alliance and a boundary by seeing her alone prior to the conjoint sessions proved fruitless. She kept on repeating: "Poor me and poor little boy." I decided to challenge the rigidity indirectly by going with the flow and prescribing the symptom.

The paradoxical "ordeal-like" intervention required that Eudora go to school every day with Frank Jr., sit with him at all times, and monitor each and every one of his activities, including lunch and bathroom breaks. Eudora needed to ask written permission from the school principal for each of the activities every day. Contrary to my expectations, not only did Eudora not balk at the amount of work involved, but she cheerfully agreed to do everything. Gradually, however, it was Frank Jr. who began to react. The other boys were teasing him and calling him a baby. He asked his mother to stop treating him so. One day Frank Jr. abruptly said that he wanted to have his own apartment with no mother, father, or wife—just two pets, a cat and a dog. He would train the cat and the dog to live together from an early age, because "if you get them old, they fight all the time, like they [his parents] do." Perhaps Frank Jr. would begin to separate and grow up a little after all. Like other breakthroughs with this family, this insight was short-lived.

The González Torres family continued to have severe problems and failed to achieve any greater degree of individuation or separation. This type of extreme overinvolvement, fusion, or symbiosis is of a different magnitude and quality than the stylistic preference for connectedness and interdependence described here for Latinos. A recent article by Robert Jay Green and Paul Werner (1996) makes a very important contribution by rethinking the concept of enmeshment into two different concepts: functional "closeness-caregiving" and "dysfunctional intrusiveness." Green and Werner argue that some family relationships have a "superficial form of closeness" (high levels of contact, high degrees of disclosure) that derive from coercion, collusion, and anxious attachment rather than from mutuality.

> Like a close embrace held too long or too hard, the inability to free each other tends to be experienced as an act of insecurity or control rather than an act of affection or support. Labeling such relationships as "extremely close" or "cohesive" masks their other qualities and potentially invalidates the experience of the participants. (p. 120)

## The Meaning of Fatherhood

In the public's narrative of cultural ideals, Latino fathers are expected to protect mother by demanding that the children obey and help her, while being only peripherally involved with daily caretaking, if at all. In reality fathers may be playful, affectionate, and do quite a bit of caretaking, particularly of young children (Gutmann, 1996).

The traditional pattern of father in the role of disciplinarian and mother as mediator between father and children may become more evident and rigid during the child's adolescence. Further, the stresses of migration and culture change may contribute to a weakening of the father's authority. Sometimes a father who appears controlling and intrusive with his adolescent children may simply be trying to be included in the family in the only way he knows how. I asked Elena's father, Mr. Morales, a Mexican immigrant, if this might be the case.

> A congenial, feisty man, Mr. Morales, rapidly answered me in the third person (with an *indirecta*): "He who appears to have military manners has in fact suffered a civilian 'coup d'état' years ago and has never been able to regain the presidency of the country." This metaphor for the ousted father became a central theme in the therapy. Mr. Morales explained that he felt guilty toward his wife because in spite of great effort he couldn't offer to the family the financial stability he had originally envisioned. Mr. Morales recalled that because of complications after Mrs. Morales had their fourth child, the lack of medical insurance led

to medical bills that took many years to pay. To compensate for his failure, Mr. Morales tried to enlist the older children's cooperation in housework, hoping to make Mrs. Morales's life easier. The more the father insisted, the more the adolescents resisted, rendering him frustrated and ineffective. Now Mr. Morales could see that some of his attempted solutions had become part of the problem.

While some theories regard Latino men's dominance as based only on traditional cultural values (Mirandé, 1988), other theories (Baca-Zinn, 1982) see it as a response to structural factors in society. Male dominance may take on greater significance when social stratification systems exclude members of a minority from public roles, access to resources, or fair recognition for effort or other social rewards. This issue would seem to be particularly relevant to immigrant Latino men. The father who remains a disciplinarian in a culturally isolated situation is less acceptable to the children because he no longer represents a community of adults who uphold the same views.

The aloofness may be increased if he migrated first and his wife and children came later. The spouses may have never totally recovered from the separation, or the father's promise of a better future may never have materialized, decreasing permanently his prestige and influence. This situation may be excerbated if the wife has joined the work force to help out financially. The husband may forcefully assert his authority with his wife, who in turn signals to the children that their father is domineering and unfair. The children may see the mother as victimized and begin to protect her, or they may feel bound by gratitude to her. This type of family triangle may present special difficulties with adolescents who become scornful and distant from the father, perhaps irreversibly. (For an analysis of the meanings, positive and negative, of family triangles from a cross-cultural perspective see Falicov, 1998.)

The widespread cultural stereotype of the Latino father as the dominant, authoritarian figure who makes all the decisions, is master of the household, and uses corporal punishment to discipline the children is contradicted by other images, views, and research data. Even as early as 1970, two studies supported a more egalitarian perspective on decision making for Mexican migrant farm families in California (Hawkes & Taylor, 1975) and a more equal division of household labor in Los Angeles and San Antonio (Grebler, Moore, & Guzman, 1970). In Mexico, Bronstein (1984, 1988) found no differences between mothers and fathers in scolding and criticizing or other exertions of authority. And while mothers were more physically nurturant in caretaking that comprised feeding and grooming, fathers were more emotionally nurturant in their playfulness and verbal instruction of school-age children. Another recent study found that Latino fathers, when asked, believe a family works better when husbands make the major decisions and wives support them, but agree that husbands should share in household responsibilities (Powell, 1995b).

These findings coincide with my own observations, although I have also encountered the more traditional authoritarian father and self-sacrificing mother, particularly in my clients' genograms of their families of origin. My interpretation is simply that with any large group of people considerable diversity will be found to support a variety of patterns. The fairest statement seems to be that Latino families are in transition, perhaps no different than families everywhere, and they display a mixture of traditional and egalitarian preferences.

## The Sibling Bond

### Fraternal Solidarity

Within the collectivistic Latino ideology, sibling ties are strong. Fraternal solidarity is an ideal that parents instill in their children from an early age. During childhood, siblings—along with cousins, or *primo hermanos*—may be constant companions. Parents prefer that their children have their own brothers, sisters, and cousins as playmates, and children seem to be happy to do so. Competition and fighting among siblings is sometimes tolerated while cooperation, sharing, and even sacrifice for a brother or sister is stressed. These values, and the sibling bonds they support, endure throughout life. It is interesting that many adult, nondocumented immigrants live with a brother or a sister (Chávez, 1985).

The strength of this family tie provides a rich therapeutic resource, especially in multiproblem, underorganized families (Lewis, 1988). Sibling therapy eases generational, language, and value differences at any point during the life cycle and with members of any social class. It can be part of an effective method of cultural-generational mediation for immigrant families. The therapist can first interview the parents separately, then the siblings, and later bring the whole family together for a feedback session. In separate interviews, siblings can negotiate issues they might not bring up with their parents present. Or their cooperation may be enlisted to extricate an overprotected or a parental child from the parental subsystem.

As a separate modality, sibling therapy provides a good alternative when conventional family therapy is difficult or impossible, a frequent dilemma when family members are separated or disrupted because of migration, economics, or other struggles.

One of my first cases of sibling therapy was with the Robledo brothers— Gilberto (13), Rafael (11), and Chui (9). These three Puerto Rican boys were inhaling airplane glue together to get high. After numerous failed attempts to engage their mother, grandmother, or any other adults at home, we resorted to asking the boys' probation officer to bring whomever he could get. He came in with the three boys. With my cotherapist, an American man in his mid-30s who had learned Spanish in the Peace Corps, we spent the first two sessions building trust, discovering the individuality of each youngster, and understanding their relationships.

We spared them talking about their home situation. Their mother was functionally and emotionally unavailable—engaged in drug abuse and prostitution. Their daily home life seemed dismal and utterly hopeless. We talked about their neighborhood, their experiences with school, and what it meant for each one of them to be Puerto Rican in Chicago. John and I talked about our own ethnicities, gender, race, migrations, our sibling group and birth order, about the good things and the bad things in these categories and experiences. We were friendly, genuine, and even shared some of our own questionable youthful experiences.

The five of us managed to feel a little closer to each other and were able to diffuse the hierarchies and the differences somewhat, but inevitably they were there. And so John and I decided to face the three youngsters as squarely as we could, by talking about our differences. We started with our differences in age, race, and gender. John and I stepped out of our roles as therapists briefly and talked about our roles as parents, in contrast to the boys' roles as children. I mentioned that I was a rather strict parent who did not like it when my children escaped their obligations to themselves, such as when they watched TV before doing their homework. Somewhat in jest I confessed that I went around telling my children that if they watched too much TV their brains would turn into mashed potatoes. The roaring, cracking, writhing laughter that followed went on and on until Gilberto intervened forcefully saying, "Yeah! Hey, hey!! Listen listen listen to this: can the stuff [airplane glue] turn your brains into mashed potatoes? Can it, can it? Hey, tell the truth, the truth!" We said we thought it did.

In the remarkable process that followed, Gilberto, the oldest sibling, became inspired to be almost primitively controlling of himself and his younger siblings. He instituted a system of surveillance and organized each brother to become "a cop" for the other, in a fashion reminiscent of William Golding's Ralph in *Lord of the Flies*. Anyone going near a hardware store or a parking lot was punished by the other two. Once when Rafael and Chui teamed up and violated both rules, Gilberto abandoned them in the streets, did not talk to them for days, and came to a session by himself. Gilberto taught me about the power of sibling love and leadership when adults cannot nurture or control, but he also taught me about the human wish to care and be cared for, whatever it takes.

## The Influence of Birth Order

Parents accord clear authority to older siblings and usually delegate some supervisory and caretaking functions to them. In large families, complex allocations of roles, division of labor, and individual compatibilities stimulate the formation of subgroups. Traditional gender role assignment encourages girls to do household chores for the boys, who in turn are supposed to chaperone and protect their sisters outside the home.

The oldest child tends to be parentified, in part a consequence of migration (the child acts as cultural and language translator) and a common pattern in large families from collectivistic cultures. The parentified child's role as intermediary may persist throughout life, especially for daughters. This situation may work well but can also present difficulties during important life transitions, as happened in the following case.

Mariana Valdez brought her family of origin to therapy when she was 28 years old. She felt that her parents needed to develop a better relationship with her 16-year-old sister, who had become defiant and disrespectful. Although there were two older brothers, they had both moved to the East Coast when they got married. Mariana lived with her second husband next door to her parents who, in spite of being in this country for 19 years, did not speak English or drive a car. Mariana took care of many of their public obligations and those of her two younger sisters who were now 16 and 14 years old. Although this was not clearly stated as the reason for the consultation, Mariana had been recently diagnosed with advanced ovarian cancer. She feared for the well-being and social survival of her family as much as for her own life, and she knew that some drastic shifting of responsibilities had to take place.

Mariana was painfully ambivalent about her power in the family. On the one hand, she was proud of having been such a fundamental part of their adaptation. Yet she was also deeply resentful about the constraints that this role entailed. Her first husband was a Mexican man who was abusive to her, yet he had been approved by her parents because he was of the same culture and kept Mariana close to home. Another source of frustration for Mariana was that her sisters didn't speak Spanish and used her as a translator and advocate to obtain freedoms, such as going out to movies and dances, that the parents didn't allow. The parents and the two younger sisters constantly turned to Mariana to mediate, causing her the stress of trying to be fair to both cultures and languages. Now she was very ill, and very sad, and very tired, and she needed a replacement.

Mariana thought that if her role was indeed indispensable, somebody else should assume it, perhaps a therapist. This was a structural trap for me, given my own very parentified role in my immigrant family of origin. Instead, I believed that a reshuffling of roles, more direct communication between the parents and younger children, and greater flexibility to make room for coexisting values seemed more appropriate therapeutic goals. (For an extensive description of this case see Falicov, 1997.)

The influential position of an older sibling, particularly with immigrant parents, can be used to help a less favored or scapegoated sibling. In Chapter 4 I introduced Margarita Alonso, who had migrated to the United States from Mexico, and was later joined by her mother and children. We revisit this case in more detail here to show how an older brother's intervention alleviated an interdependent, conflictual relationship between his mother and sister.

Soon after Margarita's mother and children joined her in San Diego, the young mother found herself struggling with the consequences of years of estrangement from all of them. Margarita was especially distressed by conflictual feelings toward her mother, Alma. She felt gratitude over the crucial role Alma played in taking care of her children while Margarita sought a better life in the United States. But Alma was critical of her daughter's lifestyle and her relationships with men. Margarita had been raised with values of *familismo y personalismo. Respeto* had stopped her from responding to Alma's criticisms until Margarita couldn't take it anymore and exploded in anger.

Gender issues played a definite role in that Alma relied on and respected the opinions of her sons, particularly the oldest, Agustín, while she treated Margarita like a second-class citizen. When Agustín visited San Diego, I seized the opportunity for a sibling interview, and presented it to Margarita as a way to obtain information about the family and enlist her brother's help.

Agustín's input was very enlightening. He was very supportive of Margarita, had a lot of empathy for her predicament, and offered his own perspective by telling Margarita a family secret. Agustín's theory was that Alma's pressure on Margarita over issues such as a woman's honor and reputation stemmed from her own shame regarding, what Agustín called, her own "questionable past." There were many indications that, during her youth, Alma had worked as a barmaid and prostitute in a tiny Mexican town. Apparently one of Margarita and Agustín's siblings, Ramona, had died of an acute infectious disease in her adolescence. Agustín had heard that their mother interpreted this death as punishment for her own "low life," and that's why she intensely returned to the Roman Catholicism of her childhood. Thus Agustín attempted to dispel Margarita's anguish over her mother's accusations by shifting the blame and by promising Margarita that he would talk to Alma about relaxing the controls and criticisms, and stressing instead all the good things one should recognize about Margarita's hard work and accomplishments in the United States.

Continued emotional support, advice, and practical help among adult siblings is a tribute to the enduring connectedness of family ties among Latinos. Perhaps because of this closeness, quarrels and resentment among adult siblings are also common. These may occur because some siblings attempt to establish a more egalitarian relationship with each other during adulthood, but birth order and age hierarchies continue to be compelling. Sibling quarrels may also be caused by parental favoritism, disagreements about inheritance, unpaid debts, or the persistence of a controlling attitude on the part of an older sibling toward a younger one. Rifts among siblings, however, are seldom permanent. New family transitions often serve as points of reunion and pathways to rejuvenate brother and sister ties.

## COMMUNICATION STYLES, CONFLICT RESOLUTION, AND EMOTIONAL EXPRESSION

Ideologies about connectedness and hierarchies as reflected in the cultural meaning systems of *familismo* and *respeto* significantly shape the Latino family's style of communication, conflict management, and emotional expression—three areas that receive frequent emphasis in therapy. In this final section I explore some of the nuances of Latino communication and their implications for treatment. An extensive case study demonstrates how interactional styles affect family functioning and guide the therapist toward specific culturally congruent interventions.

### Language and Politeness

The *amabilidad* (amiability), gentility, and civility of the Spanish language no doubt contribute to a politeness of demeanor, deportment, and address. The Mexican American writer Sandra Cisneros (1995) offers a sharp contrast between these pleasing forms and the direct, business-like messages conveyed by the English language, which sound so painfully inhuman to her father's ears:

> Because Uncle Fat-Face had been in the United States longer he gave Father advice. Look, when speaking to police always begin with, "Hello, my friend."
>
> In order to advance in society, Father thought it wise to memorize several passages from the "Polite Phrases" chapter. *I congratulate you. Pass on, sir. Pardon my English. I have no answer to give you. It gives me the greatest pleasure.* And—*I am of the same opinion.*
>
> But his English was odd to American ears. He worked at his pronunciation and tried his best to enunciate correctly. *Sir, kindly direct me to the water closet . . . Please what do you say? May I trouble you to ask for what time is? Do me the*

*kindess to tell me how is.* When all else failed and Father couldn't make himself understood, he could resort to—*Spic Spanish?*

*Que* strange was English. Rude and to the point. No one preceded a request with a—*Will you not be so kind as to do me the favor of . . . ?*—as one ought. They just asked. Nor did they add—*If God wills it*—to their plans, as if they were in audacious control of their own destiny. It was a barbarous language. Curt as the commands of a dog-trainer. *"Sit." "Speak up."* And why did no one say *"You are welcome."* Instead they grunted— *"Uh-huh"* without looking him in the eye, and without so much as a *"You are very kind, mister, and may things go well for you."* (p. 70)

In short, from early on Latinos are raised with the notion that much can be achieved interpersonally if people talk nicely, explain a lot, and give compliments.

## Maintaining Harmony: *Indirectas, Choteo,* and *Dichos*

In keeping with their desire to preserve family harmony and avoid interpersonal conflict, collectivistic cultures favor indirect, implicit, and covert communications. People publicly agree—or at least do not disagree—with each other in order to "get along" and not make others uncomfortable. Conversely, assertiveness, open differences of opinion, and direct demands for clarification are seen as rude or insensitive to others' feelings.

The use of impersonal third-person rather than first-person pronouns is one aspect of this style. For example, by stating "One could be proud of . . ." rather than "I am proud of . . ." the Latino individual is viewed as appropriately subtle and selfless. The use of allusions, proverbs, and parables to convey an opinion is commonplace, especially among Mexicans. Cubans seem more adept than Mexicans and Puerto Ricans at directness, softened by a mordant, piquant, and sometimes even outrageous sense of humor. The result of all this is an apparent harmony, sometimes at the expense of a clear understanding of the other's intent. *Indirectas* are also used to maintain harmony when the emotion at hand is anger. A Mexican saying states, "The one who gets angry loses." So criticisms often take the form of allusion (e.g., "Some people never change"), diminutives used in a sarcastic way, and belittlement. Similarly, Boswell and Curtis (1984) describe a Cuban's use of *choteo* (humor) as a way of ridiculing or making fun of people, situations, or things. *Choteo* may involve exaggerations, jokes, or satire to modify tense situations.[4]

Harmony is also maintained by the formation of "light" triangles. Rapport-based alliances, especially when based along gender lines, provide an emotional outlet in the form of gossip and secrets. Rather than being detrimental, these light alliances may enhance the stability of a marriage (Komarovsky, 1967). As in other cultures, women's proclivity to "trouble talk" may be a basic ingredient of Latina intimacy (Tannen, 1990). In fact,

Mexican working women consider it permissible to be disrespectful about their husbands' traits when talking to other women (Benería and Roldán, 1987).

In addition to the use of *indirectas* and *choteo*, positive emotional expression is highly valued in the Latino culture. Words of endearment and compliments about a person's appearance, dress, or smile or support for his or her positive qualities spice up conversations among intimates. Indeed, closeness is demonstrated not only by these verbal expressions but through physical proximity and gestures. A couch in my office that accommodates only one American parent and one child comfortably seats one or two Latino parents with two or three children! Touching, kissing, and hugging are other manifestations of close family relationships, particularly between Latino parents and children. But they extend to other friendly relationships too—in Mexico, Puerto Rico, and Cuba, teachers kiss pupils, hairdressers kiss their clients, and children kiss the parents of their friends.

In setting examples of *indirectas* and emotional closeness, Latino parents teach their children to have a "proper demeanor" and a considerate, helpful, and warm approach toward others. Later they will be praised and liked for displaying *simpatía*—the ability to create smooth, friendly, and pleasant relationships that avoid conflict (Comas-Díaz, 1989; Levine & Padilla, 1980).

## Implications for Therapy

The Latino culture's emphasis on smooth relationships, social graces, and *personalismo* has significant implications for family functioning and family therapy. On occasion communication styles that emphasize indirectness and civility in the name of avoiding conflict can become excessive and lead to concealment, lies, and intrigues. At other times they may provide veiled messages sent on circuitous routes. We again consider the case of Margarita Alonso, her mother, Alma, and Margarita's brother Agustín:

> Margarita's brother Agustín had suggested his mother might be having difficulty in her relationship with Margarita because of a "secret past" in which Alma, their mother, had worked as a barmaid and prostitute. But the story didn't end there. Two weeks after that sibling session, Margarita asked to see me alone. She started by telling me that she believed the story Agustín had told—she now vaguely recollected hearing rumors about their mother's past. But Margarita's main fear was that perhaps Agustín also meant the story as an indirect communication toward her. Margarita started weeping, pouring forth a confession about her own involvement with prostitution. In fact, she never could have paid for the three airplane tickets to the border, the "coyote" (smuggler) that crossed

them through, or the rent for their apartment had she not supplemented her meager salary with prostitution.[5] I will never know if the brother really knew, or just suspected, these events in Margarita's life, but the type of indirect communication, by allusion, is not atypical of a style that avoids direct confrontation.

Distinguishing the degree to which such patterns of indirect communication are maladaptive for a particular family is part of the therapist's task. Attention to style of communicating between client and therapist also has important implications at different points during treatment.

An initial social phase that transmits the therapist's interest rather than focusing on procedures (such as referral sheets and appointment schedules) is critical when joining with a new client family. Manifesting real interest in the client, the problem, their theories about why the problem exists, and the attempted solutions is essential given the Latino emphasis on *personalismo,* or building personal relationships.

A tone of acceptance that avoids direct confrontation or doesn't demand greater disclosure is essential throughout treatment. The therapist's use of humor, allusions, and diminutives soften the directness of treatment and are often more effective forms of delivery because they mirror preferred cultural transactional styles. Disclosure can be facilitated when the therapist becomes a philosopher of life through storytelling, anecdotes, and metaphors. Use of analogies, proverbs, popular songs, or a mysterious, unexpected communication that transmits an existential sense of the absurd or the reversals of life is consonant with Mexican cultural themes. A therapist's knowledge and timely use of *dichos* (proverbs) is an invaluable and aesthetic communicational resource (Dow, 1986; Fischer, 1988) for many groups, but Latinos are particularly adept with these metaphorical statements.

An intense emotive style and person-centered approach is more appealing than a businesslike, structured, or task-oriented approach. When feelings are subtly elicited by the therapist, Latinos respond much more openly than when they are directly asked to describe or explain their emotions and reactions. An experiential approach that emphasizes "telling it like it is" or "baring one's soul" and interpreting nonverbal language may well inhibit clients.

Similarly, while contracts and behavioral treatment goals might be too task oriented—most Latinos wouldn't be comfortable scheduling certain times to be intimate or to resolve problems—the therapist can assign "conditional homework," perhaps asking the family to think about how it would feel to engage in a particular task should the occasion arise. Such a technique is not only more collaborative and less presumptive, but it is also consonant with a culture that values serendipity, chance, and spontaneity in interpersonal relationships.

Whatever the theoretical orientation or type of intervention used, therapists should invite the family's feedback about the process of treatment. In a culture that emphasizes cooperation and respect for authority, clients may feel that it is impolite to openly disagree with the therapist. Encouraging the family to express both their positive and negative reactions to the therapist's opinions helps to establish a tone of mutuality.

## Communicational Styles and Generational Culture Clashes

The tendency to maintain harmony and avoid conflict in a large, complex family network were aggravated by an adolescent who challenged her mother to be a "modern" woman, a challenge that is on the rise among Latinas (Gil & Vásquez, 1996) and other immigrant groups (Akamatsu, 1995). The case also illustrates helpful techniques for dealing with large families that live in collectivistic, extended family settings.

> The Aldrete Mujías were a traditional, middle-class, business-oriented, practicing Catholic family. The nuclear group consisted of mother, Marta (35), father, Robert (36), and four children, Jennifer (14), Andrew (13), Chris (9), and Silvina (5). Two very large extended families lived close by. Robert was the second of eight siblings, all of whom lived with their spouses. Many of the spouses also had extended family nearby. Robert's mother, Dolores Aldrete, lived eight blocks away from him in a home that was the hub of many family activities. Robert, Marta, and the children had for years enjoyed *la comida semanal* and a game of lotto (*lotería*) at Dolores's house every Sunday afternoon.
>
> Marta Mujía was the third of seven siblings. Her mother, Lourdes, had a wonderful, large home two blocks away, where the grown children and the grandchildren spend many weekends. The house grounds became a recreational camp for the grandchildren every summer. Both Robert's and Marta's families of origin had a steady Catholic church affiliation and celebrated all religious holidays and birthdays together.
>
> During the first nuclear family interview I learned that Jennifer had been living with *Abuelita* (Grandma) Dolores for the past 3 weeks, following a particularly nasty row with her mother, Marta. In fact, Jennnifer had been fighting constantly with Marta, spreading the news on both sides of the family that she despised her and would never respect her again. Marta felt very hurt, embarrassed, and afraid of the public opinion of both families, the neighbors, and the school, all of whom were aware that Jennifer had gone to live at *abuelita's*. Robert was passive and uninvolved but was completely behind Marta. He was equally tired of Jennifer's willfullness, demands for privileges such as driving and visiting friends, and sassy retorts and provocations when her wishes were not granted immediately. There seemed to be a peer-like relationship between Jennifer and her mother rather than a hierar-

chical relationship involving parental respect. Instead, the two grand-mothers were the executive subsystem of the family.

Because so many people were involved, piecing together a coherent story was as fascinating as it was frustrating. For example, I learned from Jennifer that Marta had hit her several times, and that unbeknownst to her parents, Jennifer had sought revenge by reporting her mother to the school counselor. However, she begged school authorities not to report her mother to child protective services, so the school decided to maintain close observations and regular meetings with Jennifer until they understood the situation better. Building my therapeutic alliance with Jennifer also required that I kept this secret confidential, at least temporarily. Meanwhile, Jennifer, who had all the entitlements that come from being the first and favorite grandchild in two large Latino extended families, had secured a lot of sympathetic supporters among her paternal uncles, aunts, and cousins, who had subtly shunned Marta by not calling her or asking how she was after Jennifer had moved to the grandmother's house. Marta was mortified. She felt that years of hard work had vanished and her reputation as a mother was tarnished forever.

She feared the family's judgment and stopped the Sunday meals with *Abuelita* Dolores. She was losing her old terrain as Jennifer invaded it. Meanwhile, Jennifer was getting situated with the paternal grand-mother, Dolores, and a paternal, single aunt, *Tía* (Aunt) Catalina (29), who was living with her mother while between jobs.

I interviewed *Abuelita* Dolores and *Tía* Catalina alone. Much to my surprise, *Abuelita* Dolores seemed to speak with two sides of her mouth. She catered to every one of Jennifer's wishes, cooked every one of her meals, let her talk for hours on the phone, and had frequent conversations with her in which she criticized Marta with venom, wondering for example if her unkemptness and emotionality were connected to Lourdes's (the other grandmother) upbringing of Marta. Yet behind Jennifer's back, Grandma Dolores expressed quite a different opinion. She was critical of how willful, poorly mannered, and inconsiderate Jennifer was. She was even somewhat sympathetic of how difficult it must be for Marta to raise Jennifer. Had the preservation of harmony and indirect communication gone awry, I wondered? The intrigues of the extended family and Marta's self-imposed ostracism were escalating and needed attention.

Of all the family members I had met, Catalina impressed me as the most level headed and psychologically minded. She seemed to have a more balanced appraisal about issues between parents and adolescent children and understood the dangers of taking sides. Catalina believed the family should have come to therapy a long time ago. She also felt it was time for her brother, Robert, to be less peripheral to his family and not delegate so much of the parenting on the women. After asking the Aldretes permission, I invited Catalina to be my "link cotherapist."

The indirectness of communication in a Latino family can compound the obvious difficulties of assessing many interrelated issues. With large families, therapists can obtain the necessary information to initiate and monitor a process of change in two ways. One is to convene the entire family network and obtain as many opinions and stories as possible. The use of comparative, circular questioning is particularly helpful in this process (for example, the therapist might ask, "Who is the most concerned about Jennifer living with *abuelita?*" or "Robert, how does your mother respond when Marta declines invitations for the Sunday *comida?*"). The other method is to select a family member who is more peripheral to the problem than those in the consulting family unit but central enough that he or she can communicate or "link" with the larger group. This method was first described by Landau-Stanton (1990) for use with rigid, extended families in cultural transition that tend to close ranks and deny access to therapists. "Link therapy" is useful for many extended family issues because the tasks are usually daunting, even when the therapist is fully accepted.

> With the Aldrete Mujías family I pursued the second option. I relied on Catalina to normalize the situation in the extended setting. Her task was to reopen *Abuelita* Dolores's home for Sunday meals and reestablish routines that had been nurturing for everybody. She also was to encourage Robert to help Marta continue with "life as usual" while Jennifer remained at Grandma's house, rather than create new escalations and polarizations. Remaining calm, clear, and involved would empower Marta and raise her in the hierarchy—both would allow a shift away from her usual responses of excessive civility or angry outbursts.
>
> I met with Marta and Robert and encouraged them to become much more involved in daily decisions. Marta needed to be more effective in providing limits for Jennifer, and for the other children too, before things got out of control. Usually Marta felt overpowered by Jennifer (who had known from the time she was a young girl she could always rely on her paternal grandmother's backing). Following a confrontation with Jennifer, Marta usually became ashamed of how she handled things, feared the larger family's backlash, and either gave in to Jennifer or retreated, only to receive further challenges and contempt from Jennifer. Although Robert appropriately sided with his wife, he had never been aware of how his mother's spoiling of Jennifer undermined Marta's authority. Out of *respeto* he had never talked to *Abuelita* Dolores about this issue. But now, as he and Marta were making plans to bring Jennifer home, he broached the subject. He felt that his family of procreation needed to function as a more bounded nuclear family, while remaining part of an integrated extended network.
>
> It was actually not that difficult for Robert to convince his mother to let go of Jennifer, as the girl had become reactive to any caretaking behaviors on her grandmother's part. Careful questioning of Jennifer

failed to clarify her contempt for her mother, and to a lesser degree for her grandmother. Surprisingly, she remained respectful and admiring of Catalina and of me. She often asked career-related questions and wanted to see the books in my office. I decided to explore in a joint session with all the women involved—Dolores, Marta, Jennifer, Catalina, and myself—"women's issues," which involved cultural and personal conceptions about the meaning of being a woman and future-forward questions.

"Self-possession," calmness, and self-confidence emerged as the qualities Jennifer held in highest esteem. She felt that her mother, Marta, who was alternately intimidated and submissive or rageful and irrational, was not to be respected. Catalina proved to be the invaluable bridge—as a woman in cultural transition she could blend views and values. We talked about the pros and cons of being traditional and modern. The sharp contrast between direct and indirect communication, including secrets, lies, and duplicity were brought up. Jennifer was furious at her mother's meekness and insisted on the need for openness and resolution of conflicts, particularly with the grandmother. Of course, I was the only one who knew that Jennifer was not above reproach when it came to duplicity, given her secret denunciation of her mother to the school counselor. But I only alluded to her own secret revenge with a proverb that she understood: *La que este libre de culpa que tire la primera piedra* . . . (only the person free of guilt can throw the first stone . . . ).

In conclusion, the client who said, "I do not belong to the culture of 911" was right—there seems to be little need for the assistance of 911 in the Latino community. There is a plethora of others to turn to for help, as well as many close and distant relationships that occupy one's life. Therapists usually know little about the resources provided and the constraints imposed by large nuclear and extended family arrangements.

The challenge is to be constantly aware that a different model of individual development and family relationships may be operating than the conventional, middle-class Anglo-American version. The extended family model may be in action even when families are fragmented across countries and undergo frequent expansions and contractions in family composition. The dimensions I have selected for discussion in this chapter, namely connectedness, the cast of characters with their positions in the family hierarchy, communication, conflict resolution, and emotional expression are particularly important domains, especially when one considers the degree of consonance or dissonance between the "maps" of the family and those of the therapist. These are also dimensions of family life in which cultural continuity, cultural change, temporary culture clash—with its ensuing clinical correlates—and eventual resolution through alternation or hybridization take place.

In the next chapter, family bonds figure highly again, but with an emphasis on couple relationships. Connectedness for couples may take on quite different meanings for Latino spouses who, for example, might focus on blood relationships between parent and child rather than husband and wife, or for whom cultural mystiques about gender alter both beliefs and behaviors within a marriage or other intimate relationship. Chapter 10 is designed to help therapists understand and work with some of these important organizational issues.

## NOTES

1. Some ethnohistorical interpretations of the need to protect and conceal parts of the self are based on the idea that national traits are built in response to historical events. Silence or feigned ignorance may have seen better strategies than openness for the indigenous populations interactions with their oppressors, the Spanish colonizers (Bartra, 1987; Ramírez, 1977).

2. Denise Chávez, the vibrant, uplifting Chicana writer, devotes sections of her 1994 novel *Face of an Angel* to what she calls "The Book of Services." There she sings the praise of some of those unsung Latino heroes: the maids, gardeners, and waitresses.

3. Larissa Adler Lomnitz (1995) has studied the relationship between macro and micro social systems and believes that Mexican society is a good example of verticality reproduced at every level, from political systems to family systems to dyadic relationships. Lommitz's hypothesis is that the intense Mexican emphasis on hierarchies started with the Spanish conquest. The Spanish empire was clearly a vertical, authoritarian system that allied with another vertical, authoritarian system, the ruling class of the Aztecs, in order to subjugate the Mexican people. Puerto Ricans and Cubans (who also share a heritage of Spanish conquest) also favor vertically arranged relationships with a clear asymmetry of power between parents and children, but with a greater mixture of horizontal and informal family relationships than Mexicans.

4. Boswell and Curtis (1984) suggest that *tuteo*—the informal form of addressing people—is a precondition for *choteo*. Cubans may use the informal *tú* rather than the formal *usted* to decrease distance and increase familiarity and *personalismo* in social situations.

5. Working in clubs as a bargirl may happen even among women who live with a boyfriend or a husband. It allows poor women with no education or skills to earn more than minimum wage or even the salary of an unskilled male laborer. This helps with the economic hardships, but often presents moral dilemmas for the women and conflicts with the men in their lives (see A. R. Del Castillo, 1991).

# 10

---

# The World of Couples:
# Reality and Myth

> While men can take other men to the edges of their psyche, it is
> women who can take them to their depths.
> —RODRÍGUEZ (1996, p. 130)

At the close of this millenium, the political and social discourse on the
roles of men and women in relationships, family life, and work, rages on.
Cultural differences do not remove Latino women and men from this particular evolution, and in fact, may present additional challenges as they
seek to chose or incorporate traditional ideas and mystiques with growing
trends toward egalitarianism and dominant cultural views about how cou-
plehood "should" look. In this chapter I explore the Latino couple's complex views of gender and marriage, and suggest ways to broach these subjects clinically. First I introduce some general guidelines about Latino
couples' help seeking and engagement in therapy. Then I examine the u-
biquitous triangles of son, mother, and daughter-in-law, best understood by
contrasting the collectivistic ideology of the extended family and the more
individualistic ideology of the nuclear family. Finally, I shift to a detailed
discussion of Latino gender role ideologies and mystiques, and consider
how these beliefs help and hinder couples relationships.

Throughout, I suggest ways to approach these subjects in couples
work. The complex nature of the marital bond and the multiple meanings
spouses attribute to gender are explored clinically by examining definitions of love and intimacy, power and hierarchy. The need for careful, curi-

ous, and humble questioning is stressed, as is a heightened tolerance for ambiguity. With an awareness of these provisos, therapists can readily collaborate with couples on a fascinating journey to uncover and illuminate the multiple meanings and novel interpretations for gender and marriage that so often fall prey to unspoken stereotypes.

## ENGAGING LATINO COUPLES IN THERAPY

### Parenthood versus Partnerhood

Latinos in traditional family settings seldom see happiness as the primary goal of marriage, although they are, of course, distressed by marital unhappiness. Satisfaction in marriage is seen as the result of good fortune and wise choices. It cannot be achieved just by working toward "marital improvement" or enrichment. Further, an investment in maintaining marital harmony is part of a traditional configuration that values children and family life over individual happiness and autonomy. The romanticism of courtship and early marriage shifts quickly to a focus on family formation and parenthood, in part because of Catholic values and opposition to birth control. Couples have children sooner than their Anglo-American counterparts and their familes are usually larger. The emphasis on one's role as parent, rather than as marital partner, probably correlates with large family size.

Despite a focus on parenthood rather than partnerhood, marital instability has been repeatedly reported for Latinos (see Frisbie, 1986). Although separation and divorce are still comparatively uncommon and the majority of Mexican American families remain intact, family breakup is on the rise, especially among younger Chicano couples. Abandonment and single-parent households are more prevalent among poor Mexicans, and even more so among poor Puerto Ricans. The number of Puerto Rican single female-headed households is more than double that among Cuban and Mexican families (42% compared to 19%)(U.S. Bureau of the Census, 1991). Cubans have fewer children, achieve middle-class lifestyles, and have the highest marital stability (62%). More than other Latino groups, Cubans tend to cope with divorce by maintaining a binuclear family with high involvement from the father.

Although some couples seek marital counseling, Latino families often request mental health services when they have a problem with a child. When issues of marital harmony arise, it's possible to obtain more therapeutic leverage by utilizing the family's or children's well-being before discussing the values of a good marital relationship. For example, when a 10-year-old girl worries about her parents' fighting, a therapist might be tempted to direct the conversation toward the parents' marital relationship. But because this shift may impose a value about what matters in family life, it is better to keep the focus on the child by praising the parents for their joint concern about the child's well-being and for raising a caring child who worries about them. Indeed, Latino parents appear more challenged by shortcomings in the performance of their parental obligations than by failure to be a good partner to their spouse. In fact, parents may work more readily on their relationship if it is for the benefit of the children rather than for themselves.

A recent Mexican immigrant family came for therapy with Jacqueline, a depressed 15-year-old daughter, her 16-year-old sister, Luciana, and 9-year-old brother, Jorge. During the first session it became clear that the father, an outspoken man who worked double shifts as a janitor, was loving toward Luciana, the 16-year-old, and ignored Jacqueline.

The mother, in turn, was extremely close to her own domineering older sister. Both women worked at a tailor shop for 12 hours a day. Jacqueline had once been close to Jorge, but this had changed after she entered high school. She was feisty and negative toward her father.

The father, stimulated to reflect on the various family alliances by my use of circular questions about closeness and distance among family members, concluded that he had become very close to Luciana, the oldest daughter, because she was obedient and affectionate toward him, a "good girl" with a sunny disposition. He had dealt with his wife's distance and Jacqueline's anger and rebelliousness by either blocking them or ignoring them. Through our conversation, he figured that he and his wife needed to resolve their problems and get closer to each other. Then he wouldn't need Luciana to compensate for feeling lonely and contradicted, and he could pay equal attention to Jacqueline (even if she gave him a hard time). He concluded: "We need to change. This is making Jacqueline angry and sad. Children shouldn't suffer because of the parents' fault."

In this common scenario, parents discover that the quality of their marital relationship affects their interactions with their children. Remarkable changes can take place, for the sake of the children, in just one session of couple's therapy. In this case, the couple became closer after one meeting and agreed to attend therapy together.

## Other Gateways to Work with Couples

When marital satisfaction is minimal, common solutions include resignation, and searching for compensation in other family relationsips. Marital counseling may be sought only when problems are severe—infidelity that threatens a family breakup, chronic family-of-origin problems, or wife/mother-in-law tensions. Alcohol-related problems such as domesticviolence may also bring couples to therapy. Less dramatic difficulties, including the proverbial "communication problems" of middle-class Anglo-Americans, may be disregarded by many Latino couples, although more educated, middle-class, or acculturated couples might consider this worthy of treatment.

Latino couples may also seek counseling to address the individual struggles of a spouse. Many immigrant Latinas are referred to therapists with symptoms of depression. In the assessment they may complain that their husbands are distant and indifferent to their needs, or that they are taken for granted. It may be tempting for therapists to tie the wife's depression to subservience and the husband's lack of responsiveness to patriarchal entitlement, or at least to men's stereotypical, emotional bluntness. Whether accurate or not, this hypothesis sometimes causes the therapist to intervene quickly and encourage the wife to develop her own voice, become more assertive about her needs, and demand a more egalitarian treatment.

Encouraging the wife to be assertive without creating a supportive context for such changes creates therapeutic dilemmas. First, the therapist should be aware that cultural communication styles may be at play—the indirect approaches that serve to avoid conflict and preserve harmony are, in many settings, not problematic. Therapists should make a careful assessment with the couple when nonassertion or silence blocks conflict resolution and needs to be changed, or when it is simply a cultural style that needs to be respected. Second, the wife's newfound assertiveness may cause her husband to feel blamed and become even more entrenched in his position, which in turn precipitates escalations that can threaten the marriage. A therapeutic alliance that favors one partner over the other endangers the entire treatment.

It seems best for therapists to think in dyadic terms and include the husband in therapy whenever possible. Early conjoint sessions can be used to engage the husband in discussing his wife's depression and to elicit the specific meanings each partner gives to the depressive symptoms. Often the wife's loneliness and sadness are a by-product of migration—supportive networks, familiarity of language, and shared customs are sorely missed. And while both spouses feel disappointment about the social and economic opportunities they didn't find in the United States, traditional gender socialization tells us that the wife is more likely to express these feelings. One woman, whose husband had initiated their migration, insisted that he come home early every night to be with her: "He is asking me to live with half my heart here, the other half back there, where there are mountains of love wasting away . . . I know that he cannot fill my half-empty heart, but he is not even trying."

Recounting the story of their courtship back home often increases mutual understanding. The husband may become more appreciative of the wife's losses and her depression, and in turn may be more available in therapy and at home in ways that benefit both spouses. This new perspective helps the couple to see their marital bond as undergoing a "cultural transition" toward new ways of relating. Usually when the wife's feelings of loneliness are validated and her own strengths made explicit, her ways of asking for what she needs are more assertive and less defensive. In turn, the husband gradually learns how to hear his wife and to express his own loneliness and anxiety. Mutual empathy is enhanced by the participation of both partners in treatment.

## Joining: Accepting the Couple's Terms

Regardless of the initial reason couples come to therapy—depression in one of the spouses or behavior problems in a child, among others—acceptance and flexibility during the early stages of therapy pay off. Although Latino couples may come to talk about their marriage for one or two sessions and then cancel other appointments, usually the wife, but sometimes the husband, will come back or call me to report marital tension and ask for reassurance or advice. While trying to keep the *plática* (conversation) relatively brief, I am still likely to help brainstorm about relevant issues and ways to bring the spouse to therapy, walking through alternative scenarios. With the wife's permission I might call to invite the husband, appealing to his caring for his family and empathizing with the many practical and financial limitations on his time.

Sometimes I see each marital partner alone, taking care to balance the number of sessions to avoid the formation of alliances. I always ask if there is some issue of those discussed individually that I shouldn't bring up in the couple's session. This intermediary role in which I tell each partner how I understand their spouse's problem has proven valuable in opening up difficult topics of communication and changing fixed perspectives by creating alternative views.

Regular, prolonged contact with couples is unusual, but once they have deemed therapy helpful and my stance as sympathetic, I continue to be invited into a family's life, sometimes briefly and intensely, other times sporadically. A therapist may become like a comadre or compadre, rallying clients around a familial goal. Therapy can also provide access to additional resources that provide support and opportunity for ventilation. Same-gender networking, religion, and informal pastoral counseling are some options. Further, therapists should not be surprised if Latino couples have sought help before or during traditional psychotherapy from such folk approaches as going to curanderos, or espiristas, or engaging the services of a "black witch" (see Chapter 8).

## THE CLASH OF TWO MARITAL IDEOLOGIES

### Intergenerational and Nuclear Family Models

While similar motives join women and men in matrimony everywhere, many features of the marital bond are drastically different when husband and wife are part of an extended family network than when they live in a small, relatively isolated, nuclear group.

The conjugal relationship in a collectivistic setting puts a strong emphasis on continued inclusion of blood relatives in the couple's life. As mentioned earlier, the demands of the blood tie between parent and child prevail over the needs of the marital bond at all life cycle stages. The roles of husband and wife are valued in the Latino culture but they do not take precedence over intergenerational attachments. Marital units are largely based on procreation, the mandate of Roman Catholicism. Parental love, parental obligation, and sense of family should keep a marital relationship going for a lifetime, and it often does. These are the definitions of love in an intergenerational family. This state of affairs may contribute to marital dissatisfaction but seldom to divorce, because "marriage is for life." The individualistic, nuclear-oriented couple, on the other hand, favors greater exclusion, discontinuity, and firmer boundaries with relatives on both sides. This is a more fragile bond, regulated by romantic ideals that threaten the continuity of the marriage when dissatisfaction sets in.

The marital pair embedded in a collectivistic network is in a very different field of social interaction than the isolated, nuclear couple. In the extended network, both men and women relate intimately with members of the same sex. A dense social network usually means fewer demands placed on each spouse for self-disclosure, emotional support, and intimacy with the other. There are interesting ethnographic descriptions of lifelong closeness and loyalties among Latino men in their "*amigo* system" (circle of male friendships) (De Hoyos & De Hoyos, 1966). This involvement allows Latino men greater outlets for emotional expression, sometimes aided by a few drinks, than their Anglo-American counterparts. These friendships can also have negative consequences for marital satisfaction, perhaps because men spend a lot of time away from home and from family involvement.

In contrast, the dominant American cultural ethos of rugged individualism and corporate culture emphasizes a competitive struggle between men. This version of masculine socialization robs men of close male bonds, friendships, and support and creates an expectation that all needs should be satisfied in the marital relationship, an expectation that places unrealistic pressure on the couple's relationship that can't be met. While women, socialized for relationships, have close friends, many Anglo-American men have no one other than their wife or a lover.

When husband and wife are relatively isolated from same-sex family and friendship networks, a movement toward greater gender role flexibility and a new definition of intimacy emerges. Companionship, romance, communication, self-disclosure, and mutual support are paramount aspects of love for the couple in the nuclear family. Many young couples in Latin America are slowly undergoing an ideological shift from the traditional to this contemporary definition of marital love.

For immigrant Latinos, a shift toward a more companionate marriage is often part of the desired or necessary change, and one that may bring couples to therapy. Yet a traditional model of marriage may be upheld too. Both partners may yearn for the complementarity of separate husband-wife roles, separate friendships, or contacts with family of origin. Rather than assuming that the coexistence of marital models is impossible, therapists and couples need to stretch their creativity to support hybrid models.

In fact, to some extent all couples have to negotiate the coexistence of two types of bonds, the intergenerational and the marital. But the steps in the process and the shape of the resolution may be different depending on where the family is putting the relative emphasis. In Latino families, many conflicts arise from trying to blend couple and intergenerational ties, corresponding gender ideologies, and conflicts between parental and marital love. Therapists might mistakenly aim for an acculturative solution, encouraging separation and autonomy of the couple from the family of origin.

Most immigrants strive to preserve the intergenerational bond, primarily because of traditional respect and loyalty toward one's parents. It's true that economic conditions may necessitate proximity and reliance on extended family, but even when financial autonomy is possible, loyalty bonds are powerful.

## Mothers, Sons, and Daughters-in-Law

The intergenerational loyalty bond between mother and son can complicate marital relationships and the sharing of households (see Chapter 11, the Olivia González Lara case). The transition from this tie to the construction of a marital bond is generally encumbered by the custom of "patrilocal" residence, whereby the young couple initially goes to live with the husband's family. Many young Mexican wives yearn, above all, to have a family home of their own (Bronfman et al., 1995), but migration often complicates the picture because the conflicted young husband may "resolve" his guilt about leaving his mother by offering her his own child. This process was evident in the case of Víctor and Isabel, whom you met in Chapter 2. Let's revisit this family with a view toward intergenerational versus marital ties.

Víctor had convinced his wife, Isabel, to leave their child in Mexico with the paternal grandmother because, *"No hay un amor tan grande como el amor de madre"* ("There is no greater love than a mother's love"). The young father was not speaking about his wife, but about his own mother, how much the baby meant to her, and how she might *morir de pena* (die of sadness) if they took the child away.

Víctor had no empathy for Isabel's feelings, her sadness had not entered his mind. His guilt about leaving his mother and his loyalty to her had overpowered him. But why had Isabel agreed to leave her own baby behind? "Well," she said, "Víctor is always very persuasive." He promised her it would be "for a short time"—a year or two. Perhaps "persuasive" was a euphamism for dominant, but Isabel also knew that the baby would hamper her ability to work outside the home and supplement their unstable income.

Five years later the child was still in Mexico when Isabel and Víctor had another baby. Isabel was longing for the first child to rejoin the family, but Víctor could not face breaking his mother's heart to please his wife. The family's migration had "forced" an abrupt differentiation from family and a new focus on the marital relationship and nuclear group. Changes wrought by migration were requiring Víctor to be courageous enough to shift his family model and become more empathic and devoted toward his wife than his mother. At the very least he needed to acknowledge his own child's mother and her sense of where the child should live.


Very little is known about the relationship between mothers-in-law and daughters-in-law (or for that matter, husbands and their mothers-in-law). Perhaps this is another example of psychology's neglect for any relationship that does not fall within the nuclear family. In the 1950s a family sociologist, Evelyn Duvall (1954) conducted a national survey via a radio broadcast that asked listeners to name the most problematic person in the family. Of 5,020 responding postcards, more than half (51%) named the mother-in-law. More than 75% of the respondents were women married for less than 10 years and a very large number of these women were Jewish. It seems likely that relationships with mothers-in-law either improve over time or they become less intense and important.

In the Latino family, as in the Jewish family (Friedman, 1982), one possible explanation for the common conflict between these two women is the intense mother-son attachment. It presents a formidable challenge to the young woman who, upon entering a new extended family system, finds a very powerful mother-in-law while her own role is subordinate to and dependent on her husband. The young husband is no help because in the best of circumstances he tries to appease both women, but more often defends his mother or simply refuses to intervene. In therapy he needs to become a responsible participant in the solution, which often involves a cognitive examination of family models and a way to blend or select from each to have both relationships, with his mother and his wife, in his life (see case of Olivia González Lara in Chapter 7).

Most clinical descriptions focus only on the continued mother-son bond as the "cause" of the problem. From my own observations, the mother-in-law and daughter-in-law relationship is a complex one with a reciprocal aspect that involves family-of-origin transitional issues for the young wife too. If she has a good relationship with her own mother, she experiences a conflict of loyalties when she lives with her mother-in-law. If she gets too close to her mother-in-law, she may make her own mother jealous. On the other hand, if she has a poor relationship with her own mother, she may be hopeful that her mother-in-law will become the mother she never had, most likely an unrealistic dream. In trying to disentangle these complex triangles, it's helpful to explore the meaning of the relationships for each person and to find out about the wife's relationship with her own parents. Moving the mother-in-law toward her other children and her own husband may also yield good results.

## THE SHIFTING MEANINGS OF GENDER MYSTIQUES

### Machismo

No discussion about the dynamics of marital hierarchies could avoid reference to the popularly known masculine and feminine mystiques that drive Latino cultural belief systems. Social scientists persist in their fascination with *machismo,* or the cult of manliness, among Latin men. This has become a stable icon of popular culture around the world. According to the prototypical description of *machismo,* a man should be very strong physically, indomitable in character, and potently virile. The better man is the one who can drink the most, defend himself the best, dominate his wife (even through physical force or violence, if needed to regain his position over her), command the respect of his children, have more sexual relations, and engender more sons. It is also part of the configuration to be possessive and jealous toward the wife (Ellis, 1971; Madsen, 1964; Mirandé, 1988; Riding, 1989).

Although it's expected that men be chauvinistic or condescending of women in their conversations with other men, it is curiously considered unmanly if a man refuses the advances of any woman. Perhaps this has to do with opportunity for another conquest (a "notch on his belt"). At the same time, an important part of being a good "macho" is pleasing women and behaving as *un caballero* (a gentleman). Most of all, a man is to be very devoted to the women in his own biological family, his own mother above all others. Mexican movies of the 1950s have many examples of characters à la

Rudolph Valentino with hair slicked back, nostrils flaring, gliding across a floor, courting some damsel or another. Equally prevalent are films in which the lead male character works very hard and sacrifices his own happiness to support a widowed mother in raising her children or to rescue the honor of a "fallen" sister. A good example is the 1956 movie *Nosotros los Pobres* (*We the Poor Ones*) by the famous Mexican filmmaker Pedro Infante.

Most of the descriptions, often bordering on caricatures, portray a negative, pejorative image at which even "macho-type" men poke fun. Many Latino men are aware of growing criticism of their adherence to *machismo*, and younger men may voice it themselves, while remaining unaware of patriarchal remnants in their own beliefs and attitudes.

> Recently a client volunteered, "*Yo no soy* (I am not) *machista*. I do not drink, I do not cheat on her, I have never hit her." Yet his masculinity was being tested—the wife he had left more than a year ago had not taken him back when he wanted to return. She was asking for time to think about reconciliation. She had started seeing another man and was confused about her feelings for each. My client was aware he could not exactly be considered a *cornudo* (cuckold), a label he greatly feared, but his wife's involvement with another man was very demeaning to him publicly. He felt that all his friends, men and women, would think his wife was treating him *como su juguete* (like her toy), an affront to his masculine pride. In my opinion, this man is representative of many others who maintain some aspect of *machismo* but are very far removed from the popular caricature observed in the old films.

In my experience, more and more Latino men in therapy provide an opening in the conversation for a self-critical analysis of the cultural underpinnings of their reactions, like this client did. I have found that an appeal to their sense of fairness and justice (which could be conceived as part of their masculine mystique) helps them move beyond an automatic "wounded" reactivity more effectively than ideological discussions about egalitarianism that are not heartfelt and encourage intellectual rhetoric. A therapist can help clients examine the stereotypes of men and women and encourage differentiation from the conventional or peer pressures.

The signs of *machismo* may often be subtle and sporadic, or they may appear in the context of a relationship that otherwise was bending toward a partnership model, as I experienced in my own marriage.

> When I was 18 years old and dating my future husband, we had an interesting interchange that I will never forget. We met in a café after we had both taken exams at the university. He was a brilliant student whom I'd never dreamed of surpassing. That particular day, however, I had gotten the highest possible grade and was simply ecstatic over it. His grade was

lower than mine and his knee-jerk reaction was frankly shocking to me because he had always supported my studies, and because he greatly loved and admired his mother, who was a successful professional. In a very irritated voice he said, "Don't do this to me, don't you ever do this to me . . . I could not take it. . . . " When he realized how vulnerable and upset he sounded, he began to make light of it by adding, "I can tolerate your being prettier than me, your being softer than me, but being *smarter* than me?" After recurrent references to this event over the years he recognized his *machismo* socialization in his need to be the one with the superior intelligence. Yet this isn't the whole story. My husband's oldest brother had a genius IQ and was an extremely high achiever. My husband adored and admired his brother but silently suffered the pain of always feeling inferior to him. The remote possibility of suffering unfavorable comparison in his marriage must have frightened him.

The point is that gender roles indeed bear the mark of cultural socialization, but their manifestation (often as a protective mask) may be silently orchestrated or amplified by other dimensions, such as family-of-origin dynamics or social minority status.

When the endorsement of a masculine ideology is very strong or obsessive, physical and mental health can suffer, just as excessive adherence to the feminine stereotype hurts women. According to studies conducted with white Anglo-American men (Eisler & Skidmore, 1987), negative correlates of male gender role stress are restrictive emotionality, propensity to engage in high-risk behaviors like substance abuse, outbursts of violence toward self and others, promiscuous and unsafe sex, and somatic illnesses such as cardiac problems and irritable bowel syndrome. Excessive adherence to the *machismo* mystique probably places Latino men at a similar risk. At the same time, their strong networks in and outside the family provide outlets for emotional expression and may buffer some of the effects of stress.

Another common correlate of the mystique and the negative stereotype of *machismo* is the assumption that men are emotionally unavailable or blunted. I have not found this to be the case. Close behind the veneer of bravado, many men have deep feelings for their family and friends and are proud to demonstrate those feelings and good deeds. Although it may be safer to enter a therapeutic relationship with a Latino man without an emphasis on feelings and meanings, I find that after one or two sessions of joining and problem solving, it is very possible to encourage affective disclosure. Individual sessions combined with marital sessions are also helpful in promoting a trust and openness that transfer to conjoint meetings.

Given the predominant ideas about *machismo* and the Latino masculine mystique, it's not surprising that some therapists assume Latino men will have difficulty accepting a woman in the authority role of therapist.

This is a misconception. Until recently, female professionalism was more widespread in Latin America than in the United States, and, in general, Latino men who have had very limited access to educational opportunities value the knowledge and manners of an educated person, regardless of gender. An interesting bit of old rural Mexican mythology indicates that young women from small villages who go to work in the city are regarded, upon their return to the village, as a kind of *bruja* (witch) because of their assertiveness, manners, and aspirations. To be sure, to equate a therapist with a *bruja* would show ambivalence and a touch of humor, but it also indicates considerable admiration, respect, and even fear.

It is important for therapists to recognize that the *machismo* mystique has positive meanings too, and these are very relevant to therapeutic engagement and the process of change. *Machismo* requires men to be family oriented, brave, hard working, proud, and interested in the welfare and honor of their loved ones. Viewed through this lens, *machismo* can be a bridge rather than an obstacle to engagement in therapy (Ramírez, 1979). Negative stereotypes about Latino *machismo* emphasize a man's resistance to asking for help. This may cause a therapist to hesitate in insisting a husband engage in therapy, a step that could result in a self-fulfilling prophecy. Instead, therapists would do well to remember the positive stereotype: that *machismo* also involves a father's dedication to his children and his responsibility to their mother. Indeed, many Latino men actually come to therapy because the therapist has stressed the welfare of their families.

Recent schools of thought have promoted the concept that familism may take precedence over *machismo* (Gaines, Ríos, & Buriel, 1997; Mirandé, 1985). Some authors propose that the term *dignidad* (dignity) is more accurate in capturing the feelings of paternal pride than the concept of *machismo*, which reduces these feelings to a matter of male dominance (Marín & Marín, 1991; Paredes, 1993). New programs are emerging that capitalize on "deconstructing" those meanings embedded in the "cult of masculinity." For example, in the Los Angeles area, some new self-help discussion groups for Latino men are formed around the concept of *el hombre noble* (the noble man).

Alternative helping formats (workshops, seminars, or psychoeducational classes) are particularly well received by Latino men, perhaps because they can maintain pride in their participation without experiencing the one-down position that may occur in couples therapy, regardless of the therapist's gender. These formats decrease the sense of shame at revealing problems and pain, and may give a man a sense of being part of a community of equals rather than feeling singled out as "a patient." Programs that increase paternal competence are often readily accepted (Casas, Wagenheim, Banchero, & Mendoz-Romero, 1995; Powell, 1995b). This was demonstrated in the case of Víctor Díaz Ortiz, who became much less resistant to therapy when he took the initiative to gather a group of Latino fathers to talk about problems involved in the use of corporal punishment for child discipline.

While the *machismo* mystique clearly plays a role in how Latino men respond in relationships—including therapeutic encounters—little has been written about its contemporary, multiple meanings. Despite this, a recent ethnographic study of working-class men in Mexico City (Gutmann, 1996) is elucidating for therapists. Covering questions ranging from parenting, diapers, and dishes to sex, alcohol, adultery, and violence, Gutmann beautifully describes "emergent cultural practices" that explode stereotypes, underline creative contradictions, and embrace ambiguity as a pathway for change. Therapy with Latino men can be the venue for these same explorations and processes to take place.

## Marianismo and Hembrismo

The dual images of the Latina woman are equally complex for marital therapists. As in many myths, man-woman configurations are constructed as opposites in themselves (having a negative and a positive side) and as opposites to each other.

The feminine Latino mystique is partially embodied in the ideal of *marianismo* (or the cult of Maria, Virgin Mary, or the Madonna). Women are dichotomized into two categories: the "good ones" and the "bad ones." A good woman (the Madonna) is made in the image of the sacred mother. She is submissive, self-sacrificing, religious, humble, and modest. Like the Virgin Mary, she can be sexual only in a virginal way, without much knowledge or enjoyment. Unlike men who are encouraged to gain sexual experience by leaving a trail of broken hearts and lost innocences, sex for the good woman becomes one more of the wifely duties she must endure and not refuse. Bad women (the whores), on the other hand, are seductive, sexual, and manipulative; they cannot be trusted. They use men for their own benefit, and can likewise be used. Many mothers, representing the good women, warn their sons about the bad women they should fear (A. R. Del Castillo, 1996).

Fidelity is mandatory for a wife, but infidelity can be ignored or forgiven in a husband. Her love isn't really romantic, but rather biological and maternal. In fact, his love needs are thought to be ruled by biology too—the need for seduction and sex. But his real love is probably, like hers, familial and parental, in the sense of obligation and pride in being a good father and son.

The complexity of the *marianista* mystique is compounded by another gender construction that sometimes causes conjectures about Latino culture being "covertly" matriarchal (Benavides, 1992). This is subsumed under the term *hembrismo* (femaleness), which refers to a quality of strength, endurance, courage, perseverance, and bravery. Because these qualities are associated with "macho-type" traits, *hembrismo* is a descriptor not unlike "women with balls" or "superwoman"—those females who can do it all and show determination to face and overcome every hardship. While these qualities are definite resources for many Latinas, *hembrismo* sometimes can contribute to rigidity (Zavala-Martínez, 1988) or to considerable stress for women. This is particularly so for Latinas who maintain *marianista* behavior at home and *hembrista* behavior at work (Comas-Díaz, 1995).

Research by Amaro, Russo, and Johnson (1987) found that Puerto Rican professional women experience very high self-imposed demands to balance public behavior at work with a shift to a more traditional role at home. Adherence to the *marianista* side does not help women's health. In a study of 278 Puerto Rican women in the United States, Soto and Shaver (1982) found that women who embraced traditional gender roles were submissive, self-sacrificing, and less assertive, which was associated with poorer physical and mental health.[1] This is also found in every study of Anglo-American women.

Yet *marianismo* has many positive aspects too. A woman's self-esteem is tied to her ability to be a giving, generous mother. She is respected and revered by family and community. She obtains the respect and protection of her children, particularly her sons, but often her husband too. Although younger women are taught to be submissive, as they get older, docility is no longer a prerequisite for a woman's merit. Further, the strong traditions of *familismo, personalismo, respeto, simpatía,* and communication styles that stress harmony and avoid conflict rely to some extent on *marianista* behavior.

During the past two decades more complex cultural definitions of what it is to be a woman are emerging both in Latino countries of origin and in this country. The meaning of *marianismo* and *hembrismo* are expanding, with doubts and conflicts as to what parts to maintain and which to change. This comprises a dilemma for many Latinas, and for the therapists who work with them.

A recent book, *The María Paradox* (Gil & Vásquez, 1996), provides conceptual and practical tools to aid in this endeavor. The authors' aim is to help other Latina women integrate their cherished cultural traditions and yet identify with contemporary cultural definitions that respect individual needs and desires. Rather than espousing cultural resistance to the traditional definitions, the authors encourage self-empowerment through incorporation of the positive aspects of Latina womanhood with the emerging new definitions. Although these authors insist on using a theory of acculturation/adaptation, I believe their approach dovetails well with a theory of "alternating" cultural behaviors according to social context, and finding one's own creative compromises to deal with the inevitable contradictions of transition and culture change.

## Gender Expectations and Patriarchy: Consequences for Couples

*Marianismo* and *machismo* embody the same gender ideologies and patriarchal ethos that greatly curtail the development of sexuality in women and deny access to expressions of vulnerability in men almost everywhere. In spite of evolutions away from this model, in one measure or another these cultural conceptions about womanhood and manhood tend to be present in the public discourse of almost all Latino couples, and are often reflected in literature and art. A 1986 Cuban movie by the internationally acclaimed director Tomás Gutiérrez Alea illustrates the complexities and ambiguities of the "double standard" in a climate of women's liberation in Cuba. The movie is titled *Hasta Cierto Punto . . . (Only Up to a Certain Point)*—the implicit end to the phrase is "equality between men and women." The main male character is fond of singing a verse from a Basque song that says (my translation from Spanish): "If I wanted to do it, I could go ahead and clip her wings and then she would be mine only. But . . . then she could not fly, and what I love most is the soaring bird in her." The message of this song illustrates one popular solution to the gender dilemma: Latino men, like men in many cultures, hold on to the ideal of male supremacy by believing that they are "letting" women become freer, rather than acknowledging that women are accessing this right themselves, often against men's resistance.

These fixed and limited images of masculinity and femininity are oppressive, not only because they limit individuality for both men and women, but also because they may be used as tools for oppression, manipulation, and impediments to change by each spouse against the other. It's as though people become hostage to stereotypes, submitting and shaping themselves to cultural "ideals" that mutually reinforce gender expectations. The woman fears and condemns the man's abuses of power, yet she may be secretly scornful of him if he is weak and vulnerable rather than strong and virile. The man may really not be attracted to the woman's modesty and submissiveness but suppresses her when she becomes more assertive or sexual.

For all the mythology about Latino romanticism, it can sometimes hide a rather cold-blooded contract which both spouses enforce, perhaps for security, if not for love's sake. In cases where cultural prescriptions are used as relationship weapons, "cultural resistance" becomes part of the therapy to help each person move beyond telling the other *una mujer debe* (a woman must) or *un hombre debe* (a man must) conform to the culture's gender definitions. Rather, each spouse is helped to accept the other's possibilities, limitations, or personal choices. Other times, returning to and heeding the culture may coincide with therapeutic goals, as when a husband has abandoned his responsibilities to his wife and children.

Despite changing circumstances and an awareness of the greater complexity behind their gender-made masks, men and women often continue to use cultural prescriptions as homeostatic devices (Jackson, 1965) to "correct" relationship imbalances and personal idiosyncrasies. In Chapter 7 I discussed how these mechanisms are utilized when women's work introduces a different balance of power.

In addition to their use as "corrective" mechanisms, traditional gender stereotypes support patriarchal arrangements and, in turn, a focus in relationships on power and weakness, dominance and submission. The cyclical or interdependent nature of these processes can be seen in the psychoanalytic interpretations of *machismo*. Here the dual images men hold about women are seen as related to a man's underlying doubts about his own adequacy and masculinity (Aramoni, 1972; Gilmore & Gilmore, 1979). A man is first in awe of his mother, his sisters, and the Virgin Mary and later tries to impress other men with his prowess, an inflated drama that hides his own sense of weakness and dependency.[2] This analysis assumes that *machismo* veils an underlying hostility toward women. The language of dominance and submission seems to perpetuate this view.

Indeed, language is a mirror that reflects underlying dynamics and meanings, including those related to gender. Consider some of the curious expressions Latino men use to describe their interactions with the women in their lives—one common expression is, *"le tengo que dar cuentas a ella,"* which means something like "I am accountable to her," but it also implies that she "makes him" give an account of his activities. Or in the words of a man referring to his lover, *"me tengo que reportar porque ella me lo pide,"* meaning "I have to, I am obligated to report to her because she asks me to."

It's as though a man displays the public power of a patriarch but perceives mother and wife (once she is established as a mother herself) as having tremendous influence over him and the family. It's not always clear if the veiled irritation about having to "report" to her is an attempt to keep her in her place or if he genuinely feels dominated by women, or both.

A woman is seen by a man as the enforcer of tradition, morality, and religious values, as well as the one responsible for running the household and raising the children. The husband may see her as "holding all the cards," as able to instill obligation through guilt or shame, and to define him as a "good boy" or "bad boy," as his mother did. In their circle of friends, women seem to partake of this private, demeaning evaluation of men (Benería & Roldán, 1987). They may say that men are not to be trusted, that they are like children. They concur with Gabriel García Márquez's (1995) image: "Woman creates order where men have introduced chaos." He says of Ursula Iguarán, the mother in his fascinating novel *One Hundred Years of Solitude:* "She, like all women, holds the entire order of the species with an iron grip, while men wander around the world wrapped up in the infinite follies that push history along."[3]

## The Constraints of Gender Typing: A Case Study

*Machismo* and *marianismo* create belief systems about men and women that perpetuate endless cycles of mutual reactivity and mutual control. The myths are perpetuated as dualisms of weakness versus strength, of sexuality versus purity, of romantic love versus parental love, and so on. It is in this context of mutual gender constraints that the proverbial infidelity of men, and the existence of a second, secretly maintained household and family (*la casa chica*), makes its disturbing appearance. This phenomenon is a significant occurrence in all social classes, though economically less feasible among the poor and working class.

The Ortega Blaines, an upper-middle-class couple in their early 40s, were married for 16 years and had five children. They came to marital therapy at the insistence of Gabriela, the wife, who was very depressed. They lived in close proximity to their families of origin, all of whom were involved in a large, successful corporate business. Gabriela had six siblings, her husband had ten. Martín Ortega was ambitious but his business had not been consistently successful. Gabriela came from a very wealthy family and had a trust fund in her own name. She had money and her own work satisfaction in a public benefactor's foundation. She could have left Martín when she discovered that he was having an affair with a young cabaret dancer. So why did she stay?

When they came to therapy, Gabriela had known of Martín's affair for 2 years. After she confronted him with the evidence, Martín maintained that he had broken off that relationship months ago. Yet Gabriela kept discovering proof of his continued contact with the other woman. Gabriela fluctuated between being furious at the deception and dejected at the loss. The initial marital sessions were full of recriminations on both sides; each one asserting that the other had the power to save or destroy the marriage. Martín thought the wife should stop searching for incriminating evidence. He said, *"El que busca encuentra"* (the person who searches for things finds them). Gabriela naturally claimed that what was destructive wasn't the searching, but the finding.

I interviewed them separately, as I often do when an affair is involved. Martín assured me that the telephone calls his wife had discovered were the tail end of the affair. The other woman had seduced him, pursued him, he could not say no, it would have been "unmanly." (It's curious that in these affairs men give the destructive power to the evil woman, denying their own power and responsibility.) Perhaps he had fallen in love, but that had passed. Now he only called her because she left messages asking him to "report" to her. I asked how long it would take him to finish completely, so he could give Gabriela reassurance with total honesty. He refused the private sessions I offered to help with his confusion. At the next conjoint session, Martín made a deal with his wife—she would stop the search and the recriminations, and in 1 month he would initiate a conversation about what had happened.

For a while the marital relationship improved significantly. But 2 months passed and Martín hadn't approached Gabriela as he had promised. Now she was even more furious. What game was he playing? What was he hiding? She renewed her search and found what she feared the most. Martín had a baby with the other woman. He continued to communicate with her, although it was unclear how much he actually visited his *casa chica*.

At first it looked as though his lies were a form of paternalistic deception. He thought Gabriela "could not take it if he told her the truth." Of course these benevolent motives were mixed with less altruistic ones. Shame, fear of confrontation and possible loss, desire to remain a free agent, wanting to retain control over the situation, in short, self-protection was also operative. No doubt Martín feared Gabriela's rage, but he put it in terms of being disciplined, scolded. He felt controlled by the two women.

Martín claimed that he had told the other woman that he would always stay with his wife and children. He would never marry her. Perhaps he told her this. Perhaps not. We may see here the workings of a "familial self," faithfully devoted to the idea of a "we," a family commitment. Yet this familial self is paired with the existence of an intensely "private self" to which no other has access—wife, lover, or therapist. Of course, Martín's lying gave rise to endless misunderstandings. Gabriela saw Martín's continuous lying as a confirmation that he didn't care to redeem himself and truly come back to her. Martín thought that confessing the truth would condemn him to eternal mistrust and the loss of any opportunity for future acceptance by Gabriela.

Lying leaves very little room for a collaborative relationship with the therapist. When I suspect lies, I clearly voice my concern that the marital relationship will be based on shaky ground if the husband (or wife) feels they can continue a deception. The drama of affairs that become second families is so compelling that it envelops the therapist. I suffer for the woman. I often suffer for the man too, and appreciate his impossible predicament. For all the mystique about the Latin lover, this seems like a poor state of the art of loving, choked by the constraints of Latino gender ideals. I am very careful, however, not to offer oversimplified gender stereotypes about power, with the wife as the oppressed and the husband's *machismo* as the oppressor.

Indeed, Maturana (1991) argues for a rupture in patriarchal conversations about power and control as the way out of patriarchy. In the prologue of the Spanish edition to Riane Eisler's feminist book *The Chalice and the Blade* (1991), Maturana encourages a legitimization of conversations about collaboration, conviviality, help, agreement, sharing, and security as a true counterpart to the language of domination, authority, and power, which are the only ones valued in patriarchal societies. He urges the genuine development of a counter culture based on the "biology of love" rather than confronting the patriarchal framework using the same combative words. Using the language of gender stereotypes and power in therapy may, in fact, lead to runaway polarizations and increase the chances of marital breakup. A different construction, which I label "love in the time of cultural transition," approaches Maturana's ideal and helps me discuss the same configuration of marital patterns under a more benign, less explosive frame.

## LOVE IN THE TIME OF CULTURAL TRANSITION: A THERAPEUTIC DISCOURSE

Cultural gender myths don't stand in isolation. They are part of a web of myths that are supported by, and in turn support, social and family structures. *Machismo* seems to go hand in hand with *marianismo*, and both gender myths favor parental, intergenerational love over marital love. Emergent ideals of mutuality, monogamy, communication, and self-disclosure are contributing to new conceptions about love and intimacy for the Latino couple. These new definitions coexist with traditional ones in ways that support but also contradict the definitions of masculinity and femininity of the collectivistic family.

Increasingly there are attempts in therapy to redress gender imbalances. In their book Metaframeworks, Breunlin, Schwartz, and MacKune-Karrer (1992) present a schema of five positions—traditional, gender aware, polarized, in transition, and balanced—that are helpful in introducing gender-sensitive issues in conversations with Latinos. The authors discuss treatment of a traditional Mexican couple in gender transition after they had been in this country for 8 years. Their example illustrates how therapists can work respectfully and not impose stereotypes of how Mexican, rural, traditional, lower-class families "should" behave or by imposing stereotypes about the ideal middle-class American couple.

Therapeutic conversations that involve gender imbalances may be met by the husband (and sometimes the wife) with great fear of marital breakup or family dissolution. Therapists must be cautious as to when, why, and how to introduce conversations about the connection between presenting problems and gender inequities. It is safer to work on the constraints inherent in these imbalances once the family is well established in the new country and culture. Because some families may have initiated a greater awareness of gender issues back home, it's useful to start by exploring their own perceptions of their stage of evolution toward greater gender balance. Again, it is important to assume a respectful position that allows the Latino couple to make their own choices and blends, rather than promoting either traditional or egalitarian views about gender role balance.

Borrowing from the title of García Márquez's book *Love in the Time of Cholera* (1988), in my therapy with Latino couples I often talk about "love in the time of cultural transition," and stress a discourse of gender and love (which includes fairness and justice) rather than one of gender and power. I do so fully cognizant that complex hierarchical dynamics organize multiple aspects of Latino marriages. But talking about different concepts of love in marriage as part of a process of cultural transition provides me a safer avenue to frame marital problems and to encourage a fair balance of influence between wife and husband. As I discussed in Chapter 5, utilizing the idea of cultural transition can provide a successful way to build bridges between family members, including husband and wife.

This approach poses less danger to the therapeutic alliance with Latinos and maximizes continuance in therapy. More poetic, more enduring, and less politically flavored, the discussion of gender and love is more culturally consonant for both husband and wife than a discussion about gender and power. During therapy I usually express my opinion that many Latino couples are in a process of "cultural transition" and therefore are caught in an internal clash between two different models of love in marriage (Falicov, 1992, 1995a). Each couple needs to figure out how they construct and understand the meaning of love, and find their own creative compromises and hybrid or alternating models.

Conversations about the meaning of love with Latino couples can be fascinating and touch on myriad relationships and meanings—parental love, filial love, fraternal love, romantic love, erotic love. In these stimulating conversations about difficult definitions, the men appear initially more confused than the women, but both are equally engaged. Explorations here can include questions about how their love began, how each person was seen during the courtship and early marriage, how love changed when they became parents, how job/earner status and wife's employment affected the marriage, whether there were early conversations about fidelity, and what degree of veracity was tolerable and required by each spouse. Conversations about love and sex in the context of gender expectations are always enlightening.

> Gabriela Ortega Blaines had always felt inhibited to express the intense sexual love she felt for Martín. She had been raised to feel *pudor*—to be modest and embarrassed about her own sexuality. As many Latinas of her generation, she remembered how sexually inexperienced she was, and how she feared Martín would think of her as a whore if she showed her erotic passion. Later she was too angry and too resentful to "reward" him by showing her passionate "weakness" for him. What kind of love did her sexual inhibitions allow?
>
> Martín remembered how, very early in their relationship, he had felt very close to Gabriela and let his guard down by confessing to her

that he feared that sometime before meeting her he had impregnated a young woman he had not intended to marry. He closed off again because Gabriela accused and chastised him for many years after this confession. What kind of love did he expect to get with his confession? Maternal tolerance and assistance? Or had he wished for a friendship in marriage where honesty about the past is a prelude to continuous honesty? Was he bragging like "macho" men do with their male friends?

I asked many provocative questions to explore Martín and Gabriela's own meanings about love in the context of cultural gender expectations. A nonjudgmental climate of respectful curiosity allowed me to ask "risky" questions about difficult subjects that are often taboo for Latinos, such as the danger of sexually transmitted diseases or the concealment of financial support to the *casa chica*.[4]

In the end, Martín ended the extramarital relationship and fulfilled his obligation toward the mother and her baby through mother and child support that was automatically deducted from his bank account. Gabriela's depression subsided, but only after an extended period of being able to express her anger, and after continued reassurances and reparations (encouraged by me) from Martín—he was to call daily to "report" his activities, spend more time in family activities, and disclose all financial support to the second "household." Their sexual relationship became very passionate and at follow-up 2 years ago, their family relations were stable with the five children doing well.

It is not outside of the realm of possibilities that Gabriela and "the other woman" will some day meet and establish some pragmatic relationship, if the child needs or desires to meet his biological father. Future-forward questions on my part led to that agreement between Gabriela and Martín to help alleviate the anticipated anxiety about this kind of eventuality.

No master intervention exists for problems of transition that are so complex and encompassing of cultural and personal values. Rather, therapy sessions seem more like philosophical discussions, posing questions that may help dislodge cultural meanings that are crystallized, and revealing personal and relational definitions of gender and love instead. Such conversations pave the way for needed disclosures, reparations, and anticipations of future events.

Using a language of love rather than one of power shifts the focus to emotions. It increases proximity and empathy and decreases the distance that's associated with authoritarianism and egocentric power. Talking about love increases support and collaboration and decreases the polarization, combat, and competition implicit in conversations about who is right and who has more rights, or who is up or down in the hierarchy. Fairness and justice are more readily achieved through collaboration and empathy than through power and control.

Simply put, the implications of *machista* and *marianista* gender discourses in couples therapy cannot be underestimated. Latino men and women will undoubtedly hold, within their personal meaning systems, set opinions and deep feelings about gender, whether these are addressed in an overt manner in therapy or remain a more covert, often limiting, influence on their relationships.

For therapists, an awareness that these gender mythologies exist facilitates conversations when clients directly or indirectly refer to gender. The therapist needs to be curious about each client's personal understanding of what it means to be a man or woman. It is better to avoid any formulaic approaches because the inherent favoring of one aspect of the cultural mystique over another is both ecological and idiosyncratic. Selections of meanings depend on personal history, family of origin, present circumstances, and personal ideals.

It's also important for therapists to be aware that *machista* and *marianista* discourses have positive and negative interpretations and applications. The positive aspects of each can often be used in the service of change. At the same time, research shows that men and women who rigidly adhere to traditional gender role "specifications" are negatively affected in their social, mental, and physical well-being. Further, gender stereotypes can seriously limit or obscure qualities that don't "fit" with traditional meanings about men and women—for example, *marianismo* might downplay Latina women's economic and decision-making contributions to their families, while *machismo* obscures from view men's tenderness and capacity for fathering.

Another critical point is that couple dynamics cannot be summarily reduced to either traditional or modern gender ideologies. The reality is that Latino couples have always included husbands and wives who may be domineering (Peñalosa, 1968), husbands and wives who may be submissive and dependent on their spouses for major decisions, or husbands and wives who follow a more egalitarian power structure (Hawkes & Taylor, 1975; R. G. Del Castillo, 1996). Increasingly Latino family life is characterized by an even wider range of structures and processes, from patriarchal to egalitarian, with many combinations in between (Kutsche, 1983; Vega, 1990; Ybarra, 1982). Abundant contradictions are also part of a picture that combines traditional and egalitarian aspects. For example, younger working women in the midst of cultural transition might want to divorce an unfaithful husband (something their mothers and grandmothers couldn't do), but wouldn't think of letting their husbands walk into the street without ironing their shirts or shining their shoes.

In therapeutic settings, Latino couples can reflect on these issues and move toward greater balance in their relationships. Therapists can facilitate this process by exploring both negative and positive sides of Latino gender mystiques and introducing conversations that use a framework of love rather than power to discuss gender roles and expectations. Along the way Latino couples can weave their own blends of old definitions and new conceptualizations of love into a special marital identity that is uniquely their own.

Clearly the beliefs and expectations couples have about their roles in a relationship are not static. The dilemmas and strengths of a couple early in marriage and later in life vary, as do relationships and individual experiences in other domains. In Part V, Chapters 11 and 12 enrich our understanding of life in a Latino family by examining a range of life cycle processes that clinicians are likely to encounter in their work and therapeutic approaches to them.

## NOTES

1. A number of studies associate greater mental health for women with masculine (instrumental) qualities, but poorer physical health (e.g., heart disease) with these same qualities. Unmitigated agency, at the extreme, is particularly pernicious.
2. For an entertaining and enlightening view of the *piropo*, an encapsulated representation of the psychoanalytic aspects of *machismo* and its dual images of women see Suárez-Orozco and Dundes's work (1984). The *piropo* is a verbal comment spoken by Latino men in the street about a woman, which directly or indirectly addresses her attractiveness.
3. My translation from *El Olor de la Guayaba (The Scent of the Guava)* by Gabriel García Márquez in conversation with Plinio Apuleyo Mendoza, Editorial, *La Oveja Negra*, Bogotá, Colombia, 1982. In his novel *Love in the Time of Cholera*, García Márquez compares unattainable romantic love with domestic love.
4. Perhaps because of the shrouds of secrecy about the *casa chica* (small house) very little has been written about it, and even less about its impact on the children of both households. Sooner or later the murmurs and tears of mothers confirm what children have suspected was behind their father's absences. The deep wounds and questioning inflicted upon children and adolescents by this realization is poignantly re-created by the Puerto Rican writer Esmeralda Santiago in the chapter titled "Why Women Remain Jamona" (*jamona* is Puerto Rican slang for spinster) of her autobiography *When I Was Puerto Rican* (1993). Therapists would do well to inquire about the emotional impact of these clandestine, long-term relationships on children and can often use this information as leverage for change.

---

# PART V

# The Latino Family
# Life Cycle

---

Given the very nature of Latino life to revolve closely around family, it comes as little surprise that family therapy is a comfortable form for many Latinos—it makes sense, particularly when emotional and other problems are regularly attributed to family conflicts and family transitions. As we try to grapple with the transitional problems of many Latino clients, an understanding of cultural aspects of life cycle stages is an intergral part of accurate appraisals of requests for therapeutic help.

Indeed, the life cycle stages of Latino families cannot be viewed in isolation from beliefs and values about *familismo, personalismo,* parental authority, and intergenerational connections, among others. In Chapters 11 and 12 I offer general descriptions of the socially expected markers, dimensions, and processes (Falicov, 1988a; 1998) of the life cycle as they are influenced by Mexican, Puerto Rican, and Cuban perspectives. The descriptions provide a broad picture of transmitted traditions, age and gender expectations, and value orientations, and are intended as guidelines to aid clinicians' work with Latino clients.[1] They enable therapists to simultaneously be aware of similarities and differences, and gradually uncover the private, idiosyncratic world of each family.

Life scripts and narrative constructions of life cycle events depend on cultural visions of what constitutes optimal human development. For example, the "leaving home" transition may have different meanings for American and Latino adolescents and thus may present distinctly different challenges for their families. Therapists who understand cultural constructions can facilitate conversations with Latino clients about the meaning of life cycle events more adeptly. Clients can be helped to identify and resolve conflicts they experience when faced with American meanings for the same life passages. In this way transitions, rituals, and developmental tasks become more intelligible, and the potential for reading pathological meanings into what is merely different is reduced.

Comparing Latino life cycles with those defined by Anglo-American social science is a critical part of this reflection. Comparisons can help therapists see the limitations of applying mainstream theories outside the realm of the middle-class, Caucasian, nuclear family upon which they are based. Most of these normative theories refer to discrete, sequential life stages with an expected timing of events and developmental tasks that rarely fit a more complex and variable reality (Falicov, 1984; Gergen, 1982). Myriad possibilities for the timing and sequence of stages become even more sharply delineated with culture and migration as the backdrop. By comparing the range and variety of differences between Latino and Anglo-American ideas about life cycle, therapists open the way for culturally consonant conversation and reflection.

Latino families share many similarities and some differences in terms of the timing, tasks, transition rituals, themes, coping mechanisms, and meanings attached to different stages of the family life cycle. Similarities include the tendency for young adults to remain with the family of origin until marriage, the connection of a woman's honor to marriage and procreation, and the tendency for the elderly to remain functionally involved with the younger generations (Falicov & Karrer, 1980). Life cycle differences among Latinos can be traced to each country's and subgroup's geographical, historical, economical, political, racial, and religious influences. Other differences can be attributed to variations in the migration experience and the present ecological context for each group in the United States.

Inherent in Latino life cycle stages is the endurance of traditional rituals, which have important consequences for mental health and acquire particular poignancy for immigrants. Rituals within the family and those connected to societal institutions will be described fully here because they carry considerable therapeutic value both as spontaneous and as therapy-induced events (Bennett, Wollin, & McCavity, 1988; Imber-Black & Roberts, 1992; Schwartzman, 1983).

Life cycle stages and transitions clearly intersect with other domains that are addressed by the MECA model. Family size modifies developmental stages and processes. Small families experience stress during launching, but accept the need for separation. Large families emphasize togetherness, tend to induce parentification of older children, and rely on sibling solidarity. The meaning of life cycle transitions seems to be intimately connected with family organization. Public or "prescriptive" views of the Latino life cycle are consonant with extended, three-generation families or with large nuclear families. But the values of smaller nuclear families are making greater inroads among Latinos. Whether families adopt a traditional Latino structure or organize along modern Anglo-American lines (or some blend of both), each arrangement has inherent strengths and vulnerabilites that appear at different points in the family life cycle.

Migration also influences a family's experiences in life cycle changes. When living in its country of origin, the family approaches such transitions against an institutional backdrop that defines similar developmental expectations and an "ecological fit" is in place (Falicov, 1988a). Conversely, when a family moves to another country, such meanings may differ from those of the dominant culture. Migration disrupts the family's ecology and requires new adaptations: first, to preserve continuity of cultural identity, and second, to develop new patterns that insure survival in a different ecological situation. For racial and ethnic minorities, these survival skills require preparation for dealing with Anglo-American cultural values and with discrimination and bigotry (Harrison, Wilson, Pine, Chan, & Buriel, 1990; Padilla, 1994). Normal developmental stresses are thus intensified by migration and cultural dissonance.

At each developmental stage, then, the family reorganizes in response to the combined effects of developmental events, the inherent pressures of migration, and the need to change or maintain family structure and organization. In Chapters 11 and 12 I examine the predominate and unique processes of the Latino family life cycle, while keeping in mind these other domains.

# 11

## Childhood and Adolescence

Child psychology is itself a peculiar cultural invention that moves
with the tidal sweeps of the larger culture in ways that we understand
at best dimly and often ignore.

*interesting*

—KESSEN (1979, p. 815)

### THE FAMILY WITH YOUNG CHILDREN:
### PROPER DEMEANOR OR SELF-MAXIMIZATION?

### A Grand Welcome

When a Latino child arrives into an intergenerational and extended setting, the interpersonal effects are more far reaching than when a new baby
comes into an isolated nuclear family—more people, and more relationships, are altered by this momentous event. The *bautismo* (baptism) that initiates the infant into membership in the Roman Catholic Church is an especially important ritual. It crowns the acceptance of the new family and
serves as an extended family reunion, even if the marriage had been accepted reluctantly by the elders. The infant is sponsored by godparents or
*padrinos*, who are selected from among the social network of relatives,
friends, and prestigious acquaintances of the family for their capacity to
supplement economic and other parental functions in case of need. Indeed, a new baby captures the essence of *familismo*—preceding generations
of kith and kin turn their attention to this newest member who, from the
outset, is immersed in the many hopes, dreams, values, and ideas of his
generous, extended family.

## Infant Attachment and Developmental Ethnotheories

The quality of infant attachment to a primary caretaker is the most widely studied, initial step in child development interactional research (Ainsworth, Blehar, Waters, & Walls, 1978). Although secure attachment appears to be valued across cultures, the constructions or "ethnotheories" of the mother-infant bond are not culture-free. Research on mother-infant interaction suggests that Latino mothers may be more indulgent and show more affectionate and talkative behavior (Escovar & Lazarus, 1982; Fracasso, Busch-Rossnagel, & Fisher, 1994) than African American mothers, who respond in a more restrictive, discipline-oriented, and less stimulating way. This is consistent with the African American mother's fear of "spoiling the child" and her expectation that earlier autonomy might help children cope better in a hostile world (Field, Widmeyer, Adler, & de Cubos, 1990).

An illuminating study comparing middle- and low-income Anglo-American and Puerto Rican mothers focused on the qualities mothers associate with an infant's sense of security and optimal growth (Harwood, Miller, & Irizarry, 1995). Each group's construction of these qualities promoted very different socialization goals based on different "cultural meaning systems." Anglo-American mothers stressed "self-maximization," or the capacity to express and assert oneself in order to get one's own needs met. Mothers acknowledged that tensions would arise between a youngster's striving for self-maximization and emotions that contradict this striving. The goal—to achieve a balance between autonomy and relatedness—would require some mastery over anger and frustration, selfishness and egocentrism.

Puerto Rican mothers, on the other hand, had a much more "sociocentric" set of developmental goals for their infants and toddlers. They focused on their child's ability to engage in appropriate intimate and nonintimate relatedness, what the authors called "proper demeanor." This involved the mother's belief that a child should be *bien educado* (well taught, well brought up), obedient, and respectful. Proper demeanor includes an internal capacity to feel *vergüenza* (shame), or to be always conscious of the possibility of being embarrassed or losing face in an interpersonal situation. A shameless person (*un sinvergüenza*) not only brings shame on themselves but on their parents who failed to bring them up as honorable and worthy of trust. Honor is summarized in the description *una persona de provecho*, an ethical quality that connotes a person of moral goodness and one who readily fulfills obligations to family, friends, neighbors, or coworkers.

Like Anglo-American mothers, Puerto Rican mothers were concerned about their child's ability to control his emotions, an ingredient of proper demeanor. But for Puerto Rican mothers, emotional control was seen as enhancing or limiting the regard of others in the community. Being affectionate and sweet (*cariñoso*) is a quality of warmth that, together with *respetuoso* (respect for others), will gain you the acceptance and admiration of the community.

   *Confianza* (trust) or the capacity to maintain confidences certainly requires control of aggression, greed, or egotism. Puerto Rican mothers did not worry that limiting these behaviors might hinder individual expression or self-maximization. They believed such limits ultimately help one develop both casual and intimate relational qualities—qualities that insure the acceptance and love of the community, the highest individual fulfillment a Latino can expect.

   While Anglo-Americans focus on the constructs of self-esteem and insecurity, Puerto Ricans emphasize respeto and shame. Similar situations may be interpreted and evaluated differently, depending on whether one's conceptual and phenomenological focus is on personal inadequacy or public loss of face. Thus social interactions themselves are mediated by the cultural constructs we use to understand both self and other. For example, a toddler's active play may be interpreted as exploration and curiosity. Or it could be interpreted negatively as the infant being *intranquilo* (restless), according to a cultural construct that places greatest value on proper demeanor and dignity in social relations. These symbolic meaning systems serve to transmit much of what we call "culture," just as children abstract the rules of their native language from relevant contexts and then begin to use those rules to generate novel sentences. In this way children learn the social norms of the cultural groups to which they belong and then reconstruct, sometimes in novel ways, those norms in their own interactions. This process entails both continuity and change (Harwood, Miller, & Irizarry, 1995).

   Latino parents may experience internal or institutional conflict regarding what constitutes "correct" child development and parenting. One way to navigate this cultural transition and bridge the differences is to initiate or get involved in a group with others who are in transition, for example, parenting groups that deal with disciplining children or discuss which ethical qualities to inculcate. Mothers who can "hold" both cultural child-rearing descriptions will ultimately help their children alternate and blend their own behaviors according to cultural contexts. In a study by Gutiérrez and Sameroff (1993), Mexican American, bilingual/bicultural mothers were better able than monocultural mothers to interpret their children's behavior as a complex interaction between temperament and environment, and to see that developmental outcomes have multiple determinants. This ability actually enhanced their parenting role.

## Child-Rearing Attitudes and Techniques

As in most families around the world, the first years of a Latino child's life are typified by a nurturing, tolerant relationship with parents and extended family. The baby is especially close to the mother and other women in the family. Since the world is a given, not an object for change or mastery, as it is for those raised with the Protestant work ethic, Latino parents across socioeconomic groups adopt a relaxed attitude toward the achievement of developmental milestones or of skills for self-reliance. They appear less pressured than Anglo-American parents to correct minor deviances from the "norms" described in professional parenting books. Weaning from breast to bottle, for example, takes place at about the same time in both Latino and Anglo-American families, but Latino children are allowed to drink from a bottle or use a pacifier for a long time before being encouraged to drink only from a cup. Occasionally a child becomes so attached (for as long as 3 or 4 years) to the bottle or the pacifier that drastic weaning methods are used, such as putting some bitter substance on the bottle's nipple.

Variations in weaning and toilet training are dependent on family customs rather than prescribed social norms. As long as they are achieved within a "reasonable" length of time, there is no pride or shame attached to them. Yet many therapists have internalized developmental expectations that coincide with Anglo-American parent's worries about bed-wetting, clinging, whining, and wishes to sleep in parents's bed past the second year. They may be less sympathetic of a Latino parent's "indulgent" attitudes toward similar behavior. There is no reason, however, to be alarmed by or label as "infantilized" a Latino 3-year-old sucking a pacifier, or a 4-year-old sitting in his mother's lap, or a young child whose mother cuts up and feeds him his meat. At these early stages, a "good" Latina mother socially constructs her role as gratifying the child's needs rather than stimulating autonomy.

I have sometimes observed abrupt shifts between indulgence and restriction, and the latter may include mild physical punishment. I have also speculated whether a relaxed and accepting attitude may result in a "soft boundary" between parents (particularly mothers) and young children that ultimately requires the parents to seize drastic control. Many 5- and 6-year-old Latino children appear confident and exploratory physically and verbally. They may be reluctant to wear a seat belt, to stop watching TV, to get up in time for school, or cease from interrupting adult conversations. These children don't seem concerned when parents reprimand them, even though mother or father may resort to smacking or other forms of corporal punishment. Many Latino parents consider this pattern of softness and hardness to be normal. When asked about corporal punishment for misbehavior, many parents respond: "This is how children are. We have to spank them because we love them—to teach them right from wrong when they are still little. By age 11 or 12 years they behave themselves, and there is no need to spank them anymore." When patterns of indulgence and harsh discipline become entangled with other life cycle events, escalating, problematic processes may be set in motion.

Ernestina Garza Martínez illustrates this dialectic of intense nurturance and intense discipline. Ernestina, 31, was born in Chihuahua, Mexico. She moved to San Diego, California, with her parents and her three siblings when she was a teenager. When she was 22 years old, she married Alberto Garza, a successful, professional man from Guadalajara with whom she had two children, Kevin and Michael. When Ernestina came to therapy, she had been divorced for 5 years, and her sons were 7 and 8 years old. Child protective services had sent her to counseling after suspicions of child abuse were raised by the youngsters' school. Both children were absent from school one Monday, and when questioned by school authorities, their answers were vague. The counselor concluded that Ernestina hit the children on their buttocks about once a month with a wide belt from which she had removed the buckle, that she yelled at them frequently, and on two occasions she made them get out of the car while she pretended to "abandon" them because they were "bad" (usually she went around the block and came back). In addition, the child care worker thought the mother might be very disturbed because a home investigation disclosed that Ernestina and her two boys slept in the same bedroom. Usually they took turns, one child sleeping with mother on her full size bed, and the other on the floor in a sleeping bag, even though the boys had a perfectly nice bedroom. Most alarming was the fact that Ernestina often put diapers on the boys before going to bed, more frequently on Michael, the youngest.

When I was called to the therapeutic team, I interviewed this family, including Alberto Garza (who was a good father and provider) and the maternal grandmother, in all combinations of conjoint and individual sessions. I was surprised to see how free and comfortable, alert, sassy, and articulately bilingual the children were as they told me in great detail everything good and problematic about the family. They spoke freely in front of all the adults, and were comfortable sitting very close to their mother. Nowhere was the fearfulness one expects from strictly disciplined or abused children. Ernestina confessed, amid giggling and with a twinkle in her eye, that she didn't want her children to grow up very fast and that her own mother had been very nurturant and attached to her children, wanting them to remain little forever. Her father, on the other hand, had been the disciplinarian and often used a similar belt to the one she herself now used. Ernestina considered this polarization of parental roles "totally normal" and felt that as a single mother, she was obliged to be a "sweet angel" like her mother and also wear the "male gorilla suit" to discipline her boys when needed.

She fed the boys home-cooked, healthy Mexican food that took a long time to prepare, and had them always beautifully dressed and groomed. She herself was always impeccably dressed, with high heels, coiffure, and elaborate make-up all in place by 6:30 A.M., when she had to take the kids to school and go off to her full-time job. Her social life was very child oriented—she took the boys to movies, video arcades, and restaurants, and she never left them with babysitters.

She also felt that the physical punishment was necessary up to age 10 or 11 so that the boys would "learn right from wrong." She continued to dress the boys in diapers at night because they sometimes refused to go to the bathroom before bed. They both slept soundly and Ernestina wanted to avoid waking up in a wet bed. But this mother seemed to have an unfulfilled need for closeness herself. An important piece of information emerged—a few months after the birth of her second child, Ernestina underwent open heart surgery for heart valve replacement, an operation designed to correct a heart condition caused in early adolescence by rheumatic fever. Soon after, Alberto, who had promised eternal love and whom Ernestina and her parents "worshiped," fell in love with another woman and asked Ernestina for a divorce. Ernestina's heart surgery had been successful and her health was very good now, but her operation, the divorce, and her rivalry with her ex-husband's girlfriend intensified her mother-son attachment, as well as her motivation to be a superwoman and a supermom.

Family therapy focused on helping Ernestina decrease the perfectionistic demands on herself, learn to request and accept offers for help from her mother and ex-husband, and become better able to set limits on the children's demands. This meant learning to blend and modulate sweetness and closeness with distance and firmness less abruptly, in part by responding to the children's misbehavior earlier. She also had great interest in reading and taking parenting classes and cooperated with having a child educator from Child Protective Services come to her house for a few sessions.

Finally, individual sessions focused on Ernestina's adult needs and the knowledge that her attachment to her boys was not just cultural. Not only did Ernestina expand her cultural vocabulary about men, she also expanded her vocabulary about motherhood. She realized that there was no danger that Alberto's girlfriend would replace her in her own children's heart. Kevin and Michael would always be hers, even if she indulged them less and allowed them to spend more time away from her.

## Shaming

Latino parents challenge their children to behave better by using the same range of child-rearing techniques used by most Anglo-American parents. Perhaps what varies is the degree, and a preference for some types of discipline over others. Active shaming, which includes teasing and mocking, humiliation, threats, ridicule, and punishment, including corporal punishment, appear to be more widespread and accepted than in Anglo-American families, even when social class differences are considered. Children are made to feel small, stupid, or clumsy when their parents use labels that signify essential character flaws rather than target specific, situational behaviors.

In a Mexico City supermarket I once heard, to my dismay, a parent scold a little boy as she yanked him away from the cookies he had touched, "*Payaso* (clown), how many times do I have to tell you not to touch? If you continue to be such a clown, I'll never take you out again." Right after, I was caught in a traffic jam and watched as another driver furiously got out of his Mercedes Benz and strode up to the driver of a stalled truck. "You *payaso!*" he yelled, "What are you waiting for? Are you scratching your testicles, or what? Can't you see the line behind you, idiot?"

Even in the upper and middle classes, shaming may be considered an appropriate way to control others, particularly those of lower status. Feelings of embarrassment, excessive conformity, numbness, envy, the tendency to cover up rather than acknowledge an error or wrongdoing, and outright lying are all negative outcomes engendered by shaming. Despite this, shame may have some important adaptive functions. Nichols (1991) offers a contextual view in which shame has a useful controlling influence on behavior, a sort of domesticating effect, within tightly knit groups. As Nichols aptly points out: "Shame does double duty, reflecting the dualism of human nature. . . . Shame preserves the integrity of the individual—shielding the self against exposure—and enforces allegiances to the norms of the group"(p. 51).

## Discontinuities in Parent-Child Attachments

Let's return for a minute to the relationship between parents and children during the early years. The baby or young child enjoys a close relationship with mother and a special position in the family until either a new child is born or until he or she enters nursery school or kindergarten. These external markers define the child's passage to a new stage much more powerfully than signs of "internal readiness." Parents may expect more or demand more based on these markers than on the interior realities of the child. Thus children may experience abrupt discontinuities at the time of a transition. If there is a problematic aspect to the Latino family's relaxed attitude toward child rearing, it may be in trusting that adaptation will prevail when concrete preparation for developmental challenges is needed.

Fortunately, extended family often provides compensation for the inevitable discontinuities or losses during normative transitions. For example, even if parents haven't prepared a child for the arrival of a new sibling, their older youngster receives more attention from grandparents, uncles, and aunts. This helps free the mother to care for a new baby, but it also provides comfort to the one who might feel displaced.

During migration (and without the benefit of extended family) children often acquire new roles and changes in status by default. Sibling rivalries may grow, and when not resolved, give rise to developmental impasses. Some of these impasses are in turn aggravated by the fragmentation of the nuclear family. The following example illustrates several problematic intersections between parent-child attachment and migration.

The family consisted of 30-year-old Mr. Peralta, 25-year-old Mrs. Peralta, their 5-year-old son, Rodolfo, and their 5-month-old daughter, Marcia. Rodolfo was referred to the clinic by the kindergarten teacher because of frequent crying, fearfulness, and school absenteeism—a picture that suggested an evolving school phobia. Mr. Peralta had been living in the United States for 7 years, while his wife and son had remained in Mexico surrounded by family and friends. Because commuting between Chicago and Mexico was very tiresome and expensive, Mr. Peralta often urged his wife to come live with him in the United States. A year before they came to the clinic, Mrs. Peralta reluctantly agreed to join her husband in America.

Although he worked long hours and was underpaid, Mr. Peralta had a stable job. On weekends he spent time with his male *amigos* (friends) having a drink or two. With his wife and child now nearby, Mr. Peralta's happiness was complete. He could not understand why his wife was depressed. He felt the house and the children should keep her happy and occupied. He had no insight into her sense of loss and feelings of isolation and confusion. When Rodolfo entered school, the vacuum and loneliness in Mrs. Peralta's life grew. She responded anxiously to Rodolfo's somatic complaints, and kept him from going to school on cold days. Mr. Peralta, who valued education, had no tolerance for what he called Rodolfo's absenteeism and *flojera* (shaming word for weakness), a very negative trait for a Mexican boy.

Marcia was the first baby both parents were raising together. Mrs. Peralta was afraid of bringing up an infant on her own, without her family's help, and this propelled her to overprotect Marcia. Meanwhile, Rodolfo was sorely missing his doting relatives in Mexico and was disconcerted by the birth of Marcia, who was taking so much of his mother's time and attention away from him.

The recent immigration, the birth of a new child, and the kindergarten entry had all contributed to Rodolfo's and Mrs. Peralta's unhappiness. Had they remained in Mexico, the family would have had many available adult figures to offset an early sibling rivalry and provide Mrs. Peralta with additional support.

I felt a great deal of empathy for Mrs. Peralta's loneliness and isolation. I thought it was crucial to help her establish a supportive network. A school community representative was contacted, and she encouraged

Mrs. Peralta to attend a women's social group where she could learn to speak English and discuss the many adaptational issues of migration. The women brought young children with them and frequently compared notes about their development.

Mr. Peralta, however, voiced objections. He did not think it necessary for his wife to leave the house twice a week just to "talk with a bunch of women." I felt torn about convincing Mr. Peralta that his wife needed support feared that I might be robbing Mrs. Peralta of her own voice. She needed to develop her own capacity to make herself heard. I chose to work primarily with Mrs. Peralta, but to include Mr. Peralta in the sessions. We reviewed details of her physical, social, and cultural uprooting in her husband's presence so he could hear about her losses and she could tell him what she needed to better adapt to her new life.

Focusing on their strengths and resources, I expressed to the Peraltas my genuine admiration for their parenting abilities and their desire to improve the family's economics and education. As part of this positive appraisal, I encouraged Mrs. Peralta to reward Rodolfo for growing up, which included his attending school. This supported Mr. Peralta's conceptions of preparing Rodolfo for a successful life. It also increased his empathy toward his wife's loss of a supportive network, and he agreed that he would have to supplement this support in some measure.

The issue of Rodolfo's attachment to his mother, separation from his relatives, and rivalry toward his new sister were dealt with through a storytelling technique with photos, another way of developing the catching-up life narrative described earlier. Mrs. Peralta and Rodolfo were encouraged to spend some time after school (when Marcia was napping) looking at baby photographs of Rodolfo. The snapshots were organized chronologically, beginning with Rodolfo's birth in Mexico and moving through the migration to America. The emphasis of this task was on showing Rodolfo his own growth.

Mr. Peralta agreed to regularly take pictures of the children that would show their continuous growth. He occasionally participated in the storytelling too. This increased his nurturing involvement and his collaboration with Mrs. Peralta, but it had a much larger, unplanned, positive effect. By virtue of their separation during Rodolfo's first years, Mr. Peralta had missed many events and opportunities for bonding with his son and wife. The catching-up life narrative served not only to address developmental needs, but bridged the individual and family relations that were fragmented by migration.

Rodolfo's reluctance to attend school disappeared in 2 weeks. He was happy with the idea that his "mother was also going to school" to learn English. The teacher reported no crying or fearfulness once attendance became regular. Mrs. Peralta found her meetings with the women in the group very supportive and she established some friendships. Mr. Peralta was particularly happy since his wife stopped looking depressed and was more supportive of his plans for the children's education. At the end of 6 months, Rodolfo felt proud to be Marcia's big brother. The parents were proud of Rodolfo's school attendance and of Marcia's growth.

The photo storytelling technique, similar to the catching-up narrative, is especially helpful in working with immigrant children who suffer separations from significant others, such as a parent or grandparent. It is nonthreatening, heals relationships between parents and children and between spouses, and helps maintain a continuity of identity in the face of multiple uprootings of meaning. Photos, home movies, or even drawings depict evolving stages, continuity, and change, and create a warm, comfortable tone in the therapy.

In developmental terms, the transition to school is made smoother by a narrative re-creation of family bonds and by a shared understanding of the migration experience. This also paves the way for a family's increasing contact with the dominant culture. As a child enters school, he helps open the family's boundaries to the unfamiliar society's cultural constructions and treatment of minorities.

## THE FAMILY WITH SCHOOL-AGE CHILDREN: BRAVE IN A NEW WORLD

For Latinos, school entrance brings a fundamental transformation of the family's ecology, with implications for its internal and external functioning. For families of Mexican and Cuban descent, school may be the first direct, sustained, and structured contact with American institutions. Puerto Ricans, given their greater exposure to U.S.-style institutions, may have more experience with how the school system functions. The transition from home to school is a difficult one for families the world over, but more so for families whose parents have no formal education. For immigrants, this transition requires flexibility at a time when parents and children may still be weakened by the uprooting, as we saw in Rodolfo Peralta's case.

### School Entrance

Children of Latino descent enter primary school at the same age as Anglo-American children, but they may differ significantly in their social and emotional readiness to enter the autonomous stage expected by the American school system. Immigrant children are further handicapped by differences in language and communication styles and skills. These limitations create learning barriers that are often associated with behavior problems (Aronowitz, 1984).

School entrance may also be the child's first excursion outside her ethnic enclave and the first time she encounters prejudice and racial discrimination in full force. These are difficult issues for young children to verbalize and play therapy may provide a useful avenue.

Martínez and Váldez (1992) offer a model of play therapy with Latino children that actively introduces cultural and contextual elements and reinforces a positive sense of cultural identity. The model also elicits issues related to the child's stressful minority status, such as prejudice and shame or anger reactions to discrimination. A structured approach might involve setting up a play situation between a brown and a white doll. The therapist initiates an "as if" scenario in which the brown doll is ostracized by his or her peers because of skin color. Empowering coping strategies that emerge during the play therapy's "pretend" situations are reinforced by the therapist.

Immigrant parents may also be anxious about releasing their school-age child into the unknown American school system. They have no familiarity with the educational system and how to negotiate it. Teachers are strangers, and their expectations about acceptable behavior and forms of discipline are unknown. In a natural reaction to these fears, parents may tend to hold onto their children protectively.

For stay-at-home mothers, reluctance to separate may be aggravated by loneliness and isolation. As long as they have young children at home, their role is clear and their activities continue in a fashion reminiscent of their native town. They may be reluctant to relinquish their first or their youngest child, who symbolizes the first child they give to a foreign system or the last child they could raise without interference from a new culture. Including the parents in structured or unstructured play therapy that deals with the emotional issues associated with school can have positive expressive and psychoeducational benefits for everyone in the family.

While some cultural differences in child rearing may account for Latino children appearing infantilized or overprotected, migration may intensify a parent's overinvolvement with children. As has been shown, parents may leave some of their children in their country of origin for practical or financial reasons, or out of loyalty toward their families. It is common for parents to send for the child to come to the United States precisely around the time of school entry. When Latino children are raised by several loving (and competing) "mothers" before school age, they enter a much harsher reality when reunion with the nuclear family coincides with entering school in the United States. The mother may quickly begin a campaign of overcompensation for lost years of affection, as in the Díaz Ortiz family—a common pattern in clinical cases. She may compete with images of her mother or mother-in-law as she strives to be acknowledged as the real mother and thus "babies" her child more than she otherwise would. She may also suffer from her own separation anxiety, and feel reluctant to be away from the child for even a few hours a day so soon after the reunion. The father may adopt a "tough-it-out" attitude that reflects his own denial of the fears and losses precipitated by migration. The child, meanwhile, is struggling with his own separations and losses, all of which could be elucidated through sensitive, careful inquiry and contextually attuned play therapy interventions.

## Preteenagers

As school-age children get older, girls and boys, particularly those in poor families, often assume responsibilities for errands, babysitting, cooking, or other forms of help to their mother. In some working-class, and in most middle- and upper-class families, the presence of live-in domestic help drastically reduces children's chores relative to their Anglo-American counterparts. Greater individual responsibility for handling an allowance or small jobs outside the family, such as a newspaper route, are not customary among Latino families, regardless of social class. This may reflect different boundaries between the family and extrafamilial environment than for Anglo-Americans, and a relative lack of preparation for the work world.

A family therapist raised and trained with Anglo-American values may see greater age differentiation and autonomy for preteens as a therapeutic goal. He might suggest to Latino parents that their 11- or 12-year-old youngsters receive an allowance for work at home or small jobs outside, or suggest that preteens need increased contacts with peers. The Latino family may regard these notions as coming from people with *otra mentalidad* (a different mentality), who want to socialize the child into American ways. It is usually better to find out how children are handling increased responsibilities or privileges within the home or according to the family's own definitions of independence, within a Latino context of obedience and good manners.

Immigrant parents may also want to define a firm boundary between home and the extrafamilial world, including their preteens' peer groups. Perceiving many dangers in the urban neighborhood, they may restrict their children's activities to indoors. Children may see few playmates after school hours because parents promote siblings and cousins as companions, even when the children are far apart in age. Maslow and Díaz-Guerrero (1960) believed that Mexican children live far more in the family and less in the peer group than their American counterparts. While this observation may still have some validity for some working- and middle-class families, many poor Latino preteens are exposed to the social influences of the street, from drugs to gangs—a by-product of the mounting poverty of Latinos in this country over the past decade.

As in previous stages, Mexican American and Cuban families may "extend" some aspects of childhood beyond the early pubescent years. For girls particularly, there is no clear demarcation between childhood and puberty. In spite of definite biological markers, a 12-year-old girl may be considered a child even after menarche. When developing girls raised in very traditional or rural Mexican families move to large American cities where more liberal behaviors prevail, they often experience extreme tension and withdrawal, unable to disagree with their parents on any issue. In one case, epilepsy-like symptoms accompanied first menses. In two others, the girls started pulling out their own hair and eyebrows following menarche. All were described by their families and others as extremely "good" girls. The degree of immigrant parents' control over preteen girls may continue to be problematic well into adolescence.

School difficulties are just as apparent among preteen children as those who are just entering the system. Many Latino immigrant and second-generation children struggle with a combined lack of knowledge of the language and the school system. They also face discrimination due to race and minority status. Interventions at the school level may be necessary. Some culturally attuned techniques such as *cuento* (story) therapy may be more appropriate with this age group (see Chapter 7).

Successfully completing elementary school is a matter of great pride for Mexican American families, and is often accompanied by a celebration that includes extended family. As a ritual celebration, *la graduación* (graduation) can be used to facilitate and mark family change during the transition to adolescence. Because underachievement, school failure, and early dropout are statistically very high among Latinos, graduation from high school is cause for even greater pride and joy.

Other important transitions during this time are embedded in religion and spirituality (see Chapter 8). Parents and children become very involved in preparation for a preteen's *la primera comunión*, the Roman Catholic First Holy Communion. Attending parochial schools provides a supportive structure for these preparations, though sometimes tinged with condescending overtones toward poor families by well-meaning teachers and priests. In his short story "First Communion," the Puerto Rican writer Edward Rivera (1982) provides a moving account of the pride poor parents feel in financing this event, and the subtle yet scarring humiliations caused when this pride is underestimated by others.

## ADOLESCENCE: BETWEEN TWO WORLDS

Anxiety, depression, and confusion are considered part and parcel of adolescence in the Western world. For immigrant families, this scenario is compounded by experiences of cultural alienation, discrimination, and poverty.

A Latino teenager's experience of growing up in the United States has been described as *entremundos* (between two worlds) (Zavala-Martínez, 1994), an uneasy coexistence between two cultural orientations, two languages, two sets of values, and two philosophies of life. The development of a coherent ethnic identity—knowing and valuing who one is socially and ethnically—is critical to effective coping and a healthy outlook on life during adolescence) (Bernal, Saenz, & Knight, 1995; Hurtado & Gurin, 1995; Phinney, 1990; Phinney, Lockner, & Murphy, 1990). But Latino teenagers face immense struggles as part of an ethnically and socially discriminated minority. Their marginalized status can affect self-esteem, institutionalized racism often engenders helplessness, and society's low expectations of them become internalized. The collisions between two social realities may explode in out-of-control behaviors such as gang and drug involvement or delinquency and depression. Yet sometimes these struggles bubble as a source of young creative energy demonstrated in "border art" or collective associations of poets such as "the Taco Shop poets" in California or "the Nuyorican poets" in New York.

Amado M. Padilla (1994) describes the positive and negative tensions of socialization and "bicultural development" as well as the complexities of shifting ethnic identifications and labels:

> I have frequently interacted with adolescents working through the crisis of whether they are Mexican, Mexican-American, American, Chicano, Latino, or Hispanic. Too many labels for anyone. Yet each of these labels has a specific usage and it is not uncommon for an adolescent to use several of these labels depending on the situational context. Ethnic identifications create serious concerns for adolescents who often want to construct their own identities free of the ethnic and racial biases imposed on them by their parents, teachers, and other authority figures. (p. 27)

## Parent-Adolescent Interaction: The Clash of Cultures

During adolescence the dominant culture is no longer safely outside the family, as one could pretend it was when the children were small. It has entered the family's inner sanctum and, like an overbearing guest, clamors for attention. Differing views of connectedness and separation, collectivism and individualism, and different conceptions of age and gender hierarchies cannot be ignored any longer. The difficulties in resolving these dilemmas often bring families to therapy.

While the axiom "be good to your parents" is probably universal, cultural meanings about transgressions and consequences vary widely. For Latinos, if adolescents "answer back" verbally or deviate from obligations to their parents or society, it is not necessarily considered their parents' fault—it may be their "bad luck" in having an ungrateful son or daughter. For Anglo-Americans, having children who deviate from society's norms is an indictment of their own ability to raise good and healthy citizens. Whereas the Latino adolescent is often the guilty one, shamed by his parents for breaking rules or not maintaining "proper demeanor," the American adolescent can more often blame his parents for being either too strict or too permissive. And while Anglo-American parents accept that young people need autonomy to define themselves ("self-maximization") and thus may rebel against authority, Latino parents expect *respeto* and obedience throughout life. An adult client told me that she could never conceive of opposing her parents because all parents were like saints, in the sense of being closest to a life-giving force.

The clash of values between immigrant parents and their teenagers is manifested in many areas: attitudes toward sexuality, gender definitions, interpretations of hierarchies, standards for curfew, alcohol use, and dating. In addition, much has been written about the parentified mediator role of children who speak the new language and understand the new society better than their parents. Teenagers are essentially forced to identify with their parents' experience in order to represent them in the larger, dominant culture. Yet adolescents also wish to reject, or at least not identify with, their parents' generation, culture, and immigrant status. The depression experienced by parents as a result of this cultural clash and loss of authority has been documented with Cuban mothers in Miami (Szapoznick & Kurtines, 1980).

The culture clash between Latino teenagers and their parents may also stem from divergent cultural meanings about adolescence. Inclán and Herrón (1989) suggest that in the older, agricultural economy of many Latin American countries, a family's economic survival depends on the children staying and expanding the productivity of the previous generation. The apprenticeship model of passage into adulthood thus fosters family cohesion and devalues individuality. According to these authors, Puerto Rican parents on the mainland operate within this apprenticeship framework and so consider children to always be children, regardless of their age or responsibilities. Contrary to this view, teenagers of immigrant parents often expect an "adolescence" of the Anglo-American variety. Demands for greater freedom come at the worst possible time for the parents, whose ignorance of the language and culture limit their ability to supervise and guide. The resulting struggles between repressive, "old-fashioned" parents and acting out "liberated" youth are ubiquitous in mental health clinics—the family is indeed between realities, divided by two cultures and languages within.

While Latino adolescents are granted less individual freedom than their Anglo-American peers, they also manage greater responsibilities toward parents and younger siblings. Although this a natural occurrence in large families, migration often complicates the situation. Parents who might otherwise work out a gradual separation from their teens find the task especially difficult because of their long-standing dependency on the older child to act as translator of language and culture. The younger children may also cling to the older sibling, who appears less old-fashioned and more understanding than the parents. The older child may find herself in the confusing but influential position of parent to her parents and parent to her siblings. As mentioned elsewhere in this text, this position can pave the way for independence, or it may result in an instrumental and emotional entrapment.

## Peer Group Identification

Like adolescents everywhere, Latino youngsters want to participate less in their nuclear and extended family network and more in their own peer group. Latino parents don't easily approve and may "tighten the reins." Some adolescents passively rebel against this, others openly assert themselves, but many come to accept the parents' position. First-generation Puerto Rican parents (Inclán & Herrón, 1989) and Cuban parents (Bernal & Gutiérrez, 1988) often see their acculturated children as being less caring of them, showing less proper demeanor, and exhibiting more selfishness in their wish for autonomy.

In situations of rapid culture change, where a veritable "experiential chasm" between one generation and the next exists, the peer group often assumes a crucial and controversial socializing role. The Chicano poet Luis Rodriguez poignantly describes how the lure of gangs for Latino teens intersects with the life challenges of parents. Rodriguez, who broke free from gang life, wrote *Always Running; La Vida Loca: Gang Days in L.A.* (1993) when his own 12-year-old son joined a gang several years later. Economic marginality, family fragmentation, and adolescent identity confusion converge to make street gangs increasingly attractive to Latino youth as a surrogate *familia* and a source of ethnic pride (Vigil, 1988).

## Sexual Practices

Sexuality is a fundamental issue of adolescence. But in Latino families, conversations about sexuality (if any) are almost always indirect and focused on restrictions. This is true even of mother-daughter talks, in which more intimate conversation might be possible. *Pudor* (a shyness and modesty surrounding sexual issues), the strength of Roman Catholicism, and the practice of confession greatly influence the equating of sexuality with sin and the restriction of sex to reproductive purposes. Likewise, homosexuality often meets with cultural prohibitions. I know of two middle-class Mexican families who sent their gay adolescent sons to live in the United States to escape intense stigmatization. Homosexuality and lesbianism are repressed, hidden, and shunned among first-generation immigrants, while second and third generations are likely more open about sexual orientation.[2]

Tied up with issues of adolescent sexuality is the prospect and practice of dating, a topic that frequently comes up in family therapy. Casual dating without marriage as a goal has become more common for both sexes after age 15 or 16. Many parents expect experimental dating for girls to begin around age 16 and for boys somewhat later. Boys are supposed to take the direct initiative among Mexicans, but young Puerto Rican and Cuban women appear to be much more forward and flexible about approaching young men than they used to be. It is better for therapists to be respectfully curious rather make assumptions about family members' views on the appropriate time or age for dating.

In the past 10 to 15 years, premarital sex has become more common among Puerto Ricans, Cubans, and Mexicans across different socioeconomic levels, although some stigma remains. Mexican immigrants have been slowest in catching up with this trend, perhaps due to their adherence to Catholicism, or because parents fear they can't monitor their teenager's sexual life without the extended family networks of home. Occasionally adolescents learn during trips to Mexico that their parents in Los Angeles are stricter than their uncles in Zacatecas and thus they chose to spend summers in their parents' native and supposedly traditional setting.

## Teenage Pregnancy

Latino adolescents tend not to use contraceptives when they do engage in sex and are less inclined to have an abortion once pregnant. Young Mexicans, for example, may be less likely than others to be sexually active before marriage, but they are more likely to give birth (Solis, 1995). As with other groups, early out-of-wedlock childbearing is related to poverty, few educational possibilities, unemployment, and bleak surroundings. Although the proportion of births without marriage has been increasing, Mexican and Cuban adolescents are more likely than Puerto Ricans and other very poor groups to use pregnancy as a step toward marriage and independent living. These youngsters are more commonly involved in long-term relationships with partners who accept the pregnancy and endeavor to support baby and family. The cultural value of a young man's "honor" and pride in the virility of conception may act as motivating forces to legitimize fatherhood (Horowitz, 1983).

A recent *New York Times* article (Mydans, 1995) contained an interviewed with Angel F., a violent, "tough," 18-year-old gang member who was sweet and devoted to his newborn baby boy. He also respected his girlfriend, unconditionally worshiped his mother, and occasionaly relied on her for protection on the streets. Angel told the reporter that he planned to get out of the gang eventually to take care of his "new *familia.*" This strong cultural obligation can be used therapeutically as a path for family decision making, as the following case illustrates.

A 33-year-old single mother from Oklahoma, newly moved to California, came to consult about her willful and rebellious 16-year-old daughter. The teenager had been disobeying curfews, was truant from school, and had become sexually active. The mother was extremely worried because the girl had already had one abortion and was pregnant again. The mother didn't want to bail her out of her predicament again and was leaning toward making the daughter raise the baby with her help, repeating in some ways her own life story. I asked many questions about the girl's boyfriend. He was a 17-year-old boy, the son of Mexican immigrants, who lived with his parents but spent many nights in my client's home sleeping with his girlfriend. I told my client that perhaps the culture was in her favor—she could help her daughter save her honor and teach the young couple responsibility by visiting the boyfriend's parents, telling them about the pregnancy, and asking for their help in "doing the right thing." I am happy to report that the young couple got married, the young father is working, and the baby is gorgeous.

The strength of the adolescent girl's immigrant family usually prevails. Parents may initially be furious about the pregnancy, but they eventually look forward to the birth and may even afford special status to the young mother (Becerra & de Anda, 1984; de Anda, Becerra, & Fielder, 1988; Felice et al., 1987; Kay, 1980), perhaps because parenthood is a somewhat collective, highly valued aspect of the culture. Luisa, a Mexican American mother of two, divorced her Anglo-American husband at 28 and was furious that her parents were more condemning of her decision to divorce than of her 16-year-old sister's out-of-wedlock pregnancy.

Despite this acceptance, prevention is crucial in addressing the alarming increase in Latina teen pregnancies around the country. In San Diego, the Barrio Logan Health Center has supported a program called *Hablando Claro: Con cariño y respeto* (Plain Talk: With affection and respect). It aims at empowering a community of "askable adults" by providing sex education classes to small groups of Latino parents. A bilingual community health educator meets with five or six parents in the casual setting of someone's living room and offers information on topics ranging from learning about sexual anatomy and contraceptives to talking with your child about sexuality. The latter is a particularly difficult undertaking for most Latino parents, given their limited formal sex education and taboos surrounding a topic they never discussed with their own parents or relatives. The program includes similar meetings with gender-segregated teen groups. Therapists who become familar with such psychoeducational programs in their areas can provide a valuable resource to their clients.

## THERAPY RESOURCES FOR ADOLESCENCE

Therapists can help Latino families navigate adolescence by finding culturally consonant ways for parents to see and accept their teenager's growth while maintaining parent-child bonds. This final section explores such therapeutic interventions as the flexible use of cultural rituals and traditions, psychoeducation, and the role of the therapist as family intermediary, all in the service of connecting immigrant parents and their adolescents.

## Rituals

A ritual that accompanies a girl's entrance into the romantic, premarital arena is the *quinceañera*. At her 15th birthday, parents and relatives host this elaborate party, which includes a religious ceremony, a dinner, and a dance for 100 to 200 people. Protocol demands formal dress for the girl, her escort, and 14 other couples. The tradition tends to be preserved among Mexican Americans (Horowitz, 1983), and has become an extravagant, lavish affair for traditional Cubans in Miami (Bernal & Gutiérrez, 1988). Therapists may observe that as an initiation rite, the *quinceañera* is similar to the American tradition of the debutante ball or "sweet 16" party, but its celebration is common among all Latino social class levels.

The *quinceañera* marks the transition from girl to young woman. The 15-year-old's virginal reputation and potential availability for formal dating are affirmed through this ritual. The persistence of the *quinceañera* among established immigrant families is a good example of the alternation or hybridization theory of culture change—traditional customs often coexist with more contemporary views about premarital sex or less hierarchical parent-child relationships. Recently a Mexican mother asked me to help convince her resistant 15-year-old daughter to let her parents plan a *quinceañera* party. The daughter knew her parents worked tremendous hours to earn a very modest living and could hardly afford the financial burden of such a party. The intensity of the mother's emotions about her daughter's refusal surprised me—the girl had an older boyfriend who visited her home almost daily and with whom she was probably involved sexually, so the party's symbolic meaning hardly applied. When I asked the mother why the celebration was so important to her, she said, "A *quinceañera* is the most unforgettable event (*inolvidable* is the romantic Spanish word she used) in a woman's life and a memory that all parents dream of bestowing, from the time of their birth, upon their daughters."

The absence of a comparable initiation rite for boys can sometimes be corrected for therapeutic purposes by "inventing" a party (perhaps less elaborate than a *quinceañera*) or using graduation from junior or senior high school as a "maturation celebration." During this time, teenagers can negotiate with parents a number of privileges that may by gained through these passages.

A teenager's need for racial and ethnic identification and the therapeutic value of cultural rites of passage is dramatically illustrated by the following case.

The Harris family consisted of parents Bob and Rachel, well-meaning Anglo-American elementary school teachers in their mid 40s, and their three corpulent, talkative children: 14-year-old Betty, who was Mexican, 10-year-old Tony, an Afro-Cuban boy, and Milagro, a 7-year-old girl from Costa Rica. The children were adopted at birth and raised with as minimal an exposure to Latino culture as is possible in a border city like San Diego. The Harrises were very caring parents, dedicated to enriching their children's lives and invested in their education. Yet Betty was not doing well in school and had unexpectedly become very drawn toward other Mexican American adolescents. She was attracted to the routines of many talkative Mexican people living in small apartments, late nights of TV and laughter, lavish Sunday picnics, and adults that tolerate children's naughty pranks.

As conversations unfolded I learned that Betty (who was Hispanic looking but did not speak a word of Spanish) was profoundly ashamed to be in a "lily white" family with somewhat older parents, to the point of displaying reverse discrimination. I normalized this situation, citing my own experience, by noting that children often discriminate against or are ashamed of their parents because they are "foreign" or simply "different."

The dilemma was how to understand Betty's behavior. Sometimes it appeared that a return to her original culture was motivated by a genuine need for an identity that would fit her external appearance and to add a wished-for cultural flavor to her life. At other times it seemed that her adolescent rebellion against parental control was a rejection of white culture, which brought her closer to Latino friends, who themselves had negative attitudes about white culture. Her friends were young Chicanos who were also doing poorly in school and who rejected white values of achievement and conformity. Paradoxes were abundant. Even though Betty's rebellion strived toward things Mexican, her defiance of authority (as well as the parents' preoccupation with respecting Betty's needs) had an individualistic, American flavor. And the Harrises, out of fear of drugs, gangs, and sex, had become much more controlling than the parents of Betty's Mexican friends.

The issue of connecting with the youngsters' biological parents was broached. The five family members denied any wish on anybody's part to find out more or connect in some way. Yet it seemed possible that Betty's pull toward her cultural heritage represented a deeper search for roots and not just a passing rebellion. I encouraged them to think about what form the reconnecting might assume. From then on much of the therapy consisted of building bridges by positively Mexicanizing Bob and Rachel Harris and legitimizing Betty's attraction to the strengths and colors of her heritage. Although the Harrises were Unitarian, they became curious about Betty's interests and visited a Catholic church that she had gone to with another family.

When they were reporting the results of these Mexican-oriented adventures, I humorously wondered if they may end up throwing a *quinceañera* celebration instead of a "sweet 16" party. Everybody's first reaction was a little diffident. It seemed important to distinguish the material, external aspects of a culture from the symbolic, ideational ones, and we all talked about the meanings of symbols and rituals. But as Betty got more and more animated with the "as if" details of a future *quinceañera*—to the point of asking for mariachi music—there was no turning back. She had symbolically found herself. Betty teased the parents warmly rather than angrily, "Don't worry, Mom and Dad. I'll take you home at 10:30 P.M., tuck you in bed and go back to dance until 2 A.M.!"

Family conversations and rituals that address in a light tone a teenager's ethnic identity facilitate such cases as the Harrises. But the shifts needed in school performance and the negative influence of peers on school achievement usually necessitate something more. One was the introduction of school consultation, which required Betty to report regularly to her counselor about her school progress and homework. The other was to link Betty with a community program of group support where Latina teenagers could explore their own issues. The weekly group, like many of its kind, was led by role models who shared how to be in charge of one's life choices, how to have a boyfriend and get married, and how not to drop out of school, especially given the value of education for women.

## Building Bridges between Worlds

Much of family therapy centers on creating bridges between the worlds of parents and adolescents. The therapist often acts as a family intermediary, clarifying expectations, justifying conflict, translating family members' cultural behavior, and encouraging compromise and negotiation when the developmental clock for dating, curfews, and other freedoms is out of sync between the generations. The following case illustrates the tremendous utility of the family intermediary role in families with severe presenting problems, such as adolescent suicide threats or attempts.

Elena, a 15-year-old girl, was referred after she took a bottle of aspirin and two boxes of Sudafed, and left a suicide note. The family consisted of the parents, Mr. Morales (38) and Mrs. Morales (35); an older brother, Tonio (17); a younger sister, Cecilia (13); and three other youngsters. Mr. Morales had left Monterrey, Mexico, when Cecilia was born, and stayed in the United States for 5 years before he was able to bring his wife and children to their new home. The younger children were born in California. It was readily apparent that Mrs. Morales and the older children formed a very close, cozy group ("her children"). The father was isolated from them, but was affectionate and playful with the three younger children ("his children"). When the father talked, the three adolescents quietly mocked him or muttered disparaging comments.

Mr. Morales worked as a bus driver many hours of the day and night, during the week, and on weekends. At home he was tired and did nothing but watch TV. Yet he constantly asked the older children to do more to help their overworked mother. The teenagers passively opposed him by using delay tactics, while relying on mother's tolerance.

The precipitating event for Elena's suicidal gesture was her father's refusal to allow her to take the bus to visit a friend who had moved recently to another neighborhood. What at first appeared as anachronistic rules were later evidence of caring concern on Mr. Morales's part: the bus stop was in front of a tavern, "not a place for a girl" (an uncle had seen Elena around the tavern on several occasions); Mr. Morales was upset by the loud and wild behavior he witnessed every day by adolescents who rode the buses in the inner city and he was trying to delay exposing his daughter to these bad examples; and as a concerned father, Mr. Morales checked on all of his children's activities. These were legitimate concerns that developed into a rigid and ineffective stance, no doubt compounded by years of separation and the fact that Elena was the first girl to undergo adolescence in the United States.

Unhappiness and intense depression, including suicidal thoughts, are not uncommon among Latino adolescents, particularly among girls who are very strictly raised and closely supervised. In a study of Puerto Rican adolescents in New York City (Canino, 1982), six out of nine girls suffered some type of psychiatric symptoms that seemed to be related to conflicting cultural expectations about sexuality and problems establishing a sense of identity.

A suicide attempt in a rebellious 16-year-old Puerto Rican girl, Nancy R., is described by Canino and Canino (1982). Nancy's feelings of being overly controlled and her wish to protest were augmented by her identification with Mrs. R. Nancy's mother was depressed, socially isolated, did not speak English, and spent her days cooking and cleaning, while Mr. R. took her for granted and spent his free time at the bar playing dominoes with his Latino *amigos* (male friends). Nancy's behavior was caught in a repetitive cycle of unresolved marital issues between the parents. When she came in late, her father imposed excessive restrictions while her mother undermined her husband's discipline by siding with the girl.

In a similar case, Bernal and Gutiérrez (1988) richly describe Lisa Gómez, the 15-year-old daughter of a Cuban family. The Gomezes came to therapy when the mother read Lisa's diary and found out that she had tried to kill herself by taking a bottle of antibiotics. Lisa felt stifled by her "old-fashioned" parents who treated her "as a prisoner" when it came to curfews, parties, and dating. The first therapist who saw the family quickly confronted the "backwardness" of the parents' values, stating that in the

United States a girl's virginity is not "such an important matter," and encouraged the parents to allow Lisa more freedom. The parents felt insulted
and did not return.

It's not uncommon for young therapists to feel sympathetic toward
Latino teenagers and attempt to "rescue" them by speaking in favor of
granting them greater freedom. Needless to say, this stance only alienates
the parents. Probably suspecting that this is what happened, another therapist proceeded to call their home and interview the parents and daughter
separately. This second therapist carefully mediated and negotiated a gradual series of very small compromises and more flexible controls. The
Gomezes were reminded about Lisa's good qualities, they were praised for
having the best intentions as parents, and they were warned about the dangers of escalation that have led girls in Lisa's cultural predicament to become totally rebellious, lose interest in school, and even become involved
with drugs and teenage pregnancy. Bernal and Gutiérrez report that sharing of information about their cultural family problem alarmed the parents
and made them more amenable to make certain concessions, which in
turn increased Lisa's cooperativeness and happiness.

## Psychoeducational Conversations

Sharing statistics, results of studies, and other information relevant to adolescence and the parent-teen relationship is a useful technique to normal-
ize, diffuse, and facilitate conflict resolution. Initiating conversations with
teenagers, in front of their parents, about the cultural tensions they experience in school usually increases the emotional resonance parents feel
rearding their own immigrant or minority experience. Such conversations
provide other views of the problems of youth and new avenues for change.
In therapy, Latino parents may be amenable to suggestions that teenagers
need a sympathetic ear from their parents so they can confide or speak
honestly. Suggestions that teenagers need the freedom to experiment and
learn from their own experiences can be made as well. Nonetheless, it is
very important to stress to the whole family that a modified equivalent of
*respeto* for parental authority remain in place. This stance helps assuage parents fears that the therapist may be siding with what they regard as the perils of American permissiveness.

Living in large nuclear and extended families may naturally facilitate a
move away from an excessive focus on adolescent troubles to other developmental transitions that require parental attention: the birth of a new baby, a
younger sibling's entrance into school, an older married sibling's entrance
into parenthood, the need for attention to aging parents. Therapists can direct attention to these new events and relieve pressure for the adolescent.
Siblings, grandparents, aunts, cousins, and godparents are an invaluable
therapeutic resource always, but particularly during adolescence. The large

family offers a wealth of alternatives not open when the therapy is prag-
matically limited to the parents and the adolescent in conflict.

Immigrant parents, and sometimes first-generation parents, extend
their calls for help to their country of origin when they find themselves unable to deal with an unruly adolescent. They may simply send the adolescent to live with relatives in Mexico or Puerto Rico. Often this is a desirable
move; certainly preferable to a life of drugs and crime in the streets, or jail.
A mother I know in San Diego saved money to take her two gang-involved
sons back to her Mexican hometown, albeit using the excuse of a family vacation. As a calmer young adult, the removed person may later be integrated back into the nuclear family in the United States. Other times, the
adolescent does not reform in the extended setting, or never returns to his
nuclear group. As we have seen, an increasing number of "solo" teenage
immigrants come to the United States to escape dismal poverty and terrible
home situations, only to enter a dangerous and equally dismal street life in
this country.

In this chapter it is possible to observe that the ecological niche of Latino children, adolescents, and parents comprises unlimited variability. Differences in meanings about developmental paths, parenting, and growing
up intersect at every turn with issues of migration, family structure, and minority status. The same holds true for the experience of Latino adults,
whether they are just starting out in the world of grown-ups and of marriage, are launching their children as they travel through middle age, or
face losses and generational conflicts in their later years. In the next chapter I traverse the domain of adulthood and glimpse the many meanings attributed to particular stages of adult life.

## NOTE

1. Some aspects of these life cycle descriptions appeared in a previous chapter by
   Falicov and Karrer (1980).
2. An interesting illustration of the social construction of homosexuality is the fact
   that among Mexicans, the label of homosexual is applied exclusively to one of
   the two partners of a homosexual encounter. The homosexual is only the passive
   partner who is penetrated and is thought to be more effeminate. The aggressive
   one who penetrates is often bisexual and heterosexually married. He is thought
   to be manly and therefore not homosexual (Bronfman et al., 1995). This construction has many dangers for women whose husbands may not take precautions in practicing "safe sex" with men on the basis that they are not "really"
   involved in a homosexual encounter.

# 12

## Adulthood across the Lifespan

> In principle theories of human development constitute . . . a science
> whose intrinsic object is not only to describe but to prescribe . . . we
> create an implicit world such as we think it *ought to be*.
> —J. BRUNER (1986, pp. 20–21)

### YOUNG ADULTHOOD: STAYING HOME AND MOVING ON

Late adolescence and early adulthood in Latino families differs from that in Anglo-American families in that there is an emphasis on staying home rather than leaving home. Staying home often implies financial dependence or interdependence—status that is expected, acceptable, and very much a part of the familism of collectivistic cultures. Contemporary developmental theory, however, emphasizes separation/individuation as the hallmark of healthy development, clearly favoring the values of middle-class, Anglo-American families.

This striking difference suggests that therapists should question the cultural bias of most developmental theories. Some studies have found a very large discrepancy between therapists' judgments of normality as equated with separation from family of origin, and the continued wish of many clients for closeness with their families (Kazak, McCannell, Adkins, Himmelberg, & Grace, 1989; Rogers & Leichter, 1964).

The cultural norm among many Anglo-Americans is to leave home as a solo act, proving themselves capable of autonomy, decision making, and self-sufficiency in emotional and financial realms. Indeed, young Anglo-American adults separate geographically from their families more than Latinos of all socioeconomic levels.

When Latinos leave home, they generally do so in the context of forming a new and connected family of their own—dating and courtship provide the "launching" phase and marriage the preferred means of separating from the family. This is partly because other avenues for leaving home, such as going to college, getting a job, and living independently or with a roommate, are limited for many Latinos.

While separation/individuation tends to occur in the context of a developing bond with a prospective mate, many deep loyalties to one's parents and siblings remain active during this period, and new challenges arise. Launching siblings may pave the way to emancipation for younger brothers and sisters, or when an older parentified child leaves, parental dependency may shift to the next in line. Other children may be "recruited" or "elected" for these roles with various degrees of success. Among siblings themselves, launching rarely precipitates the waning contact found between Anglo-American brothers and sisters—this bond remains strong (and sometimes complicated) despite courtship and marriage.

## Separation and Gender

Gender expectations also shape the separation process. Sons may stay away from home for increasingly longer periods of time, coming home only at night to sleep. Parents may occasionally complain about not seeing him often enough, but his peripheral role is acceptable. Marriage, work, or school eventually send him on his way. For young women, participation and visibility at home continue to be expected. Further, daughters are perceived as far more vulnerable than sons to external influences, and therefore in need of protection. A young woman's time in the company of a boyfriend or male peers is likely to be closely monitored, if not chaperoned in some fashion.

In spite of greater openness toward sexuality, double standards still make a woman's reputation dependent on her chastity and later her fidelity. A young man's sexual dalliances, on the other hand, are accepted and often encouraged. Two of my current female Mexican clients are in their late 20s, have had exclusive long-term relationships with boyfriends, yet were both virgins at marriage. A third client, described below, also demonstrates the powerful influence of cultural prescriptions regarding courtship and sexuality.

Josefina Canedo, a Puerto Rican middle-class professional in her early 30s, regretted her two premarital sexual relationships and attributed her "looseness" to the bad influence of an American coworker. The client had been raised Catholic but was not practicing in adulthood. Interestingly, she came to therapy for treatment of vaginismus—a recurrent, persistent psychosexual problem in which spasms of the vaginal muscles are so strong that penetration during intercourse is impossible. Therapy for the client focused on "cultural resistance," in this case, a recognition that her guilt and conflict about sex was more the product of social religious recruitment than her own personal conviction.

As always, it was important to reflect internally, define and compare my own attitudes to those of the client—as an Argentine, Jewish, political liberal, I feared that my inclination toward greater sexual liberation might differ from hers enough to create dissonance and even imposition of my values in the conversation. To facilitate a greater ideological and emotional connection for Josefina, I suggested she read short stories by Latina writers such as Sandra Cisneros, Julia Álvarez, Denise Chávez, Angeles Mastretta, and Esmeralda Santiago, whose work could be used to enhance therapeutic conversations about sexual issues in Latina women's development. The client's ecological niche, that is, her age, ethnicity, Catholic upbringing, and educational aspirations mirrored the dilemmas of traditional upbringing in a sexually freer culture so clearly expressed by the female writers of her own culture.

During treatment, Josefina became able to practice progressive vaginal dilation and take hot sitz baths, behavioral treatment she had learned in a sexual dysfunction clinic but had been reluctant to follow. All these techniques may have contributed to her success, but a change in her attitude was essential in giving her "permission" to use these mechanical aids. Josefina Canedo became free enough and motivated enough to date again. She eventually married a Cuban man who "respected her" (abided by her wish to not have sex) up until the wedding night. Her request of him showed how deeply she had internalized a cultural value on premarital chastity, even if at this point it was only symbolic.

## Courtship as Launching

In comparison with mainstream American culture, Latino courtship forms a significant life cycle stage and is taken very seriously, even among youth. In part, this is because marriage is a weighty decision for Roman Catholics, a commitment for a lifetime. Parents in Latino families often check out potential candidates for steady dating whenever a daughter appears to be seeing a young man with some frequency. Good manners, financial prospects, and education level all enter into consideration in this covert assessment process. Once an opinion has been formed, parents exert considerable pressure for or against the selection of a particular mate.

In spite of, or perhaps because of, mounting intermarriage (Murguia, 1982), Latino parents who want to preserve their ethnic identity may disapprove of their children dating people of other ethnic backgrounds, including Latinos from other cultures. Therapists who believe a Puerto Rican woman and a Mexican man make a good match based on similarities of language and culture may assume that their problems are purely related to personal conflicts. Rather, the couple may be struggling with prejudices against each partner's racial and ethnic background, as well as an ambivalent permission to marry from both families of origin.

Once approved, steady courtship is usually legitimized by a *compromiso*, or an engagement party, which involves a public announcement, elaborate festivities, and formal exchange of rings. The *compromiso* may take place even after the wedding date has been set to symbolize the seriousness of the commitment. After the *compromiso*, both extended families often begin including each other in their get-togethers.

For the courting couple, family ties continue to play a significant, occasionally problematic, role. The young man may experience conflicting demands from his mother and his fiancée. The young woman may feel confused or resentful that her "ownership" has been transferred from her family to her husband-to-be. And as families of origin incorporate their future in-laws, new relationships and hierarchies are worked out. The challenge may be particularly great if parents cling excessively to their son or daughter, or if the engaged young adult is extremely involved with the parents, as is common among recent immigrant families. If these issues are unresolved during early adulthood, they may reappear at later points in the family life cycle.

## Taking a Different Path

For growing numbers of Latinos, courtship and marriage is not the only pathway from their parents' home. Education and job opportunities may beckon for young men and women—a fact that has particular repercussions for grown daughters and their families. A college-educated Latina who decides to get her own apartment may be considered disgraceful by some parents, or at least frowned upon.

Elisa García, a 23-year-old Cuban woman, decided to get her own apartment with her salary as a medical secretary while she was taking night courses in medical administration. Her angry father's comment was, "There's only one reason a young woman gets her own apartment!" This was the beginning of Elisa's break with her family. After she married, she moved east—another decision that violated the family's expectations. Meanwhile, her brother played the devoted child and stayed nearby, and then took care of his parents when they got old. Elisa, who only did what middle-class Americans take for granted, had to break with her family to follow first her career and then her husband.

If courtship never takes place or doesn't lead to marriage, the unmarried Latino man or woman tends not to move out of the parental household. But if both parents die, it's more acceptable for unmarried adults to live with married siblings than to live on their own. These family members often play a significant role in the dynamics of their brother's or sister's home. Yet therapists need to be careful not to assume their presence is a problem or that a solution lies in urging the unmarried adult toward greater autonomy. When an unmarried brother or sister is part of a problematic triangle (perhaps diverting marital conflict, and marital solutions), sibling therapy can be a helpful way to address old ledgers and loyalties from the family of origin.

## Marriage: Returning to the Fold?

Marriage combines two important firsts for many young Latinos: it is likely their first intimate relationship outside of family and their first experience in setting up a separate household. As we have seen, a collectivistic culture may focus on formation of a familial self rather than emphasize differentiation or individuation at this time. Yet gradual individuation may take place in the less hierarchical context of marriage, as the couple creates common goals and negotiates values, priorities, and everyday routines.

The late teens and early 20s is considered a socially acceptable age for marriage in most Latino families, although later marriage is more tolerated for men. Eighteen- and 19-year-old Latinos have much higher marriage rates (24%) than African Americans (5%) and non-Hispanic whites (12%) (Duany & Pittman, 1990). This discrepancy may be because many Latinos are more likely to consider people under 21 years of age ideal for marriage and child rearing (Erickson, 1990).

The Latino wedding itself—the *casamiento*—is a colorful and joyous, collective celebration. From working-class to upper-class settings, a casamiento is an elaborate church and dinner affair with formal attire and hundreds of guests. Many adult relatives and family friends become financially and instrumentally responsible for various aspects of the wedding—godparents of *cojines* put the pillows to lean at the altar, godparents of *flores* buy the flower arrangements, and godparents of *pasteles* provide the cakes and sweets. Occasionally a *casamiento* may be complicated when a younger, perhaps more bicultural or modern couple rebels against a traditional wedding ceremony. While grown children may protest, often to save their families huge debts, parents often insist on an elaborate celebration. In Francis Ford Coppola's film *Mi Familia* (1994), José Sánchez's daughter gets married 22 years after he came on foot from his small town in northern Mexico to Los Angeles. Although he and his wife work very hard to make a modest living for their six children, they throw a magnificent *casamiento* with mariachis, lavish food, great dresses, and joyous dancing. One of José's sons later recalls it took his father years to recover from the debt, still "Father had to show the world how much his daughter meant to him . . . but that is what money is for!"

The early stages of a new marriage may seem especially harmonious—
sometimes due to family-of-origin legacies to suppress anger and communicate indirectly about differences and conflicts. But this time can also be a
tumultuous one. It may be the first time a young man or woman expresses
more individualistic desires—desires that may reflect an expanding bicultural self. In a commentary about the limitations of developmental models
based on the progressive resolution of discrete life cycle tasks (Falicov,
1983), I described a dilemma I experienced soon after my wedding. Just as
I began to share a bed and a life with my husband, I pleaded with him for
the room of my own I never had growing up. Although the paradox was obvious, my battle for both rooms (a single room of my own, another for us as
a couple) enhanced my personal and my relational development simultaneously.

Overlapping tasks and double meanings of self—becoming an independent woman and a married one at the same time, for example—often
need to be taken into account when working with immigrant Latino clients. They may be struggling with coexisting or conflicting developmental
frames of reference and cannot neatly follow some prescribed sequence of
life cycle events.

Financial limitations and family interdependence often slow down the
process of setting up a truly separate household. The newly constituted
family may live with or nearby the husband's family and receive temporary
economic support. Occasionally couples live with the wife's family, but this
dependence may be perceived as a lack of masculinity on the husband's
part. While physical proximity and emotional involvement with families of
origin can be helpful, it may limit the couple from exploring their separate
identities as husband and wife, particularly if one of the spouses performed
valuable functions in his or her family. The following case illustrates several
of these points.

Mrs. Olivia González Lara, a 23-year-old Mexican woman, was referred
for individual treatment. She had been married for 6 months when she
developed intense fluctuations in mood, ranging from depression to a
psychiatrist's diagnosis of paranoid ideations, including feelings of being
persecuted by other people. For example, she accused her husband, Mr.
Federico González, of intentionally ruining her plants by blowing a fan
in front of them for prolonged periods.

Federico González Lara, 26, had been working for a house painting
company in the United States for 10 years. After achieving some modest
success, he decided to find a wife. No suitable Mexican American woman
could be found, so he began exploring the possibilities of finding a wife
in Guadalajara. He came across a magazine containing ads for pen pals
and began a letter-writing relationship with Olivia. This correspondence

went on for several months. In the language formalities of the culture, the letters expressed, in flowery Spanish, highly romanticized and idealized feelings that made both fall "madly in love."

After some time, Federico went to Mexico to marry Olivia and bring her back to the United States. He neglected to mention to his new wife that they would be living in his mother's home. He was certain that Olivia would have no objection. Federico's four sisters lived in the house as well and ever since their father had suffered a stroke, Federico had stepped into his father's shoes.

Olivia was confused. Not only had she not been told about the living arrangements, but she had also sensed a veiled hostility from the other women in the household. Every time she attempted to discuss her feelings with Federico, he would forcefully defend his family, denying they were hostile in any way. At the same time, Federico was often approached by his mother and his sisters with complaints about Olivia: "She is too dreamy" or "She keeps too much to herself." They even hinted at a "possible drinking problem." Federico would only feebly defend his wife. He began listening to the women's advice on how to deal with Olivia, and ultimately took their suggestion to send her to a psychiatrist.

The newly arrived daughter-in-law felt that "as a daughter in my mother-in-law's home I could never become a wife, especially of her favorite son. I feel I am the lowest, the one with the least power among the women in the house." Because generational and territorial hierarchies did not allow Olivia to express her resentment directly to her in-laws, she turned this resentment toward Federico.

In order to find an area of private and more effective communication, I suggested that rather than talking the couple write to each other three times a week, especially since this had proven to be so successful in the past. The letters were to date from the time just before the wedding and then continue. Federico was to explain exactly what Olivia could expect while living in his familial household, including what his relationship was like with his mother and sisters. Olivia was encouraged to ask him for details and clarification. This exercise created a temporary truce by assigning each partner responsibility for creating more open and specific communication. It also clarified many issues for Federico, who began to express more empathy for Olivia's difficult predicament. In turn, Olivia began to appreciate Federico's efforts. She became more willing to help him create some emotional boundaries that helped to define himself not just as a son and brother, but as a husband as well.

I was tempted to take an Anglo-American perspective and push, however gently, toward an independent living arrangement for this couple. However, I recognized the intensity of the Mexican mother-son bond, and the time it takes for a new marital bond to parallel the strength of this connection. Further, neither spouse mentioned moving from Federico's mother's house—theirs was an ethnically consonant and economical arrangement for the first stage of marriage.

The fact that this is a culturally and economically based pattern doesn't make it a healthy one in all cases and for all involved, and it may be even less so in a new ecological setting where the pattern is less common and acceptable. Wives in this kind of patrilocal arrangement are often stressed and disempowered and frequently complain, nag, or show anger and depression. They often harbor an intense wish to have their own married dwellings (Bronfman et al., 1995). This knowledge influenced me in the next stage of therapy.

> I explored each spouse's feelings about living separately and asked whether future plans included moving from Federico's mother's home. I also asked who would be most affected by staying and by moving. Both spouses answered that they planned to move when finances allowed. I suspected but did not say that Olivia, like other women in her position, would be more likely to gain power and influence when she became a mother herself and acquired a different status in the family's eyes.
>
> The unfairness of this situation needs to be questioned, yet solutions are not easily found. I have seen cases in which the wife succeeds, after many threats, in obtaining a separate house, only to be defeated by a husband who visits and eats at his mother's home almost every day, or secretly confides his problems to his mother and relishes her unconditional support. Two years after their therapy ended, the González Lara family came back for a few sessions. They were expecting a baby and used the therapy sessions to problem solve a transition to a home of their own.

A therapist may consider eliciting, perhaps privately, the cooperation of the wife when couples and families are faced with these kinds of dilemmas. This intervention blocks the wife's usually ill-fated attempts to gain her husband through escalating criticisms of her mother-in-law. While this may seem to Anglo-American therapists an unfair burden on the young wife, the goal is to empower her within an already established family model rather than support her unproductive attacks or cutoffs.

Even when a young Latino couple doesn't live with extended family, they may have more contact with kin after marriage than during their courtship, when they were left somewhat alone to explore their relationship. Thus marriage, paradoxically, may signify a return to rather than a separation from the fold. Couples therapy for newly married Latinos will undoubtedly involve complex interconnections with families of origin.

## Entrance into Parenthood

The young Latino couple's entrance into parenthood may not be experienced as the major crisis many Anglo-American couples encounter. With less emphasis on romantic privacy, a Latino couple may not perceive the loss of time and activities together as keenly as many Anglo-Americans. Young Latino parents, including single mothers, may have a network of grandparents and relatives who provide relief from full-time caretaking and provide lots of coaching and advice. Having a baby in the house is less draining than for the isolated couple who is managing alone.

Anglo-American, middle-class women regard motherhood as a symbol of emancipation from their parents and a passage from being a daughter (or a girl) to being a "coequal" with mother (Falicov, 1971). In contrast, motherhood does not change the status of Latinas in relation to their parents. To prove their self-sufficiency, Anglo-American women often limit their mother's visits postpartum. Aware of rapid ideological and technical changes, they will use other young mothers as role models and get their information about child care from pediatricians, books, and magazines. The young Anglo-American mother's reactivity to her mother's advice often makes it hard for the two of them to feel close and deepen their connection through their mutual connection to the baby. Young Latina mothers, on the other hand, are usually in less conflict about relying on the wisdom of their mothers, grandmothers, and other older women both for advice and regular caretaking of their baby. Nevertheless, they also incorporate new media and professional information about child care.

Entrance into fatherhood for the young Latino father is a fundamental milestone. Negative cultural stereotypes of Latino men circumscribe their investment in procreation exclusively to a desire to confirm and to publicly display their male potency. The idea that men only want to engender male offspring is also part of the cultural myth. The reality of fathers' attachment to their children, both boys and girls, is far more textured and emotionally complex. Fathering greatly enchances male identity in a culture that values parenting so highly. Most Latino men take great pride at becoming a father. Being a good father means, above all, loving and doing well by their children. There are some differences in the attitudes and fathering practices in upper- and lower-class settings, and between rural and urban areas. How directly the father is involved in holding, changing diapers, or playing is mostly related to whether women work oustide the home and whether extended family help or hired maids are available. Recent generational changes also alter, and may contradict, the traditional notion of a father's peripheral role in parenting. Men spend less time and do less infant care than women but they are not necessarily seen as less tender, affectionate, or caring by both sexes (Gutmann, 1996).

## The Effects of Divorce

While divorce can occur at any time in a marriage, we briefly touch on the subject here to reflect the fact that marriages are at particular risk for breakdown when children first arrive on the scene and during middle age, when those same children are launching. Divorce is more traumatic and less common for Latinos than for Anglo-Americans. The criticism and judgmental disappointment about the decision to divorce is most intense among first-generation immigrant Mexican parents. Since marriage is for life, a divorce on the basis of marital incompatibility may be alien to cultural and religious beliefs. Divorce bears a social stigma, and extended family members may play a role in shaming the separating couple (Wagner, 1988). Adjustment to the divorce process and much needed emotional support may be compromised by these prejudiced attitudes.

The open condemnation and intense feelings of loss that accompany a divorce are not circumscribed to the older generation. I have seen 9- and 10-year-olds as well as teenagers become very vocal, upset, and angry at their parents when there is a threat of divorce or separation. Children dread hearing about an impending family breakup, an outcome they may criticize sharply in families of their friends or of American children. Children hate the prospect of losing the joy of shared birthdays, family dinners, and picnics or other outings with both parents and both extended families. For Latino children more than Anglo-Americans, contact with both sets of grandparents, uncles, aunts, and cousins is constant—contact that may be severely disrupted by divorce.

Given the Latino family's connectedness, emotional expressivity, and in some cases, permeable generational boundaries, children may have witnessed marital quarrels. They often have many feelings and thoughts about what their parents could have done to save the marriage. A forum-like therapy in which the children can create a narrative that the therapist documents in writing, and which includes their views about the family's past, present (predivorce), and future (postdivorce) is very helpful.

Although divorce is not common among Mexicans of any social class, single parenthood is ubiquitous in lower socioeconomic ranks due to teenage pregnancy and spousal abandonment. Puerto Ricans and African Americans share similar statistics for divorce and single parenthood. Cubans divorce more than Mexicans, but they tend to remain in two-parent or binuclear households more than functioning as single parents.

Latino stepfamily formation often follows divorce after some period of time. Stepfamilies among Latinos face similar problems to blended families everywhere—difficulties between stepparent and the spouse's children or rivalries between the stepparent and the spouse's former partner. The content of the problems, however, may reflect cultural preferences in family values relating to connectedness and separation or age and gender hierarchies.

A family I saw in therapy exhibited considerable tension between the new stepmother, a 53-year-old middle-class Mexican woman who had raised her own biological family in Mexico, and a 50-year-old Anglo-

American physician who was the father of three adolescent children. His children spent half the time with their biological mother, and the other half with their father and stepmother. The Mexican stepmother was very nurturant, cooked many foods, and sewed dresses for her 14-year-old stepdaughter. Yet she also complained to her husband about the children's lack of respect toward her, their poor eating habits and table manners, the degree of neatness of their rooms (she called them *cochinos* [pigs]), lack of affectionate gestures ("cold"), and their lack of gratitude ("selfish") for all she was doing for them. She was completely oblivious to the cultural differences implied in her labels. She believed that "good" children are the same everywhere and assumed I would support her definitions. The therapeutic goal was to help the couple integrate two sets of cultural meaning systems, which were easy to categorize under the summary labels of "proper demeanor" and "self-maximization." These cognitive frames eased the negotiation of stepparenting boundaries.

## MIDDLE AGE: A FULL NEST

Middle-aged Latino parents, like most Western middle-age people, face the tasks of facilitating the separation of their young adult children, renewing their marital relationship, and assuming the role of grandparents. Outcomes depend on their ability to redefine relationships with grown children and find new meaning in their marital bond.

Cultural values on blood relationships and parent-child bonds may have prepared the couple for parenting, but not for creating marital happiness. A compromise is usually reached by finding an acceptable, more disengaged manner of parenting the married children, focusing on grandchildren, and increasing contact with relatives, in-laws, and other significant kin. Sometimes this transitional stage creates an impasse that brings the couple into treatment. A kind of emotional separation is common—both spouses may be living together and carrying on their family duties, but they hardly relate to each other directly.

Many middle-aged people from Latin America were raised with the notion that one must be married for life. This prohibition against divorce, plus strong family obligations and finanaical dependencies, bring a nonelective element to the marriage that may contribute to inertia and resignation. Depression and an emotionally distant marriage may be expressions of this predicament. Sometimes there is actual physical, long-term separation between the spouses without divorce. The man may be living with another woman with whom he may have children. This arrangement may also be called *la casa chica* even though it is not a secret affair or double life. This is because the man is still legally married and presumably has obligations to his first family. Without denying the financial and emotional impact caused by spousal desertion, Gutmann (1996) believes that among multiple meanings *la casa chica* could be interpreted as a creative "social invention in defiance of the church's ban on divorce" (p. 141) and a way of coping with marital dissatisfaction.

Exposure to Anglo-American expectations of greater personal fulfillment and marital happiness may stimulate self-questioning during middle age. It is interesting that conversion to Protestantism serves many functions, one of which may be a more permissive attitude toward divorce. But consistent with their family orientation, middle-aged parents may be attentive to and involved in pursuing happiness for their children's marriages. In some of my couples therapy cases, it is the middle-aged parents of the husband or wife who have insisted that the young couple go for therapy and who often offer to pay. The driving motivation is to prevent the young couple from divorcing, but there are other reasons as well. In one case the mother was critical of the son because he treated his wife in a domineering and disrespectful way. She was supportive of her daughter-in-law, encouraging her to challenge the husband's rudeness in the way that she wished she had done early in her own marriage. This vicarious attempt at reparation is born of personal unhappiness and a most likely mistaken resignation that it is too late to change the older couple's marriage. In my experience it is possible to suggest to the younger generation that they reciprocate their parents' favor by encouraging the older pair toward couple's therapy, where they can rethink the meaning of their marriage.

## Exits and Entrances

The separation of grown children is accomplished with various degrees of conflict, but because of cultural values that stress family interdependence, considerable connectedness remains. The "empty nest" phenomenon described for upwardly mobile, Anglo-American families is not as visible in the Latino family regardless of social class.

Although developmental milestones such as weaning, school entrance readiness, and launching occur later in Latino families than in most Anglo-American families, Latinos marry and have children earlier than their Anglo-American counterparts. This means they become parents at a relatively early age. The offspring also marry young, sometimes outside their ethnic group, a situation that gives rise to initial conflict and gradual accommodation to a culturally dissonant relationship with Anglo-American or other in-laws.

Middle-aged grandparents assume an important role in child rearing. Their influence is felt and usually accepted by the new parents, and they don't experience the peripheral role and fear of intrusion that middle-class, Anglo-American grandparents often feel. Regular involvement with the two younger generations contributes to a relative prolongation of middle age relative to old age and a swelling rather than attrition in the family ranks. A sense of vitality and continued usefulness among middle-aged Latino grandparents contrasts with the "empty nest," existential, and marital renewal issues typically described for middle-class, Anglo-Americans in this age group.

Incorporation of older, widowed parents often takes place while young married adults are being launched to live in their own dwellings. A middle-aged couple that had migrated 25 years earlier may now be forced to bring one or two of their aging, widowed, or ill parents who had originally remained in the country of origin to live with them. The adjustments are multifaceted. The elderly person does not speak English, may feel lonely and lost, and may tax the resources of the middle-aged children who feel a strong obligation to create a happy situation for the parent. Traditional moral responsibility falls on the oldest daughter to become the caretaker of a widowed parent, but financial considerations modify this guideline to target the most affluent and less overburdened offspring.

Considerable accommodation must take place as families cope with the overlapping stresses of launching and marriage of children, new relationships with in-laws, and illnesses or death of one's own parents—all happening virtually under the same roof.

## Double Dilemmas

In Latino families, it's not unusual for hierarchies among husband and wife or parent and child to alternate between excessive complementarity and some manner of symmetry. When couples in mid-life face the double transitions of reestablishing their marital relationship and launching grown children, these fluctuations can exacerbate the process, polarizing family members further. Wives may be more vocal about their frustrations with their husband's behavior, without taking action. The younger generation may find it difficult to accept their parents' lifestyle, question their marital arrangement, and rebel against parental values. The following example illustrates many of the conflicts between parents in mid-life and adult children slowly leaving home.

> Mrs. Zapata, a 46-year-old Mexican woman who had lived in the United States for 23 years, was referred because she had psychosomatic complaints and was talking about divorcing 48-year-old Mr. Zapata, her husband of 25 years. The couple had six children: Araceli (23), Marta (21), Rebeca (20), Michael (17), Elizabeth (16), and Gloria (15). All were living at home. Araceli was finishing school in social work at a city college, Marta was working as a postal employee, Rebeca had plans to enter medical school, Michael had dropped out of high school and was erratically employed, and Elizabeth and Gloria were both attending a neighborhood high school.

Mr. and Mrs. Zapata were trapped in a long-standing feud. Mrs. Zapata and the oldest daughter, Araceli, had formed a stable coalition that maintained a muffled conflict between the spouses. Araceli's proposal to leave home to attend graduate school precipitated a family crisis. Marta, the second daughter, was feeling pressured but was unwilling to assume Araceli's vacant spot as marital mediator. Becky was defiant, clearly stating to the family that her plans to attend medical school were a priority. She openly challenged her parents' marital arrangement and supported her mother's talk of divorce. Elizabeth and Gloria had elected to be passive observers as the family's drama unfolded. Michael, meanwhile, avoided open conflict by being absent from most family activities, coming home late at night, and getting up in the morning after other family members had left the house. He appeared to be the most vulnerable person in the family. When Michael dropped out of school, Mr. Zapata had shown his deep disappointment by disengaging from his only son. Initially the father had attempted to guide his son, but he did so in an ineffectual, lecturing manner which Michael adeptly turned off.

The sibling group and the parental couple were organized around two main themes: individual achievement and a family/marriage orientation, which represented cultural polarizations. Araceli, Rebeca, and the two youngest girls (together with father) represented the achievement orientation in the family. Michael and Marta, on the other hand, were backed by their mother in their wish to marry and settle down. Marta was particularly critical of her parents' marriage and expressed a desire to find a meaningful relationship where communication could be free and open. Michael could not state his preferences clearly but he felt marriage was the only way for him to leave his family.

Mr. and Mrs. Zapata, unprepared for their children's separation, and tenuously allied by their attack, feebly defended themselves and spoke of filial ingratitude. Both attempted to entrap Marta as the new mediator between them, but Marta did not accept this role. Mr. Zapata, who worked as a laborer and was keenly aware of his own unfulfilled aspirations, identified with his daughters' desire for education. Although a traditional man, he could defend his girls' education as a way to get ahead in the world, but he could not accept their leaving home to get that education. Mr. Zapata was a bright and sensitive individual, but he appeared to be frozen in time, rigidly unable to update the worldviews he had incorporated as a young man. On the other hand, Mrs. Zapata had recently begun to work as a seamstress—her first job outside the home. The experience awakened in her a desire for an independence that could provide a much needed respite from home life.

Family therapy sessions focused on conversations about the dilemmas of a cultural transition that included gaps in age, cultural values, and education between parents and children, husband and wife. The tone I used was philosophical. Future-oriented questions encouraged everyone to entertain "as if" models and options for family relations. Sibling issues were discussed in separate sessions. Sometimes the parents sat behind the one-way mirror to observe their children at work. This setting provided a new closeness for the spouses, and some needed distance from the children.

Mr. and Mrs. Zapata remained married, but different working shifts minimized their involvement and made the relationship tolerable. Araceli left for college. Marta continued to live at home and to hold a job. Becky was accepted at medical school. The younger girls continued to attend high school, relieved to have the option, pioneered by Araceli and now accepted with pride by the parents, to go away to school. Michael got married and brought his wife, a 16-year-old girl, to live with his parents, perhaps a necessary transitional step toward autonomy for him.

## THE LATINO ELDERLY: LOSSES AND A SHARED LIFE

The developmental tasks of this period, common among Anglo-Americans and Latinos, include adjustment to the physical and psychosocial concomitants of old age: grandparenthood, retirement, illnesses, and death. Stresses of cultural transition appear in two forms. The older Latino may have migrated in early adulthood and therefore incorporated traditional cultural expectations about aging. These do not fit the changing norms of his or her children and grandchildren or their urban-egalitarian setting. Alternatively, and in increasing numbers, the older person may be a new immigrant.

Many parents of these first-generation adult immigrants remain behind in their countries of origin. When they become ill, widowed, isolated, or too old to work they are encouraged to move to the United States to live either with or nearby their offspring. The elderly parent arrives in an unknown setting, without knowledge of the language or the skills necessary for independent living. She or he may or may not find a useful role. An older woman may be easily integrated in her customary tasks of housekeeping and babysitting. But an older man may be limited to babysitting, reporting on the grandchildren's activities, and running small errands. He may sit long hours on the porch or watch Spanish programs on television all day, deprived of his country's lifelong associations. The elderly may have traded the losses of uprooting for a shared life with their children, but the balance is often questionable, and even those who have been in this country for many years may long for their roots.

Elderly Latinos who have been in the United States for many years retain important roles when they live with their adult children. Their presence helps reduce anxiety for the younger nuclear family when stressors loom large—sick children, a husband's overtime at work, a wife's struggle to deal with employment and child care. Wisdom, and even sorcery, are attributions given only to the old. Their knowledge and experience, coupled with the younger generation's respect for authority, allow older people to exert considerable influence on their married or single children through criticism and reminders about "proper demeanor." They may even screen suitors for grown-up, divorced daughters. The ability to become a "tough old bird"—energetic, involved, and self-confident—and perceive old age as arriving later than for Anglo-Americans, seems to be preserved among the Mexican American elderly (Clark & Mendelson, 1975). This finding may stem from Latino values on collectivism, conservation, cooperation, and continuity. Growing old does not require the dramatic shifts in life orientation suggested by Anglo-American standards. The latter emphasize many aspects of "self-maximization," including financial solvency, that are harder to obtain or maintain in old age.

## Multiple Jeopardy

Latino elderly experience "multiple jeopardy" (Dowd & Bengtson, 1978)— their ecological niche, including their age, minority status, lack of knowledge about language and institutions, and lack of transportation and support networks, make them especially vulnerable as they face the stresses of old age (Bastida, 1984). Most do not receive pensions, Social Security, or Medicare (Gallegos, 1991). It is difficult to imagine a more excruciating uprooting than the one that occurs in old age. The multiple jeopardy of this stage is known to be a source of chronic stress and emotional longing for elderly Puerto Ricans (Mahard, 1989). In spite of the prevalence of extended family caregivers (Greene & Monahan, 1984; Merkides, Boldt, & Ray, 1986), it is probably a disservice to the Latino elderly to assume, as the stereotype of close family ties invites us to do, that the family can meet all their needs (Gallegos, 1991).

Exploring and developing alternative support networks is the most constructive solution to the problems of the elderly. A natural network that involves reciprocity and mutual assistance appears to work much better than simple charity or help for the aged (Miranda, 1991). In the case that follows, a young mother and her elderly neighbor exchange favors and services, transportation and babysitting. An exchange-oriented approach resonates with complementary cultural patterns that maintain the vitality of the old in extended families.

The brief sections that follow highlight some of the special challenges faced by elderly Latinos and their families.

### Hard Reality Issues First

Economic hardship, language difficulties, social isolation, and limited adaptation to the unknown environment outside of the home are the bane of this generation. These hard realities, or some derivative thereof, often bring elderly Latinos in contact with mental health services.

Mrs. Corrales, a 70-year-old Puerto Rican, was referred to a mental health clinic by her local priest. She had told him that she was depressed, irritable, and losing weight. Mrs. Corrales had no friends within the urban barrio. She had migrated from Puerto Rico 8 years earlier to live with her two sons and her 45-year-old single and mildly developmentally impaired daughter. Two years before she came to the clinic, her sons had moved to a nearby city in search of better jobs. Mrs. Corrales remained behind with her daughter, who spoke no English and did not work. Among other questions, the Latin American therapist asked her if she was losing weight because she had lost her appetite, to which she quipped: "No, I've lost my teeth, not my appetite! That's what irks me!" Indeed, Mrs. Corrales had almost no teeth left in her mouth. Apparently, her conversations with the priest (an American who had learned to speak Spanish during a Latin American mission and was sensitive to the losses of migration) had centered on the emotional losses she had suffered with her sons' departure. The priest thought this was the cause of her "anxious depression." Though well meaning, he had failed to consider practical issues. Mrs. Corrales had no dental insurance, did not know any dentists, and had no financial resources.

For humane reasons, the therapist made various efforts to secure free dental care for Mrs. Corrales. Finally, a university dental clinic agreed to have her seen by practicum dentistry interns under supervision. This required a long trip to another part of the city to be seen at an institution that had no Spanish-speaking personnel—and she had no transportation.

The next step for the therapist was to explore through an "ecomap" Mrs. Corrales's natural and neighborhood network. The client was then encouraged to enlist the cooperation of a bilingual neighbor, Rosa, to accompany her to the dental clinic appointments. Rosa was a willing helper, and to reciprocate (with only a hint on the therapist's part) Mrs. Corrales began to do some babysitting for Rosa's infant.

This example illustrates that simple, practical, hard realities should be examined as causes (and needed as solutions) of an elderly Latino's problems before searching for complex psychological sources. With good intentions, the priest had not been alert to his own preconceptions, a generic tool in all therapy, but critically important when working with minority clients (Montalvo & Gutiérrez, 1989). Further, it is often necessary for therapists to assume an advocacy role and act as social intermediary between the elderly client and appropriate institutional, neighborhood, and network resources.

## Retirement

Retirement from their usual occupation may not represent as a significant turning point for older Latino men or their families as it does for Anglo-Americans. Productive work in one's occupation is not as central a life task as it is for those raised in the Protestant ethic, although middle-aged Cubans in Miami may be now steeped in a similar work ethic. Various anchors outside of work and home are found in male friendship groups and in extended family relationships. In their Latin American countries of origin, few people retire in a prescribed compulsory manner. The only exceptions are government employees who retire between age 60 and 65 and receive pensions. A retirement date that signifies passage to a new stage may not be specified because older men continue to work as long as possible. They gradually reduce their output and begin to move closer to the family orbit. There an older man joins a houseful of people, rather than a wife who has learned to live alone for the past 20 years. In fact, retirement does not demand very significant shifts for the wife or adjustment for the couple, since they often maintain separate gender spheres of social contact and leisure, as well as common interests in grown children and grandchildren.

In Latino culture, being old doesn't strand people on an experiential island—it allows them to remain in the mainstream of life. The need to appear young or to pretend to be younger than one's age, to deceive oneself and others about aging, and fearing the inevitable is not as present as among older Anglo-Americans because Latino culture does not idealize youth to the same extent. These cultural values and family practices mean that retirement is potentially a smoother transition than for Anglo-Americans, though migration may painfully alter this picture.

## Nursing Homes

Self-sufficiency isn't expected from an old or sick person in Latino culture. The expectation is that the young will take care of the old until the end and not place parents in nursing homes. The entire family tends to respect cultural values that emphasize filial love, or at least obligation, over efficiency and practicality. In Anglo-American culture, an emphasis on justice often includes the belief that older people "get what is coming to them" according to how they lived their lives. Americans believe that those who worked hard, saved, planned ahead, or raised a good family deserve a more comfortable old age than the derelict or the alcoholic, who never provided adequately for his family or abused them.

Among Latinos, grown children are obligated to care for and respect their parents whether the elderly person rightfully deserves it or not. The notion that family members owe one another loyalty, or that they acquire merit by supporting one another, is helpful in understanding Latino values (Bernal & Florez-Ortíz, 1982; Boszormenyi-Nagy & Krasner, 1986; Boszormenyi-Nagy, Grunebaum, & Ulrich, 1981; Goldenthal, 1996). One must take into account that a relational ethic of intrinsic duty and obligation toward one's own parents moves Latinos to obey this mandate regardless of whether the ledger of debts is reciprocal, balanced, and fair, or whether it is unilateral, imbalanced, and unfair. Age and parenthood themselves provide sufficient merit.

In situations involving intergenerational loyalties, often the task of therapy is to disentangle the personal relational history from the cultural mandates and arrive at compromises that are acceptable to the client. However, it is important to remember that the immigrant case involves the additional loyalty and deep emotional connections to cultural roots, legacies, and the country itself, which may assume proportions similar to deep family attachments.

The three Latino groups differ in their readiness to incorporate elders in the nuclear households of the younger generation. Cubans appear to be the most assimilated to the middle-class American mentality of segregating the elderly in retirement communities or nursing homes. Puerto Ricans and Mexicans will protect parents and grandparents routinely, but even more so in advanced old age, and they are very unlikely to rely on nursing homes, even if they have the financial means.

## Somatization and Maintaining Influence

In situations of rapid social change, the Latino elderly may find themselves losing some of their influence among the younger generations. The familiar (and expected) deference and respect paid by grown children and grandchildren wanes, and the wisdom and advice of the old is given less weight than tradition requires. When this happens, somatic symptoms may be the most respectable way of maintaining some measure of influence and attention.

Nervousness, illnesses, and ailments are sometimes "called upon" to remind adult children of their obligations to their parents. One should not automatically assume pathology such as overpossessiveness or egocentrism. Inducing guilt in grown children is more acceptable in Latino families than in most Anglo-American families. When this occurs, therapists can coach adult children toward greater differentiation while protecting the old—a particularly useful tack when generational differences in acculturation are marked.

Occasionally the aging parent becomes the center of attention and activity in a large extended family—everyone rallies around the elderly's psychosomatic complaints, "sinking spells," and agitated calls to the family. The parent may attribute folk explanations to the illness and may seek the help of a folk healer. The weary, grown children and grandchildren may come to see the ailments and spells as mere attention-getting manipulations. Yet the elderly "identified patient" may be doing the double duty of bringing attention to themselves and to some unresolved issue in the family.

Mr. and Mrs. Juárez, both in their late 60s, came to the United States from Jalisco, Mexico, after their 10 adult children had immigrated over a period of 20 years. The Juarezes went to live with their youngest son because his wife had returned to work after the birth of their first child and the grandparents could babysit. In the same apartment building lived a widowed daughter, Beatriz (46), and her six children. In a third apartment lived a divorced daughter, Claudia (39), and her two children, plus two single brothers, Bernardo (29) and Ezequiel (25).

People were constantly in and out of the various apartments amid considerable conflict and accusations about responsibilities. Many of the grown children went to dance and drink on the weekends. Initially the newly arrived *abuelitos* (grandparents) disliked what they saw as their children's Americanization. They used questions and criticisms in an attempt to control the outings and visitors of their adult offspring. The older parents were particularly critical of their two daughters, whom they saw as "too old" (notice they were not "too young") to go out at night. The *abuelitos* also installed themselves on the porch or by the window and scrutinized anybody who walked in and out of the building. Nothing changed in their children's and grandchildren's behavior. Then on weekends, Mrs. Juarez began to suffer *ataques*—dizzy spells and palpitations (for a discussion of this syndrome, see Chapter 8). She panicked about getting cancer or dying. Her children were forced to cooperate to decide what to do, and to call the ambulance during her *ataques* and faintings. The doctors consistently told her the symptoms were due to "nerves." Mrs. Juárez, or her husband, always responded that her nerves would not calm until the children cooperated with each other, or at least "behaved."

The older parents' insistence on controlling their grown children's behavior was clearly anachronistic, the result of freezing the clock through many years of separation. The children continued to do as they pleased but maintained a shallow appearance of *respeto* for the traditional hierarchies and their mother's cultural preference for "taking care of all of us." I met with the adult children alone. They often used the word *respeto*, so I asked what this meant for them. It was clear that nobody believed the mother had any real authority, and they rather "rubber stamped" her words. By pretending that mother was in charge, the children supported a cultural tradition. But pretending also provided a convenient way to avoid responsibilities for managing a complex household, with its many schedules and obligations and conflicting ideas about family life.

Discussing with the children the contradictions of living with two sets of cultural values about individual freedom and strict parental controls proved enlightening. It pointed to the dilemmas and duplicity created by their interpretation of American individual freedom and democracy without clear individual responsibilities. It also highlighted their complicity in perpetuating their parents' frustrated and dramatized demands for traditional Mexican values.

Predictably, once the siblings could no longer rally around their mother's latest *ataques*, they began to criticize each other. This was more constructive, however, because it initiated processes of assuming individual and collective responsibility for change.

Conflicts of loyalty between obligations to aging parents and to the nuclear family can surface in anyone and cause considerable stress. As in the Juárez case, intergenerational stresses can be resolved without insisting that the older generation be present. In fact, most Latinos are likely to resist the idea of leveling hierarchies in "public" or using assertive communication, particularly between parents and children. If, for example, an older mother still controls too many affective areas of her married son's life, a more effective approach than encouraging confrontation would be to help him weaken the ties with his mother in a thoughtful, gentle, and gradual manner.

## The Power of Small Gestures

The almost inevitable loss of purpose and meaning in old age, so prevalent in the United States, occurs eventually with Latinos too. But ongoing connections with two or three other generations makes a difference. Therapists can capitalize on this by encouraging in others the small heartwarming and reassuring cultural gestures that pamper the elderly a little.

Earlier in this book I introduced Mrs. Santos, a 75-year-old, Spanish-speaking, Puerto Rican woman. She and her husband followed their 55-year-old daughter, Juana, from New Jersey to Canada where Juana had gone to live with her third husband. Mrs. Santos's husband died suddenly and she became depressed and displayed symptoms of senility, confusion, dizziness, and lapses of memory. Juana's new husband was very reluctant to have Mrs. Santos move permanently into their home, and Juana did not want to "rock the boat" with him. Rather, she asked her 32-year-old daughter, Maggie, a legal secretary in San Diego who loved her mother and grandmother very much, to have Mrs. Santos come live with her.

Maggie consulted me a few months after her grandmother arrived. Now she wanted to move the elderly woman to an apartment down the block, but feared that Mrs. Santos might have trouble handling the gas stove and other chores related to her self-sufficiency. Maggie planned to moonlight as a legal typist to rent an apartment for her grandmother so that she could have a little more of a young single woman's life. Our consultation included some practical case management: network building, medical and mental evaluation, and supervision by county home services to meet Mrs. Santos's needs. Yet we also talked about a system of daily routine checks between Maggie and Mrs. Santos, and one or two shared, preferably ethnic meals a week which would satisfy the emotional attachment between grandmother and grandchild.

Half-humorously, I remembered seeing many elderly men and women who went with their families to dance *el danzón* in the town square in Veracruz, Mexico, or of seeing the elderly watch their adult children and grandchildren dancing in the night clubs of Bogotá, Colombia. I asked Maggie what she thought about taking her grandmother along when she went out salsa dancing on Friday nights. We both laughed at the cultural impossibility. Instead, Maggie came up with the idea of pampering her grandmother every week by taking her to an inexpensive salon to make her feel pretty—a ritual Mrs. Santos would likely have kept had she remained in Puerto Rico.

## DYING AND GRIEVING

Memories of the homeland and feelings about uprooting may return with force when an immigrant faces death or bereavement in a foreign country. As a final "recovery of belonging," the aged may fantasize about returning home to be buried. The presence of supportive compatriots that share language, history, and values can provide invaluable support when dying or grieving a loved one's death.

As therapists we need to become aware of our own field's narrow cultural assumptions about "good" and "healthy" mourning. The cultural gulf that often lies between Anglo-American and Latino is probably at its deepest when the two face death and dying: for the Anglo-American, there is the impersonal and bounded culture of cold hospitals and austere cemeteries; for the Latino, there is a more direct, intimate, and expressive tradition around death. Sad and tragic misunderstandings may deepen this gulf further, as was shown in the case of Ricki's great aunt and the hospital staff (see Preface).

The physical and emotional support of the extended family and community provide nurturance for the bereaved. Emotions may be vented, perhaps because they are better tolerated and contained within a large, closely knit group. Equally possible are stoic resignation and acceptance. Cultural norms dictate in part how and when one must publicly display the depths of one's sentiments. The unexpressive son or daughter may raise suspicions and be labeled as having a *corazón de piedra* (stone heart). Who can mourn and how much is partly dictated by the degree of family connectedness. If someone is a distant relative but cries profusely, he or she may be criticized as not having sufficient reason to *para encender velas en este entierro* (to light the candles in this wake).

Religion also plays a role in helping family members deal with an impending loss, or in providing guidance or consolation for the ill, elderly, or bereaved. Two rituals provide a sense of involvement and encourage resignation to accept the inevitable: the first, to request a small, private mass to pray for the recovery of a seriously ill person, and second, to organize a *velada* or community mass to pray for recovery or for the salvation of the soul. Both act as anticipatory mourning rituals. The Catholic belief in the immortality of the soul may work to ameliorate some of the most frightening aspects of death.

When a person dies, the presence of the body in the home, the open casket, the quiet atmosphere, and the whispering voices during the wake encourage emotional expression. Events of the life and the death of the deceased are openly shared, and sensitivities are high. Traditionally the wake was conducted at home, but the use of funeral parlors and Protestant rituals are increasing among Latinos. Aside from their excessive expense, burials in a foreign land are emotionally very difficult for immigrants.

The Latino custom in which the oldest son is responsible for the funeral arrangements may be maintained in the United States with the requisite expenses shared among siblings and other relatives. Varying degrees of acculturation may provide an additional stress for those in charge of decisions. Family members who immigrated as young adults may not have been exposed to the cultural practices and conduct expected at times of illness and death. Feeling alone and confused, they can benefit from active contact with the extended family or substitute networks—the best sources for the preservation of healing traditions during the family's life cycle.

This chapter marks the completion of our extensive journey across the domains of MECA—migration, ecological context, family organization, and family life cycle. While this volume has focused on Latino families from the perspective of the MECA model, this new way of acknowledging and exploring the multiple, cultural contexts of our clients is applicable to all the individuals and families we see. Clearly the field of multiculturalism abounds with ideas and approaches that may be harmful or helpful to our clients. The implications of working with culture and cultural issues from the perspective of MECA and other stances is addressed in Chapter 13.

# PART VI

---

# Conclusion

---

# 13

## Current Trends and Future Directions in Multiculturalism

> The first thing you do is to forget that I am black.
> Second, you must never forget that I am black.
> —PARKER (1990, p. 297)

Our emphasis on psychotherapeutic inclusions of culture is a part of larger sociocultural trends that affect generic and particular applications of cultural frameworks in mental health. In a world in which distinguishing separate cultures is becoming increasingly difficult, this chapter addresses the changes necessary to reflect this growing complexity of collective identities.

### CONTEXTS FOR MULTICULTURALISM: A BRIEF REVIEW

Grappling with mental health and therapy issues for Latinos, or any other minority group, requires a critical understanding of the complex social forces subsumed under the rubric of multiculturalism. Indeed, as the United States increasingly becomes a society of many peoples, cultural diversity has gained unprecedented importance in literature, political science, education, philosophy, and psychology—it is, in fact, a central concern of public life. Terms such as "multiculturalism" or "identity politics" are commonly used to refer to collective movements that demand inclusion, respect for differences, and equal rights for the values and worldviews of Native Americans, African Americans, Latinos, Asian Americans, women, gays and lesbians, and many other groups that lack the power and privilege of full participation and political representation in mainstream America (Taylor & Gutmann, 1994).

The call for cultural sensitivity in mental health services isn't new. The civil rights movement demanded that institutions be more responsive and less discriminatory toward minority clients, and the nationwide development of community mental health programs in the 1970s attempted to expand services to economically disadvantaged and culturally marginalized groups (Padilla, Ruíz, & Alvarez, 1976; Rogler, Malgady, Constantino, & Blumenthal, 1987). The multiculturalist movement of the 1990s has revitalized these concerns, even while funding cutbacks threaten many public sector programs.

Despite, or perhaps because of, its vast influence, multiculturalism hasn't been without its critics. They point to the irony that the multiculturalist call for diversity is sometimes accompanied by intolerance for diversity of opinion and a rigid promotion of "political correctness," what Richard Berstein (1994) has called the "dictatorship of virtue." Indeed, if multiculturalism leads to divisiveness, culture wars, and "balkanization," with each minority against the other claiming greater oppressed status, the original purpose of multiculturalism, of creating an inclusive, humane, and just society, is defeated (Friedan, 1996). The challenge of true multiculturalism is in working toward a cohesive society while understanding, respecting, and protecting cultural differences.

Family therapy has emphasized contextual issues since its earliest days and continues to be very much a part of the multicultural movement. With its foundation in systems theory, mainstream family therapy has always regarded the behavior of families as contextual and ecological (Auerswald, 1968). Early research and scholarly writings that focused on minority families enriched the field and highlighted the importance of sociocultural context in understanding family life (Aponte & Van Deusen, 1981; Minuchin et al., 1967; Montalvo & Gutiérrez, 1983, 1988; Scheflen, 1976; Sluzki, 1979). Other notable early contributions include the work of Papajohn & Spiegel (1975) and Spiegel (1971), which compared the value orientations of various ethnic groups. The work that followed included McGoldrick, Pearce, and Giordano's (1982) examination of ethnicity and families; Boyd-Franklin's (1989) multiculturalist approach in *Black Families in Therapy;* the feminist critique of family therapy (Goldner, 1985; Hare-Mustin, 1978; Luepnitz, 1988; McGoldrick, Anderson, & Walsh, 1989; Walters, Carter, Papp, & Silverstein, 1988); multiculturalism as an organizing framework in work (Breunlin, Schwartz, & MacKune-Karrer, 1992); the inclusion of ethnic and migration variables in family therapy (Saba, Karrer, & Hardy 1989); the idea of "cultural consultants" in the Just Therapy approach in New Zealand (Waldegrave, 1990); and my own work, which proposes a more comprehensive definition of culture and challenges the assumed universality of family therapy theory (Falicov, 1983, 1988b, 1995b; Falicov & Brudner-White, 1983).

Clearly a renewed interest in minorities and in "differences that make a difference" permeates society. This emphasis on multiculturalism poses myriad challenges and dilemmas for family therapy theorists and practitioners, not the least of which is defining minority and ethnic groups.

## COLLECTIVE IDENTITIES AND CULTURAL EXCHANGE: A WORLD OF VARIATION

Defining specific ethnic groups, or describing "collective identities," is at first glance both possible and practical. We look at the worldviews, values, and customs of certain groups and assume these traits to be normative and stable. We talk about how Latinos value family closeness and interdependence, Anglos are time conscious and schedule oriented, the Irish like to tell stories and drink. However, as shown throughout this book, on close examination, deciding about sameness and difference isn't so simple.

Even if one could describe characteristics that make up something like Jewishness or Mexicanness or Blackness, ethnicity is profoundly modified by other variables that affect behavior, experience, and worldviews. The cultural experiences of African American women are very different from those of African American men. A millionaire Mexican executive with a home in Beverly Hills and another home in Mexico City has a different position in his culture than a poor peasant from a small, isolated place in Oaxaca who lived in a border Mexican city and later entered the United States illegally and he now waits every day to pick up inconsistent, underpaid jobs. A Puerto Rican elder who practices *espiritismo*[1] to deal with the loss of her daughter to cancer has a different connection to her heritage than the Puerto Rican mother who only trusts her Roman Catholic priest for advice about her drug-addicted son.

Collective cultural identities are not essential attributes—they are historically and socially constructed within ethnic and cultural groups themselves. Gender, race, class, religion, nationality, and even cohort (the historical generation into which a person is born) all contribute to one's cultural meaning systems and worldviews, and must be taken into account when describing an individual's or family's culture. Consistencies of thoughts, feelings, and behavior lend a sense of familiarity and community for people who share the same culture. But inconsistencies, variabilities, and novelties exist as well.

Cultural identities are also influenced by the constructs supplied by the dominant society (and often by its narrow, denigrated, or self-serving views about particular groups). Furthermore, collective identities are sub-

ject to evolving ideas, socioeconomic change, and shifting world conditions, such as globalization.[2] Understanding these influences, and the myriad blendings of culture that result, helps us avoid treating original cultures
as static. But how do we address in therapy this incredibly complex, moving
construct we vaguely call the "culture" of a person or a family?

## MULTICULTURALISM AND PSYCHOTHERAPY

### The Role of Cultural Diversity

One of the first effects of bringing culture into the therapy room is that it
upsets our theoretical applecart. Multiculturalism challenges what particular schools of thought—psychoanalytic, systemic, structural, strategic, and
so on—consider to be universal. Views about how families function, how
problems develop, and how change is facilitated by those approaches may
be local ideas originated (and unwittingly imposed as universally valid on
clients) by the professional middle-class in the United States. It follows
from this that many diverse beliefs or behavior that would be judged as dysfunctional, or at least idiosyncratic, may in fact be part of a cultural heritage of beliefs and meaning systems that are different from those in which
a psychotherapist has been schooled.

A multicultural therapist incorporates a critically questioning attitude
toward Anglo-American biases and would have a perspective on his or her
own cultural biases. Instead, a practice based on curiosity and respect for
diversity explores the healing resources within the client's culture (González, Biever, & Gardner, 1994). Cultural insights about collective identities
support representation and accommodation to new and diverse ethnic
groups. Further, critiques of mainstream theories may lead to totally new
perspectives and genuine transformations of theory and practice, rather
than only mere accommodations of taken-for-granted psychotherapy concepts and techniques (Gergen, Gulerce, Lock, & Misra, 1996; Sampson,
1993; Taylor & Guttman, 1994). Such cultural criticism at home aims to
"bring the insights gained on the periphery back to the center to raise
havoc with our settled ways of thinking . . . " (Marcus & Fischer, 1986, p.
138). Thus multiculturalism holds a transformative promise for those theories we once assumed had universal validity. In Parts IV and V, I discussed
concepts of family life that raise critical questions about the customary assumptions of mainstream psychotherapy.

### The Role of Social Justice

Multiculturalism comprises more than a respect for diverse meanings or
values and a move toward culturally based theories. A component of social
justice is essential to the movement. Members of collective identity political

movements—African Americans, Chicanos, gay rights advocates, or feminists—maintain they have been denied their own voice in determining the conditions of their lives and identities (Sampson, 1993; Young, 1990). Minority activists believe that a standard derived from the values of white Western men has been used to judge all other groups. They seek redress not only by recognizing the legitimacy of their own diverse cultural heritage, but also by obtaining equal access to resources and equal rights (or social justice) for each minority.

In the clinical arena, this social justice position directs the attention of therapists and clients to life conditions and power differentials that limit social and economic opportunities, promote internalized racism, and affect psychological development and mental health for those who are poor, actively marginalized, or fall outside of the mainstream. It is insufficient to pay respect to ethnic diversity without reference to a societal context that may downgrade precisely the same cultural diversity. (Montalvo & Gutiérrez, 1988).[3] Without a lens that includes issues of racism, sexism, and other social inequities, ethnic preferences may be used as explanations for economic failure, domestic violence, or poor school performance, while the larger negative effects of poverty and social discrimination are downplayed, as I discussed in Parts II and III.

A social justice practice connects mental health issues with experiences of social oppression and limiting cultural definitions. This practice has also called needed attention to the issues of power, powerlessness, and the need for empowerment in individuals' and families' interactions with larger systems, including therapy (Hardy & Lazzloff, 1994; Korin, 1994; Prilleltensky, 1994, 1997). Therapists who focus on social justice or responsibility often assign intentionality to cultural forces by considering them as either oppressive, when they come from the white dominant groups, or as liberating, when they are part of the native or ethnic subculture. Concepts of cultural resistance (Weingarten, 1995)[4] and Just Therapy (Waldegrave, 1990) guide these approaches.

The resurrection within clinical and social psychology of approaches whereby clients obtain an insightful, empowering awareness of the socio-economic, political, cultural, and ideological circumstances that affect their lives has been variously subsumed under social justice, and sometimes under social ethics and "psychology at the service of social change" (Prilleltensky, 1990). For the sake of consistency I use the term social justice here, but I find social ethics, social responsibility, and even social action more accurately reflect the praxis domain of therapy. "Social justice" attributes to therapists a capacity for correction and restitution of social ills that seems to me to be beyond the capacity of the individual endeavor, however praiseworthy.

Furthermore, I believe this focus on the sociopolitical aspects of a client's life problems should occur within a collaborative context, where the client is fully informed about the ideological position of the therapist rather than the therapists attributing to themselves the righteous sole capacity to administer social justice. The term ethics reflects the informed joint agreement, the term social action refers to the empowering elements of the approach. In this book I connect personal issues with social themes within a context of conjoint, client-therapist reflection about the effects of social, racial, or gender inequalities. Empowerment is often a by-product of these reflections.

Two constructs, which address the complex relationship between culture and psychotherapy and between society and psychotherapy, are central to acquiring cultural sensitivity: (1) a cultural diversity practice that respects cultural preferences and critically examines existing models of the family and Anglo-American theories and techniques; and (2) a social justice practice that focuses on the effects of power differentials (due to gender, economic, and racial inequities) on individual and family well-being. Other attempts to understand these complex dynamics have identified cultural dissonance approaches, which focus on problems that emerge because of differences between the ethnic and dominant culture, and institutional racism approaches which view the problems of minorities as stemming from experiences of discrimination (De Hoyos, De Hoyos, & Anderson, 1986; Terry & Domokos-Cheng Ham, 1994).

While cultural diversity and social justice are critical components of multiculturalism, individual and family resilience, creativity, and personal agency are also part of the equation. Therapy must not become a form of social and cultural reductionism. The client's biography is always unique, though interlaced with history and larger sociocultural patterns. To date, therapists vary widely in their adherence to the cultural diversity or/and the social justice aspect of the multicultural approach and their evaluation of its usefulness.

## CULTURAL EMPHASIS: A SPECTRUM OF CHOICE

Therapists can and have made the choice to consider cultural influences as either tangential and optional, or as central and necessary to the theory and practice of family therapy. For some clinicians, culture provides a background narrative and is seen as one of a multitude of forces that shape a family's predicament. Therapist and client have the choice to reflect upon these cultural forces or not. At the other extreme, therapists who view culture as an overpowering foreground narrative believe that many emotional problems are connected to dominant, constraining definitions imposed by socialization or causing alienation from one's ethnic identity and traditions or from disempowering social forces. For this latter group, the healing potential lies in emotionally and ideationally reconnecting clients with their cultural myths, legacies, and sense of belonging to their cultural community. Clinicians are further guided in the way they approach culture by taking certain positions—more implicit than explicit—about the relationship between culture and family therapy. The following section examines three of these positions and their implications for family therapy, and then situates a fourth approach, which has been the focus of this book.

## The Universalist

As can be expected, this position maintains that families are more alike than different. Similarities are emphasized and universal predicaments are cited: all children need love, and all parenting involves various combinations of nurturance and control. A universalist position emphasizes similarities rather than differences in both intrapsychic and interpersonal processes. Some therapists who believe in the stable universality of family processes claim that contextual variables such as race, gender, or ethnicity are irrelevent distractions from basic individual and family processes (Friedman, 1994). Indeed, most psychological concepts and theories are based on universal assumptions: object relations, multigenerational transmission, triangulation, and life cycle transitions, to name a few. Those who assume a universalist position regard culture as tangential to therapy.

It is undoubtedly correct that many shared biological and social imperatives create similarities across cultures. It is also crucial to appreciate the sameness between groups. The danger, however, lies in therapists' vulnerability to ethnocentric errors while believing their stance to be objective and impartial. An experienced Argentinian family therapist, Estrella Joselevich, told me about witnessing a young capable trainee interview a Bolivian family that had lived in the mountains but had recently moved to the capital. The family spoke about the grandparents as though they were alive and living in the household. Much to her dismay, the trainee later learned they had been talking about the skulls of their ancestors, which they kept in a closet at home. Because the trainee's repertoire of hypotheses didn't include a cultural (i.e., religious) inquiry for possible explanations, she believed the family had developed a psychotic reaction around the grandparents' death. In this case, the trainee assumed (probably correctly, to some extent) that processes of grief and mourning have universal similarities. But, in fact, the family was appropriately following a ritual cultural prescription of their peasant group, a subculture within the larger Bolivian culture.

By emphasizing universal similarities only, and minimizing cultural differences, a universalist position may cause therapists to fall in the trap of ethnocentrism, since the therapist will assume the majority view as the standard of health (Falicov, 1983; Walsh, 1983). Unwittingly, stylistic cultural forms will be seen as problematic or pathological and the therapist's hypothesis or theory will be assumed to be universally, rather than locally, valid. Ricki's case, which was cited in the Preface, is another example of this type of bias. The normative use of Murray Bowen's self-differentiation scale to judge the emotional development of family members of any culture is typical of the universalist position, and without the benefit of cultural relativism.

## The Particularist

At the other extreme is the particularist position, which states that families are more different than they are alike. Each family's idiosyncrasies make it a culture unto itself. Each family's personal themes, myths, customs, and rituals, passed on from generation to generation, become labeled as the family's culture. Jules Henry (1963), an anthropologist, moved in with families to conduct ethnographic studies of their unique, individual lives and called his work a study of families' cultures. He also studied through painstaking observation the ideas and beliefs that governed interpersonal relations at a therapeutic institution for emotionally disturbed children. He called this a study of the "interpersonal culture" of that setting.

Here the word culture refers more to the present and past beliefs of each particular family than to regularities in the broader social context. A case of anorexia nervosa may be seen as idiosyncratically linked to an over-involved mother and a peripheral father without awareness of the gender specialization of parents and the social demands for thinness in young women. Much like in the notion of an alcoholic family culture, the transmission of culture comes from the interior of the family and occurs intergenerationally rather than from the family in interaction with the larger context. From a particularist perspective, no generalizations can be made about the relationship between family and the larger culture, and therefore the interior of the family becomes responsible for everything. Virtually all psychotherapy up to the 1980s falls into this category, wherein all family interactions were regarded as idiosyncratic.

## The Ethnic-Focused

This third position stresses predictable diversity of thoughts, feelings, and behavior, of attitudes toward health or illness, and of customs and rituals among different groups. The dimension responsible for this diversity is "ethnicity." It speaks to the tendency of Irish people to marry late, the inclination of Italians to draw tight boundaries around the biological family, the strange panic disease called Koro among the southeastern Chinese, the extreme fear called Susto among Latin Americans, or the acknowledgment of native healers such as *curanderos*, among myriad collective idiosyncrasies. This position, best represented by McGoldrick, Pearce, and Giordano (1982) and McGoldrick, Giordano, and Pearce (1996), has been pivotal in developing sensitivity to ethnic differences. It requires therapists to have knowledge about the characteristic traits of different ethnic groups, and provides information along those lines. In spite of its proven merit, this approach has drawbacks, as its own proponents admit.

By definition, an ethnic-focused position tends to systematize the concept of shared meanings due to ethnicity, and therefore ethnocultural groups may appear more homogeneous than they really are. This position does not address the multidimensionalities of collective identities. There is little room for cultural inconsistencies, dilemmas, or contradictions.

The ethnic-focused approach also assumes that the observer is objective. It portrays factual information about ethnic groups much in the same way that classic ethnographies described distant cultures recorded by a neutral observer (Rosaldo, 1989). Family therapists should take into account the more recent notion in anthropology that "the other" or the "former native" may not really be separate from the perceptions, goals, and the subjectivity of the observer (E. M. Bruner, 1986).

Another problem is that ethnic-focused generalizations tend to portray culture as static and stable rather than changing and unstable, which is true of most present cultures. An anthropologist studying a hunter-gatherer society (Bower, 1989) followed an aboriginal woman into the fields in order to record a song she was singing to her baby. He hoped that he could open a window to the past. As he got nearer he recognized the lyrics of a familiar English lullaby. Distressed and disappointed that he was not finding what he had set out to find, he concluded that there are no "native cultures" left. Even the most culturally isolated societies are in constant flux, largely moving toward Western ways.[5]

A related drawback is the fact that the ethnic-focused approach requires a great deal of a priori knowledge on the part of the therapist. This information is difficult to obtain, given so many ethnic groups and subgroups (Akamatsu, 1995). It also tends to homogenize and stereotype diversity because it can only be transmitted by making broad generalizations. Like the anthropologist in the example above, therapists may set out to find family traits that don't exist in their particular client families. The ethnic family may then be thought of as deviant from "its own norms" and possibly dysfunctional: a case of an iatrogenically induced diagnosis. Ethnic sensitivity may become just another version of "the tyranny of cultural correctness."

Taken altogether these limitations may cause therapists to be confident in their knowledge of the family's culture and inadvertently fall into biases of ethnic stereotyping—exaggerating differences between themselves and their clients (Falicov, 1983). After visiting an elderly Mexican woman who refused to leave her apartment, a young therapist returned to the clinic convinced that she had simply witnessed a typically Hispanic living room with walls painted in red and crucifixes with burning candles on every wall. Problematic aspects in the woman's behavior (and in her living room) and the rapidly changing, dangerous neighborhood were minimized in the name of ethnic sensitivity.

It is possible to avoid some of these pitfalls of an ethnic-focused approach; for example, therapists can learn more about a particular group by taking a hands-on approach in the community or agency where clinical practice takes place. They can become participant-observers in a specific community (perhaps through schools, agencies, churches, or clubs), learning through inquiry and experience rather than coming in as a priori experts. The constraints and the risks of the specific gang and drug subculture, the natural strengths of the neighborhood group, the particular resiliencies and new stresses of old family and church rituals are learned on site and with each specific case rather than as static descriptions of rules, roles, or customs that have either been idealized or historically constructed.

## From Either/Or to Both/And

The ethnic-focused position, which requires knowing as many details about particular cultures as possible can be contrasted to a "not-knowing" stance[6] in therapy. Not-knowing approaches are based on curiosity, and encourage a dialogue that takes into account all meanings—cultural and personal—as they emerge in the therapeutic situation. From this perspective, academic, personal, or consulting knowledge of the culture is not necessarily required. In my opinion, a both/and approach, which combines a not-knowing stance with information about specific cultures that is relevant to the conduct of therapy, can provide the most beneficial means of working with diverse client families, as the following case illustrates.

> Behind the one-way mirror I witnessed an emerging power struggle between a family therapy trainee at a well-known training institution and a Puerto Rican family which I shall call Bernal. The therapist insisted that the father's delusions should be treated with psychotropic medication. But the family politely refused pharmacotherapy.
>
> I suggested to the therapist that she ask the family if they had other health or religious resources that might be helpful (see Chapter 8). The wife said she thought her husband would get better because prayer would help him. I suggested the therapist adopt a curious stance by asking the family, "How does prayer work?" To this the mother replied that she met twice a week with her friends to pray at a local storefront church, and all of their prayers together swelled up to a powerful, luminous energy that could counteract the dark forces that had overtaken her husband's psyche. The family believed in the power of the gradual accumulation of these positive forces through prayer, and they felt that medication would drastically interfere with this process.

A therapist with knowledge of cultural details, attuned to the possibility that religion may be playing a role in the family's resistance to a "universal" medical cure for delusions, would have inquired about the family's religious resources. A therapist with a not-knowing approach toward culture might have arrived at the same place, but more likely would have stayed close to the parameters provided by the family. The family, conscious of differences with the dominant culture views, would not have volunteered their prayer practice. One might be tempted to say the first therapist would have done better. Not necessarily. The ethnic-focused therapist may have stopped at a simple respect for the family's cultural solution, while a not-knowing, curious stance revealed how prayer works in this particular subculture of religion. Weaving back and forth between these stances—one informed by cultural knowledge and the other guided by curiosity—could clarify the family's fears that medication would preclude their prayers from working. The therapist could then ask the family to better define what kind of help they needed and were willing to accept from the clinic.

This example typifies a fourth approach to culture—one that's inclusive and doesn't force a choice between two necessary and useful perspectives. In such a both/and position, the therapist must be comfortable with an ever-present "double discourse"—an ability to see the universal human similarities that unite us beyond color, class, ethnicity, and gender, while simultaneously recognizing and respecting culture-specific differences that exist due to color, class, ethnicity, and gender. This double discourse may be explicit or implicit, foreground or background, expanding or shrinking the cultural emphasis. It may come about from a basic knowledge of cultural differences or from a curious and respectful not-knowing stance, depending on the demands of the particular clinical case. This both/and position also includes at all times a particularist view that recognizes and respects the uniqueness and idiosyncracies of each family's story and choices.

MECA, or the multidimensional, ecosystemic, comparative approach, is a means of engaging in a both/and position. It encompasses the ability to hold the previous three positions. It offers a comprehensive definition of culture, a method for making meaningful comparisons, and room for multiple and evolving cultural narratives.

## A VIEW TO THE FUTURE

As mentioned earlier, one of the great dilemmas in writing a book about Latinos in family therapy is the inherent potential for reifying or stereotyping culture; in this case, the collective identity subsumed under the label Latino. This is particularly true in an increasingly global environment in which hybridizations and remarkable mixtures of cultural beliefs and practices are becoming the norm rather than the exception for Latinos and other individuals and families. Culture is, indeed, ever-changing and evolving, as is our understanding of it. These complexities are what MECA attempts to address, while acknowledging and respecting the existence of distinct meaning systems that might fall under the rubric of culture.

The framework presented offers a way of thinking about parameters of similarities and differences that are relevant to therapeutic practice. The generic parameters, namely ecological context, migration/acculturation, family organization and family life cycle can be applied to the study of diverse cultural groups and not only to Latino groups. Underlying connections between, say, the family organization or the social circumstances of different cultural groups can be discovered along with the variations across groups. This opens a different possibility from learning the special characteristics of separate and distinct groups by using a different set of categories for each group—an approach that stresses differences only and unwittingly supports separateness. Relevant to this issue is an interview about the emphasis on cultural diversity in clinical practice and supervision, in which Montalvo (1994) eloquently argues the importance of appreciating sameness between groups, the cross-cultural common ground, the perception of kinship and "the underlying core of our humanity" (p. 2). He goes further when he comments that by celebrating differences only and not solidarities, similarities and unifying shared circumstances, we may reflect in the training situation trends toward societal fragmentation and tribalism.

Rather than making culture marginal to theory and practice, a multidimensional, ecosystemic, comparative approach takes culture into the mainstream of all teaching and learning. It maintains that it is possible and desirable to integrate cultural sensitivity at every step in the process of learning how to observe, how to conceptualize, and how to work therapeutically, regardless of theoretical orientation. For example, if the issue being considered is divorce, remarriage, or stepparenting, what are the ethnic, social class, or religious differences one may expect to see reflected on these events? And what are the universals that transcend particular group variations? Culture is then discussed in the context of a specific issue rather than in the abstract.

Although suggestions and illustrations of therapeutic interventions are given, MECA does not prescribe a particular approach to conducting therapy. Rather it introduces cultural relativism that can be applied to many established schools of family therapy and practice.

With MECA, the therapist always views families in a comparative, sociocultural context. Therapists make a quick holistic assessment of all the contexts to which the family belongs and attempt to understand the resources, the constraints, and the cultural dilemmas those multiple contexts create. Since families distill and draw selectively from the groups and ideologies to which they belong, the therapist should not assume that knowing the context is knowing the family. Consistent with the reality of shifting multiple contexts, there is no list of "dos" and "don'ts" when working with Latinos or any other group. There is only one do and one don't—do ask, and don't assume. Familiarity with various contexts provides an avenue for raising relevant questions—the answers will be cocreated between the family and the therapist's impressions, which are likewise derived from being a witness and a participant in diverse cultural contexts.

Like the lines of the Pat Parker poem at the beginning of this chapter, we must relate to each other's universal humanity, while not forgetting about each other's significant and meaningful cultural contexts. The borderlands we share can be a meeting place for these conversations to begin.

## NOTES

1. A belief in invisible spirits (often the ghost of a dead significant other) that can attach themselves, or fleetingly materialize, to human beings.
2. Although globalization makes all societies increasingly more similar to each other, this notion can be overplayed. The same symbols, codes, or objects can take on different meanings in different contexts and social situations. The child able to play with a Mickey Mouse toy in a small Mexican village has a relationship of subordination and inaccessibility quite different than the Anglo-American child who enjoys this privilege and Disneyland outings as a matter of fact, although both children are indeed playing with the same toy (Valenzuela, personal communication, 1995).
3. Such is the case with school programs that teach youngsters about the great men and women in their cultural heritage without helping them discover how the same heritage can "help them deal with deteriorating neighborhoods, unemployment, and their own catastrophe—a national dropout rate for Puerto Ricans twice as great as the national average" (Montalvo & Gutiérrez, 1988, p. 182).
4. This "cultural resistance" position supports protesting culturally imposed curtailment of self-definition and thus is clearly rooted in an individualistic cultural position (see Fowers & Richardson, 1996).
5. Edward M. Bruner (1986) goes further when he says: "The Pueblo Indians are performing our theory; they are enacting the story we tell about them in our professional journals. We wonder if it is their story or ours. Which is the inside or the outside view . . ." (pp. 148–149).
6. Harlene Anderson and the late Henry Goolishian (1988) are the most articulate and philosophically grounded advocates of this position.

# References

Acuña, R. F. (1996). *Anything but Mexican: Chicanos in contemporary Los Angeles.* London: Verso.

Ainsworth, M. D. S., Blehar, M. C., Waters, E., & Wall, S. (1978). *Patterns of attachment: A psychological study of the strange situation.* Hillsdale, NJ: Erlbaum.

Akamatsu, N. N. (1995). The defiant daughter and compliant mother: multicultural dialogues on woman's role. *In Session: Psychotherapy in Practice, 1*(4), 43–55.

Alonso, L., & Jeffrey, W. D. (1988). Mental illness complicatd by the *santería* belief in spirit possession. *Hospital and Community Psychiatry, 39*(11), 1188–1191.

Alvírez, D., Bean, F. D., & Williams, D. (1981). The Mexican American family. In C. H. Mindel & R. W. Habenstein (Eds.), *Ethnic families in America: Patterns and variations* (pp. 271–292). New York: Elsevier.

Amaro, H., Russo, N. F., & Johnson, P. (1987). Hispanic women and mental health: An overview of contemporary issues in research and practice. *Psychology of Women Quarterly, 11, 393–407.*

American Psychiatric Association. (1994). *Diagnostic and statistical manual of mental disorders* (4th ed.). Washington, DC: Author.

Anderson, H., & Goolishian, H. A. (1988). Human systems as linguistic systems: Preliminary and evolving ideas about the implications for clinical theory. *Family Process, 27,* 371–393.

Angel, R., & Guarnaccia, P. (1989). Mind, body and culture: somatization among Hispanics. *Social Science and Medicine, 28,* 1229–1238.

Anzaldúa, G. (1987). *Borderlands/La frontera: The new mestiza.* San Francisco: Spinsters/Aunt Lute.

Aponte, H. J. (1976). The family-school interview: An ecostructural approach. *Family Process, 15,* 303–311.

Aponte, H. J. (1994). *Bread and spirit: Therapy with the new poor.* New York: Norton.

Aponte, H. J., & Van Deusen, J. (1981). Structural family therapy. In A. S. Gurman & D. P. Kniskern (Eds.), *Handbook of family therapy* (pp. 310–360). New York: Brunner/Mazel.

Applewhite, S. L. (1995). *Curanderismo:* Demystifying the health beliefs and practices of elderly Mexican Americans. *Health and Social Work, 20*(4), 247–253.

Aramoni, A. (1972). Machismo. *Psychology Today, 5*(8), 69–72.

Aron, A. (1992). Testimonio: A bridge between psychotherapy and sociotherapy. In E. Cole, O. Espin, & E. D. Rothblum (Eds.), *Refugee women and their mental health: Shattered societies, shattered lives* (pp. 173–189). Binghamton, NY: Haworth.

Aronowitz, M. (1984). The social and emotional adjustment of immigrant children: A review of literature. *International Migration Review, 18,* 237–257.

Auerswald, E. H. (1968). Interdisciplinary versus ecological approach. *Family Process, 7,* 202–215.

Auerswald, E. H. (1990). Toward epistemological transformation in the education and training of family therapists. In M. P. Mirkin (Ed.), *The social and political contexts of family therapy.* Boston: Allyn & Bacon.

Augenbraum, H., & Stavans, I. (1993). *Growing up Latino.* New York: Houghton Mifflin.

Azieri, M. (1982). The politics of exile: Trends and dynamics of political change among Cuban-Americans. *Cuban Studies, 7,* 55–74.

Baca-Zinn, M. (1975). Political familism: Toward sex role equality in Chicano families. *Aztlán, 6*(1), 13–26.

Baca-Zinn, M. (1982). Familism among Chicanos: A theoretical overview. *Humboldt Journal of Social Relations, 10,* 224–238.

Baca-Zinn, M. (1994). Feminist rethinking from racial-ethnic families. In M. Baca-Zinn & B. T. Dill (Eds.), *Women of color in U.S. society* (pp. 303–314). Philadelphia: Temple University Press.

Baca-Zinn, M. (1995). Social science theorizing for Latino families in the age of diversity. In R. E. Zambrana (Ed.), *Understanding Latino families: Scholarship, policy, and practice.* London: Sage.

Barsky, A. J., & Kleiman, G. I. (1983). Hypochondriasis, bodily complaints and somatic styles. *American Journal of Psychiatry, 140,* 273–283.

Barthes, R. (1974). *S/Z.* New York: Hill & Wang.

Bartra, R. (1987). *La jaula de la melancolía: Identidad y metamorfosis del Mexicano.* Mexico, D. F.: Editorial Grifalso.

Bastida, E. (1984). Reconstructing the world at sixty: Older Cubans in the U.S.A. *Gerontologist, 24,* 465–470.

Bateson, M. C. (1994). *Peripheral visions: Learning along the way.* New York: Harper Collins.

Bean, F. D., & Tienda, M. (1987). *The Hispanic population of the United States.* New York: Russell Sage.

Becerra, R. M., & de Anda, D. (1984). Pregnancy and motherhood among Mexican American adolescents. *Health and Social Work, 9*(2), 106–123.

Behar, R., & León, J. (1994). Bridges to Cuba/ *Puentes a Cuba. Michigan Quarterly Review, 33,* 477–496.

Benavides, J. (1992, October 17). Mujeres rule the roosters. *Santa Barbara News Press,* p. B1.

Benería, L., & Roldán, M. (1987). *The crossroads of class and gender: Industrial homework, subcontracting and household dynamics in Mexico City.* Chicago: University of Chicago Press.

Bennett, L. A., Wolin, S. J., & McCavity, K. J. (1988). Family identity, ritual, and myth: A cultural perspective on life cycle transitions. In C. J. Falicov (Ed.), *Family transitions: Continuity and change over the life cycle.* New York: Guilford Press.

Bergin, A. E. (1991). Values and religious issues in psychotherapy and mental health. *American Psychologist, 46,* 394–403.

Bernal, G. (1982). Cuban families. In M. McGoldrick, J. K. Pearce, & J. Giordano (Eds.), *Ethnicity and family therapy.* New York: Guilford Press.

Bernal, G., & Florez-Ortíz, Y. (1982). Latino families in therapy: Engagement and evaluation. *Journal of Marital and Family Therapy,* July, 357–365.

Bernal, G., & Gutiérrez, M. (1988). Cubans. In L. Comas-Díaz & E. H. Griffith (Eds.), *Clinical guidelines in cross-cultural mental health*. New York: Wiley.

Bernal, M. E., Saénz, D. S., & Knight, G. P. (1995). Ethnic identity and adaptation of Mexican American youths in school settings. In A. M. Padilla (Ed.), *Hispanic psychology: Critical issues in theory and research*. Thousand Oaks, CA: Sage.

Bernstein, R. (1994). *Multiculturalism and the battle for America's future*. New York: Knopf.

Berry, J. W., Trimble, J. E., & Olmedo, E. L. (1986). Assessment of acculturation. In W. J. Lonner & J. W. Berry (Eds.), *Field methods in cross-cultural research*. Beverly Hills, CA: Sage.

Berry, S. (1996). Personal communication. [Research in progress on adolescent "solo" immigrants.]

Betancourt, H., & López, S. R. (1993). The study of culture, ethnicity, and race in American psychology. *American Psychologist, 48*(6), 629–637.

Boswell, T. D., & Curtis, J. R. (1984). *The Cuban-American experience: Culture, images, and perspectives*. Totowa, NJ: Rowman & Allanheld.

Boszormenyi-Nagy, I. (1987). *Foundations of contextual therapy*. New York: Brunner/Mazel.

Boszormenyi-Nagy, I., Grunebaum, J., & Ulrich, D. (1981). Contextual therapy. In A. Gurman & D. P. Kniskern (Eds.), *Handbook of family therapy* (Vol. II). New York: Brunner/Mazel.

Boszormenyi-Nagy, I., & Krasner, B. (1986). *Between give and take: A clinical guide to contextual therapy*. New York: Brunner/Mazel.

Bourgois, P., (1995). *In search of respect: Selling crack in El Barrio*. New York: Cambridge University Press.

Bower, B. (1989). A world that never existed. *Science News, 135*(17), 264–266.

Boyd-Franklin, N. (1989). *Black families in therapy*. New York: Guilford Press.

Brandon, G. (1991). The uses of plants in healing in an Afro-Cuban religion, *Santería*. *Journal of Black Studies 22*(1), 55–76.

Breunlin, D. C., Schwartz, R. C., & MacKune-Karrer, B. (1992). *Metaframeworks: Transcending the models of family therapy*. San Francisco: Jossey-Bass.

Bronfenbrenner, U. (1977). Toward an experimental ecology of human development. *American Psychologist, 45*, 513–530.

Bronfman, M., Amuchástegui, A., Martina, R. M., Minello, N., Rivas, M., & Rodríguez, G. (1995). *SIDA en Mexico: Migración, adolescencia y género*. Mexico: Información Profesional Especializada.

Bronstein, P. (1984). Differences in mothers' and fathers' behaviors toward children: A cross-cultural comparison. *Developmental Psychology, 20*, 995–1003.

Bronstein, P. (1988). Father-child interaction: Implications for gender role socialization. In P. Bronstein & C.P. Cowan (Eds.), *Fatherhood today: Men's changing role in the family* (pp. 107–124). New York: Wiley.

Brown, L. (1995). Cultural diversity in feminist therapy: Theory and practice. In H. Landrine (Ed.), *Bringing cultural diversity to feminist psychology: Theory, research, and practice*. Washington, DC: American Psychological Association.

Bruner, E. M. (1986). Ethnography as narrative. In V. W. Turner & E. M. Bruner (Eds.), *The anthropology of experience* (pp. 139–158). Urbana: University of Illinois Press.

Bruner, J. (1986). Value presuppositions of developmental theory. In L. Cirillo & S. Wapner (Eds.), *Value presuppositions in theories of human development* (pp. 19–28). Hillsdale, NJ: Erlbaum.

Burnam, M. A., Hough, R. L., Kerna, M., Escobar, J. I., & Telles, C. A. (1987). Acculturation and lifetime prevalence of psychiatric disorders among Mexican Americans in Los Angeles. *Journal of Health and Social Behavior, 28*, 89–102.

Bustamante, J. (1995). *The socioeconomics of undocumented migration flood.* Presentation at the Center for U.S.–Mexican Studies, University of California, San Diego.

Cade, B. W., & Cornwell, M. (1985). New realities for old: Some uses of teams and one-way screens in therapy. In D. Campbell & R. Draper (Eds.), *Applications of systemic family therapy: The Milan approach* (pp. 47–57). London: Grune & Stratton.

Canino, G. (1982). Transactional family patterns: A preliminary exploration of Puerto Rican female adolescents. In R. E. Zambrana (Ed.), *Work, family and health: Latina women in transition* (pp. 27–36). New York: Hispanic Research Center, Fordham University.

Canino, G., & Canino, I. A. (1982). Culturally syntonic family therapy for migrant Puerto Ricans. *Hospital and Community Psychiatry, 33*(4), 299–303.

Canino, I. A., Rubio-Stipec, M., Canino, G., & Escobar, J. I. (1992). Functional somatic symptoms: A cross-ethnic comparison. *American Journal of Orthopsychiatry, 62*(4), 605–612.

Casas, J. M., Wagenheim, B. R., Banchero, R., & Mendoza-Romero, J. (1995). Hispanic masculinity: Myth or psychological schema meriting clinical consideration. In A. Padilla (Ed.), *Hispanic psychology: Critical issues in theory and research.* London: Sage.

Castaneda, C. (1972). *The teachings of Don Juan: A Yaqui way of knowledge.* Berkeley: University of California Press.

Castillo, A. (1996). *Goddess of the Americas, la diosa de las Américas: Writings on the Virgin of Guadalupe.* New York: Riverhead Books.

Castillo, R., Waitzkin, H., Ramírez, Y., Escobar, J. I. (1995). Somatization in primary care, with a focus on immigrants and refugees. *Archives of Family Medicine, 4,* 637–646.

Castro, F. G., Furth, P., & Karlow, H. (1984). The health beliefs of Mexican, Mexican American and Anglo American women. *Hispanic Journal of Behavioral Sciences, 6*(4), 365–383.

Cecchin, G. (1987). Hypothesizing, circularity, and neutrality revisited: An invitation to curiosity. *Family Process, 26,* 405–413.

Chapa, J., & Valencia, R. R. (1993). Latino population growth, demographic characteristics, and educational stagnation: An examination of recent trends. *Hispanic Journal of Behavioral Sciences, 15*(2), 165–187.

Chávez, D. (1994). *Face of an angel.* New York: Warner Books.

Chávez, L. (1985). Households, migration, and labor market participation: The adaptation of Mexicans to life in the United States. *Urban Anthropology, 14,* 301–346.

Ciola, A. (1996). *Estar sentado entce dos sillas: La condición del migrante.* In W. Santi (Ed.), *Herramientas para psicoterapéutas.* Buenos Aires: Paidós.

Cisneros, S. (1994). *The house on Mango Street.* New York: Random House.

Cisneros, S. (1995, fall–winter). In two humors. *Sí Magazine, 1,* 68–70.

Clark, M., & Mendelson, M. (1975). Mexican-American aged in San Francisco. In W. C. Sze (Ed.), *Human life cycle.* New York: Jason Aronson.

Cohen, L. M. (1980). Stress and coping among Latin American women immigrants. In G. V. Coelho & P. I. Ahmed (Eds.), *Uprooting and development: Dilemmas of coping with modernization.* New York: Plenum Press.

Comas-Díaz, L. (1981). Puerto Rican *espiritismo* and psychotherapy. *American Journal of Orthopsychiatry, 51*(4), 636–645.

Comas-Díaz, L. (1989). Culturally relevant issues and treatment implications for Hispanics. In D. R. Koslow & E. Salett (Eds.), *Crossing cultures in mental health.* Washington, DC: Society for International Education Training and Research.

Comas-Díaz, L. (1994). Lati Negra. *Journal of Feminist Family Therapy, 5*(3/4), 35–74.

Comas-Díaz, L. (1995). Puerto Ricans and sexual child abuse. In L. A. Fontes (Ed.), *Sexual abuse in nine North American cultures: Treatment and prevention* (pp. 31–66). Thousand Oaks, CA: Sage.

Comas-Díaz, L., & Jacobsen, F. M. (1991). Ethnocultural transference and counter-transference in the therapeutic dyad. *American Journal of Orthopsychiatry, 61,* 392–402.

Constantino, G., Malgady, R., & Rogler, L. (1986). Cuento therapy: A culturally sensitive modality for Puerto Rican children. *Journal of Consulting and Clinical Psychology, 54*(5), 639–645.

Constantino, G., & Rivera, C. (1994). Culturally sensitive treatment modalities for Puerto Rican children, adolescents, and adults. In R. G. Malgady & O. Rodríguez (Eds.), *Theoretical and Conceptual Issues in Hispanic Mental Health.* Malabar, FL: Krieger.

Currier, R. L. (1966). The hot-cold syndrome and symbolic balance in Mexican and Spanish-American folk medicine. *Ethnology, 5,* 251–263.

Davis, M. P. (1990). *Mexican voices, American dreams: An oral history of Mexican immigration to the United States.* New York: Holt.

Day, A. (1992, April 19). The transposition novelist: Interview with Carlos Fuentes. *Los Angeles Times Magazine,* pp. 16–33.

de Anda, D., Becerra, R. M., & Fielder, E. (1988). Sexuality, pregnancy, and motherhood among Mexican-American adolescents. *Journal of Adolescent Research, 3*(3–4), 403–411.

De Hoyos, A., & De Hoyos, G. (1966). The amigo system and alienation of the wife in the conjugal Mexican family. In B. Farber (Ed.), *Kinship and family organization.* New York: Wiley.

De Hoyos, G., De Hoyos, A., & Anderson, C. B. (1986). Sociocultural dislocation: Beyond the dual perspective. *Social Work,* January–February, 61–67.

Del Castillo, A. R. (1991). *Mexico City ficheras: The moral culture of the 'mala' mujer.* Paper presented at the invited session of the Social and Biomedical Labels, American Anthropological Association, Chicago, IL.

Del Castillo, A. R. (1996). Gender and its discontinuties in male/female domestic relations: Mexicans in cross-cultural context. In D. Marciel & I. D. Ortiz (Eds.), *Chicanas/Chicanos at the crossroads: Social, economic and political change.* Tucson: University of Arizona Press.

Del Castillo, R. G. (1996). *La familia: Chicano families in the urban southwest, 1848 to the present.* Notre Dame, IN: University of Notre Dame Press.

Delgado, M. (1978). Folk medicine in Puerto Rican culture. *International Social Work, 21*(2), 46–54.

Delgado-Gaitán, C. (1988). Sociocultural adjustment to school and academic achievement. *Journal of Early Adolescence, 8*(1), 63–82.

Delgado-Gaitán, C., & Trueba, H. (1991). *Crossing cultural borders: Education for immigrant families in America.* London: Falmer.

DePalma, A. (1995, June 11). Racism? Mexico's in denial. *The New York Times.*

Díaz-Guerrero, R. (1975). *Psychology of the Mexican: Culture and personality.* Austin: University of Texas Press.

Dieterich, H. (1993, November 10). Madonna y el machismo. *La Jornada,* 27.

Dossey, L. (1993). *Healing words: The power of prayer and the practice of medicine.* San Francisco: Harper.

Dow, J. (1986). Universal aspects of symbolic healing. *American Anthropologist 18,* 58–59.

Dowd, J. J., & Bengtson, V. L. (1978). Aging in minority populations: An examination of the double jeopardy hypothesis. *Journal of Gerontology, 33,* 427–436.

Duany, L., & Pittman, K. (1990). *Latino youths at a crossroads.* Washington, DC: Examination Board.

Duvall, E. M. (1954). *In-laws: Pro and con.* New York: Association Press.

Eisler, R. M., & Skidmore, J. R. (1987). Masculine gender role stress: Scale development and component factors in the appraisal of stressful situations. *Behavior Modification, 11,* 123–136.

Elkaim, M. (1982). From the family approach to the sociopolitical approach. In F. W. Kaslow (Ed.), *The international handbook of family therapy.* New York: Brunner/Mazel.

Ellis, J. A. (1971). *Latin America: Its people and institutions.* New York: Bruce.

Erickson, G. D. (1975). The concept of personal network in clinical practice. *Family Process, 14*(4), 487–498.

Erickson, P. I. (1990). Combating school-age pregnancy among Latinas in Los Angeles County. In E. R. Forsyth & J. Solis (Eds.), *Recommendations for improving the delivery of human services to Latina immigrants and their children in Los Angeles County* (pp. 25–36). Claremont, CA: Tomás Rivera Center.

Escobar, J. I., & Canino, G. (1989). Unexplained physical complaints: Psychopathology and epidemiological correlates. *British Journal of Psychiatry, 154*(Suppl. 4), 24–27.

Escovar, P. L., & Lazarus, P. J. (1982). Cross-cultural child-rearing practices: Implications for school psychology. *School Psychology International, 3,* 143–148.

Esquivel, L. (1990). *Like water for chocolate.* New York: Avon Books.

Fairchild, H. H., & Cozens, J. A. (1981). Chicano, Hispanic, or Mexican American? What's in a name? *Hispanic Journal of Behavioral Sciences, 3*(2), 191–198.

Falicov, C. J. (1971). *Interpersonal perceptions during pregnancy and early motherhood.* Doctoral dissertation, Committee in Human Development, University of Chicago.

Falicov, C. J. (1982). Mexican families. In M. McGoldrick, J. K. Pearce, & J. Giordano (Eds.), *Ethnicity and family therapy.* New York: Guilford Press.

Falicov, C. J. (1983). Introduction. In C. J. Falicov (Ed.), *Cultural perspectives in family therapy.* Rockville, MD: Aspen.

Falicov, C. J. (1984). Commentary: Focus on stages. *Family Process, 23*(3), 329–334.

Falicov, C. J. (Ed.).(1988a). *Family transitions: Continuity and change over the life cycle.* New York: Guilford Press.

Falicov, C. J. (1988b). Learning to think culturally in family therapy training. In H. Liddle, D. Breunlin, & D. Schwartz (Eds.), *Handbook of family therapy training and supervision.* New York: Guilford Press.

Falicov, C. J. (1992). Love and gender in the Latino marriage. *American Family Therapy Association Newsletter, 48,* 30–36.

Falicov, C. J. (1993, Spring). Continuity and change: Lessons from immigrant families. *American Family Therapy Newsletter,* 30–34.

Falicov, C. J. (1995a). Cross-cultural marriages. In N. Jacobson & A. Gurman (Eds.), *Clinical handbook of couple therapy* (2nd ed., pp. 231–246). New York: Guilford Press.

Falicov, C. J. (1995b). Training to think culturally: A multidimensional comparative framework. *Family Process, 34,* 373–388.

Falicov, C. J. (1997). So they don't need me anymore: Weaving migration, illness and coping. In S. Daniel, J. Hepworth, & W. Doherty (Eds.), *Stories about medical family therapy.* New York: Basic Books.

Falicov, C. J. (1998). The cultural meaning of family triangles. In M. McGoldrick (Ed.), *Re-visioning family therapy: Race, culture, and gender in clinical practice.* New York: Guilford Press.

Falicov, C. (1998). The Latino family life cycle. In B. Carter & M. McGoldrick (Eds.), *The changing family life cycle* (3rd ed.). New York: Allyn & Bacon.

Falicov, C. J., & Brudner-White, L. (1983). The shifting family triangle: The issue of cultural and contextual relativity. In C. J. Falicov (Ed.), *Cultural perspectives in family therapy*. Rockville, MD: Aspen.

Falicov, C. J., & Falicov, Y. M. (1995, Spring). Proposition 187: What therapists can do. *AFTA Newsletter*, 51–54.

Falicov, C. J., & Karrer, B. (1980). Cultural variations in the family life cycle: The Mexican-American family. In E. Carter & M. McGoldrick (Eds.), *The family life cycle: A framework for family therapy*. New York: Gardner Press.

Falicov, C. J., & Karrer, B. (1984). Therapeutic strategies for Mexican American families. *International Journal of Family Therapy*, 6(1), 16–30.

Fanon, F. (1967). *Black skin, white masks*. New York: Grove.

Felice, M. E., Shragg, G. P., James, M., & Hollingsworth, D. R. (1987). Psychosocial aspects of Mexican-American, white, and black teenage pregnancy. *Journal of Adolescent Health Care*, 8, 330–335.

Fernández-Marina, R. (1961). The Puerto Rican syndrome: Its dynamics and cultural dterminants. *Psychiatry*, 24, 79–82.

Field, T., Widmeyer, S., Adler, S., & de Cubos, M. (1990). Teeenage parenting in different cultures, family constellations, and caregiving environments: Effects on infant development. *Infant Mental Health Journal*, 11(2), 158–174.

Fischer, M. M. (1988). Aestheticized emotions and critical hermeneutics. *Culture, Medicine and Psychiatry*, 12(1), 31–42.

Fiske, S. (1993). Controlling other people: The impact of power on stereotyping. *American Psychologist*, 48(6), 621–628.

Flores, J. (1992). Cited in Cortijo's revenge: New mappings of Puerto Rican culture. In S. Indice, J. France, & J. Flores (Eds.), *On edge: The crisis of contemporary Latin American culture*. Minneapolis: University of Minnesota Press.

Fortes de Leff, J., & Espejel, E. (1995). *Cultural myths and social relationships in Mexico: A context for therapy*. Paper presented at the 7th World Family Therapy Congress, "Family Therapy: Myths and Realities," Guadalajara, Mexico.

Foucault, M. (1973). *The order of things*. New York: Vintage Books.

Fowers, B. J., & Richardson, F. C. (1996). Why is multiculturalism good? *American Psychologist*, 51(6), 609–621.

Fracasso, M. P., Busch-Rossnagel, N. A., & Fisher, C. B. (1994). The relationship of maternal behavior and acculturation to the quality of attachment in Hispanic infants living in New York City. *Hispanic Journal of Behavioral Sciences*, 16, 143–154.

Friedan, B. (1996, June 3). Children's crusade: A gathering heralds a shift toward a new paradigm. *The New Yorker*, pp. 5–6.

Friedman, E. (1982). The myth of the shiksa. In M. McGoldrick, J. K. Pearce, & J. Giordano (Eds.), *Ethnicity and family therapy*. New York: Guilford Press.

Friedman, E. J. (1994). Sensitivity to contextual variables: A legitimate learning objective for all supervisors? *Supervision Bulletin*, VII(2) 4–7.

Frisbie, W. Parker. (1986). Variation in patterns of marital instability among Hispanics. *Journal of Marriage and the Family*, 48, 99–106.

Furnham, A., & Bochner, S. (1986). *Culture shock: Psychological reactions to unfamiliar environments*. London: Routledge & Kegan Paul.

Gafner, G., & Duckett, S. (1992). Treating the sequelae of a curse in elderly Mexican Americans. *Clinical Gerontologist*, 11(3–4), 145–153.

Gaines, S. O., Jr. Ríos, D., & Buriel, R. (1997). *Familism* and personal relationship processes among Latina/Latino couples. In S. O. Gaines, Jr. (Ed.), *Culture, ethnicity, and personal relationship processes*. New York: Routledge.

Gallegos, J. S. (1991). Culturally relevant services for Hispanic elderly. In M. Sotomayor (Ed.), *Empowering Hispanic families: A critical issue for the '90s.* Milwaukee, WI: Family Service America.

García, C. (1992). *Dreaming in Cuban.* New York: Random House.

García Canclini, N. (1995). *Hybrid cultures: Strategies for entering and leaving modernity.* Minneapolis: University of Minnesota Press.

García Márquez, G. (1988). *Love in the time of cholera.* New York: Knopf.

García Márquez, G. (1995). *One hundred years of solitude.* New York: Knopf.

García-Prieto, N. (1996). Puerto Rican families. In M. McGoldrick, J. Giordano, & J. K. Pearce (Eds.), *Ethnicity and family therapy* (2nd ed.). New York: Guilford Press.

Garza, R. T., & Ames, R. E. (1972). A comparison of Anglo and Mexican-American college students on locus of control. *Journal of Consulting and Clinical Psychology, 42,* 919–922.

Garza-Guerrero, A. C. (1974). Culture shock: It's mourning and the vicissitudes of identity. *Journal of American Psychoanalytic Association, 22,* 408–429.

Geertz, C. (1973). *The interpretation of cultures.* New York: Basic Books.

Geertz, C. (1995). *After the fact: Two countries, four decades, one anthropologist.* Cambridge, MA: Harvard University Press.

Gergen, K. (1982). *Toward transformation in social knowledge.* New York: Springer-Verlag.

Gergen, K. J., Gulerce, A., Lock, A., & Misra, G. (1996). Psychological science in cultural context. *American Psychologist, 51*(5), 496–503.

Gil, R. M., & Vázquez, C. I. (1996). *The Maria paradox.* New York: G. P. Putnam's Sons.

Gilmore, M., & Gilmore, D. (1979). *Machismo:* A psychodynamic approach (Spain). *Journal of Psychological Anthropology, 2,* 281–299.

Goldberg, M. M. (1941). A qualification of the marginal man theory. *American Sociological Review, 6,* 10–20.

Goldenthal, P. (1996). *Doing contextual therapy: An integrated model for working with individuals, couples, and families.* New York: Norton.

Goldner, V. (1985). Feminism and family therapy. *Family Process, 24,* 31–47.

González, R., Biever, J., & Gardner, G. (1994). The multicultural perspective in therapy: A social contructionist appoach. *Psychotherapy, 31,* 515–524.

González de Alba, L. (1994, January 17). Todos somos blancos. *La Jornade,* 28–29.

González-Ramos, G., Zayas, L. H., & Cohen, E. (1993). [Cultural beliefs in Puerto Rican childrearing.] Unpublished raw data, available from authors.

González-Wippler, M. (1996). *Santería: The religion.* St. Paul, MN: Llewellyn.

Grebler, L., Moore, J., & Guzmán, R. (1970). *The Mexican American people.* New York: Free Press.

Green, R. J., & Werner, P. D. (1996). Intrusiveness and closeness-caregiving: Rethinking the concept of family enmeshment. *Family Process, 35*(2), 115–134.

Greene, V. L., & Monahan, D. J. (1984). Comparative utilization of community-based long-term care services by Hispanic and Anglo elderly in a case management system. *Journal of Gerontology, 39,* 730–735.

Griffith, J. (1983). Relationship between acculturation and psychological impairment in adult Mexican American. *Hispanic Journal of Behavioral Sciences, 5*(4), 431–459.

Grinberg, L., & Grinberg, R. (1989). *Psychoanalytic perspectives on migration and exile.* New Haven: Yale University Press.

Gutiérrez, J., & Sameroff, A. (1990). Determinants of complexity in Mexican-American mother's conceptions of child development. *Child Development, 61,* 384–394.

Gutmann, M. C. (1996). *The meanings of macho: Being a man in Mexico City.* Berkeley: University of California Press.

Handel, G. (1967). *The psychosocial interior of the family*. Chicago: Aldine.

Haour-Knipe, M. (1989). International employment and children: Geographical mobility and mental health among children of professionals. *Social Science and Medicine, 28,* 197–205.

Haraway, D. (1991). *Simians, cyborgs, and women: The reinvention of nature.* New York: Routledge.

Hardy, K., & Laszloffy, T. (1994). Deconstructing race in family therapy. *Journal of Feminist Family Therapy, 5*(3/4), 5–33.

Hare-Mustin, R. C. (1978). A feminist approach to family therapy. *Family Process, 17,* 181–194.

Harrison, A. O., Wilson, M. N., Pine, C. J., Chan, S. Q., & Buriel, R. (1990). Family ecologies of ethnic minority children. *Child Development, 61,* 347–362.

Harwood, A. (1981). *Ethnicity and medical care.* Cambridge, MA: Harvard University Press.

Harwood, A. (1994). Acculturation in the postmodern world: Implications for mental health research. In R. G. Malgady & O. Rodriguez (Eds.), *Theoretical and conceptual issues in Hispanic mental health.* Malabar, FL: Krieger.

Harwood, R. L., Miller, J. G., & Irizarry, N. L. (1995). *Culture and attachment: Perceptions of the child in context.* New York: Guilford Press.

Hawkes, G. R., & Taylor, M. (1975). Power structure in Mexican and Mexican American farm labor families. *Journal of Marriage and the Family, 37,* 807–811.

Henry, J. (1963). *Pathways to madness.* New York: Vintage Books.

Horowitz, R. (1983). *Honor and the American dream: Culture and identity in a Chicano community.* New Brunswick, NJ: Rutgers University Press.

House, J. S. (1974). Occupational stress and coronary heart disease: A review. *Journal of Health and Social Behavior, 15,* 12–27.

Howard, G. S. (1991). Culture tales: A narrative approach to thinking, cross-cultural psychology and psychotherapy. *American Psychologist, 46*(3), 187–197.

Hurtado, A., & Gurin, P. (1995). Ethnic identity and bilingualism attitudes. In A. M. Padilla (Ed.), *Hispanic psychology: Critical issues in theory and research.* Thousand Oaks, CA: Sage.

Imber-Black, E. (1988). *Families and larger systems: A family therapist's guide through the labyrinth.* New York: Guilford Press.

Imber-Black, E., & Roberts, J. (1992). *Rituals for our times: Celebrating, healing, and changing our lives and our relationships.* New York: Harper Collins.

Inclán, J., & Ferrán, E. (1990). Poverty, politics, and family therapy: A role for systems theory. In M. Mirkin (Ed.), *The social and political context of family therapy.* New York: Gardner Press.

Inclán, J., & Hernández, M. (1993). Cross-cultural perspectives and codependence: The case of poor Hispanics. *American Journal of Orthopsychiatry, 62*(2), 245–255.

Inclán, J., & Herrón, G. (1989). Ecologically-oriented therapy with Puerto Rican adolescents. In J. Taylor Gibbs & L. Nahme Huang (Eds.), *Children of color: Psychological interventions with minority youth.* New York: Jossey-Bass.

Jackson, D. D. (1965). The study of the family. *Family Process, 4,* 1–20.

Johnston, R. (1976). The concept of the "marginal man": A refinement of the term. *Australian and New Zealand Journal of Science, 12,* 145–147.

Kay, M. A. (1980). Mexican American and Chicana childbirth. In M. Melville (Ed.), *Twice a minority* (pp. 52–65). St. Louis, MO: Mosby.

Kazak, A. E., McCannell, K., Adkins, E., Himmelberg, P., & Grace, J. (1989). Perception of normality in families: Four samples. *Journal of Family Psychology, 2*(3), 277–291.

Keefe, S. (1984). Real and ideal extended familism among Mexican Americans and Anglo Americans: On the meaning of "close" family ties. *Human Organization, 43,* 65–70.

Keefe, S. E., Padilla, A. M., & Carlos, M. L. (1978). The Mexican American family as an emotional support system. In J. M. Casas & S. E. Keefe (Eds.), *Family and mental health in the Mexican-American community* (Monograph No. 7). Los Angeles: University of Californa, Spanish Speaking Mental Health Center.

Kelly, P. F., & García, A. (1989). Power surrendered, power restored: The politics of home and work among Hispanic women in Southern California and southern Florida. In L. Tilly & P. Gurin (Eds.), *Women and politics in America.* New York: Russell Sage.

Kerchoff, A. C., & McCormick, T. C. (1955). Marginal status and marginal personality. *Social Forces, 34,* 48–55.

Kessen, W. (1979). The American child and other cultural inventions. *American Psychologist, 34,* 815–820.

Kluckhohn, F., & Strodtbeck, F. (1961). *Variations in value orientations.* Evanston, IL: Row, Peterson.

Komarovsky, M. (1967). *Blue collar marriage.* New York: Random House.

Korin, E. C. (1994). Social inequalities and therapeutic relationships: Applying Freire's ideas to clinical practice. *Journal of Feminist Family Therapy 5*(3/4), 75–98.

Kretch, D., & Crutchfield, R. (1948). *Theory and problems of social psychology.* New York: McGraw-Hill.

Kutsche, P. (1983). Household and family in Hispanic northern New Mexico. *Journal of Comparative Family Studies, 14,* 151–165.

LaFramboise, T., Coleman, H. L. K., & Gerton, J. (1993). Psychological impact of biculturalism: Evidence and theory. *Psychological Bulletin, 114*(3), 395–412.

LaFramboise, T. D., & Rowe, W. (1983). Skills training for bicultural competence: Rationale and application. *Journal of Counseling Psychology, 30,* 589–595.

Lambert, W. E. (1977) The effects of bilingualism in the individual. In P. W. Hornby (Ed.), *Bilingualism: Psychological, social and educational implications* (pp. 15–27). San Diego, CA: Academic Press.

Lamphere, L. (1974). Strategies, cooperation, and conflict among women in domestic groups. In M. Zimbalist Rosaldo & L. Lamphere (Eds.), *Women, culture, and society.* Palo Alto, CA: Stanford University Press.

Landau-Stanton, J. (1990). Issues and methods of treatment for families in cultural transition. In M. P. Mirkin (Ed.), *The social and political contexts of family therapy.* Boston: Allyn & Bacon.

Lappin, J. (1983). On becoming a culturally conscious family therapist. In C. J. Falicov (Ed.), *Cultural perspectives in family therapy.* Rockville, MD: Aspen.

Lechner, N. (1992). Some people die of fear: Fear as a political problem. In J. E. Corradi, P. W. Fagen, & M. Garretón (Eds.), *Fear at the edge: State terror and resistance in Latin America* (pp. 26–35). Berkeley: University of California Press.

Levine, E. S., & Padilla, A. M. (1980). *Crossing cultures in therapy: Pluralistic counseling for the Hispanic.* Belmont, CA: Wadsworth.

Lewis, K. G. (1988). Sibling therapy with multiproblem families. *Journal of Marital and Family Therapy, 12*(3), 291–300.

Lomnitz, L. A. (1996). *A comparative study of political cultures in Mexico and Chile: An anthropological approach.* Research Seminar on Mexico and U.S.-Mexican Relations, University of California, San Diego, CA.

Lomnitz, L. A., & Pérez-Lizaur, M. (1987). *A Mexican elite family: 1820–1980.* Princeton, NJ: Princeton University Press.

Luepnitz, D. A. (1988). *The family interpreted: Psychoanalysis, feminism, and family therapy.* New York: Basic Books.

Madsen, W. (1964). *The Mexican Americans of South Texas.* New York: Holt, Rinehart & Winston.

Mahard, R. (1989). Elderly Puerto Rican women in the continental United States. In C. García Coll & L. Mattei (Eds.), *The psychosocial development of Puerto Rican women.* New York: Praeger.

Malgady, R. G., Rogler, L. H., & Constantino, G. (1990a). Culturally sensitive psychotherapy for Puerto Rican children and adolescents: A program of treatment outcome research. *Journal of Consulting and Clinical Psychology, 58,* 704–712.

Malgady, R. G., Rogler, L. H., & Constantino, G. (1990b). Hero/heroine modeling for Puerto Rican adolescents: A preventive mental health intervention. *Journal of Consulting and Clinical Psychology, 58,* 469–474.

Marcus, G. E., & Fischer, M. M. J. (1986). *Anthropology as cultural critique: An experimental moment in the human sciences.* Chicago: University of Chicago Press.

Marín, G., & Marín, B. V. (1991). *Research with Hispanic populations.* Newbury Park, CA: Sage.

Marris, P. (1980) The uprooting of meaning. In G. V. Coelho & P. I. Ahmed (Eds.), *Uprooting and development: Dilemmas of coping with modernization* (pp. 101–116). New York: Plenum Press.

Martínez, E. (1997). Unite and overcome. *Teaching Tolerance 6*(1), 11–15.

Martínez, K. J. (1994). Cultural sensitivity gone awry. *Hispanic Journal of Behavioral Sciences, 16*(1), 75–89.

Martínez, K. J., & Váldez, D. M. (1992). Cultural considerations in play therapy with Hispanic children. In L. Vargas & J. D. Koos (Eds.), *Psychotherapeutic interventions with ethnic minorities, children and adolescents.* San Francisco: Jossey-Bass.

Martínez, R., & Wetli, C. V. (1982). *Santería:* A magico-religious system of Afro-Cuban origin. *American Journal of Social Psychiatry, 2*(3), 32–38.

Maslow, A., & Díaz-Guerrero, R. (1960). Delinquency as a value disturbance. In J. Peatman and E. Hartley (Eds.), *Festschrift for Gardner Murphy.* New York: Harper & Bros.

Massey, D. S., & Denton, N. A. (1993). *American apartheid: Segregation and the making of the underclass.* Cambridge, MA: Harvard University Press.

Massing, M. (1996, February 1). Crime and drugs: The new myths. *The New York Review of Books,* pp. 16–20.

Maturana, H. (1991). Preface. In R. Eisler, *El Cáliz y la Espada: Nuestro Historia, Nuestro Futuro.* San Francisco: Harper & Row.

McClure, E. (1977). Aspects of code-switching in the discourse of bilingual Mexican-American children. In M. Saville-Troike (Ed.), *Linguistics and anthropology* (pp. 93–115). Washington, DC: Georgetown University Press.

McGoldrick, M., Anderson, C., & Walsh, F. (1989). *Women in families: A framework for family therapy.* New York: Basic Books.

McGoldrick, M., Giordano, J., & Pearce, J. K. (Eds.). (1996). *Ethnicity and family therapy* (2nd ed.). New York: Guilford Press.

McGoldrick, M., Pearce, J., & Giordano, J. (Eds.). (1982). *Ethnicity and family therapy.* New York: Guilford Press.

McKay, M., & Fanning, P. (1991). *Prisoners of beliefs: Exposing and changing beliefs that control your life.* Oakland, CA: New Harbinger.

Merkides, K. S., Boldt, J. S., & Ray, L. A. (1986). Sources of helping an intergenerational solidarity: A three-generations study of Mexican Americans. *Journal of Gerontology, 41,* 506–511.

Mindel, C. H. (1980). Extended families among urban Mexican Americans, Anglos, and Blacks. *Hispanic Journal of Behavioral Sciences, 2*(7), 21–34.

Minuchin, S., Montalvo, B., Guerney, B., Rosman, B., & Schumer, F. (1967). *Families of the slums: An exploration of their structure and treatment.* New York: Basic Books.

Miranda, M. R. (1991). Mental health services and the Hispanic elderly. In M. Sotomayor (Ed.), *Empowering Hispanic families: A critical issue for the '90s.* Milwaukee, WI: Family Service America.

Mirandé, A. (1985). *The Chicano experience: An alternative perspective.* Notre Dame, IN: University of Notre Dame Press.

Mirandé, A. (1988). Chicano fathers: Traditional perceptions and current realities. In P. Bronstein & C. P. Cowan (Eds.), *Fatherhood today: Men's changing role in the family* (pp. 93–106). New York: Wiley.

Mirandé, A. (1988). *Que gacho ser macho:* It's a drag to be a macho man. *Aztlán, 17,* 63–69.

Moll, L. C., Rueda, R. S., Reza, R., Herrera, J., & Vásquez, L. P. (1976). Mental health services in East Los Angeles: An urban community case study. In M. R. Miranda (Ed.), *Psychotherapy with the Spanish speaking: Issues in research and service delivery* (Monograph No. 3, pp. 52–65). Los Angeles: University of California, Spanish Speaking Mental Health Research Center.

Montalvo, B. (1994). Editorial: A conversation about diversity. *Supervision Bulletin, II*(1), 2–7.

Montalvo, B., & Gutiérrez, M. (1983). A perspective for the use of the cultural dimension in family therapy. In C. J. Falicov (Ed.), *Cultural perspectives in family therapy* (pp. 15–30). Rockville, MD: Aspen.

Montalvo, B., & Gutiérrez, M. (1988). The emphasis on cultural identity: A developmental-ecological constraint (pp. 181–210). In C. J. Falicov (Ed.), *Family transitions: Continuity and change over the life cycle.* New York: Guilford Press.

Montalvo, B., & Gutiérrez, M. (1989). Nine assumptions for work with ethnic minority families. In G. W. Saba, B. M. Karrer, & K. V. Hardy (Eds.), *Minorites and family therapy.* New York: Haworth Press.

Moore, J., & Pachon, H. (1985). *Hispanics in the United States.* Englewood Cliffs, NJ: Prentice-Hall.

Mull, J. D., & Mull, D. S. (1983). Cross cultural medicine: A visit with a curandero. *The Western Journal of Medicine, 139*(5), 728–736.

Murguia, E. (1982). *Chicano intermarriage: A theoretical and empirical study.* San Antonio, TX: Trinity University Press.

Mydans, S. (1995, September 11). Hispanic gang members keep strong family ties. *The New York Times,* pp. 1, 8.

National Opinion Research Center. (1989, January 8). Study points to increase in tolerance of ethnicity. *The New York Times,* p. 24.

Navarro, E. M., & Carrillo, E. (1997). *Delivery of public mental health services to the Latino population: An inpatient and community based model.* Presentation at the Third Annual conference of the Latino Behavioral Health Institute, Los Angeles, CA.

Nichols, M. (1991). *No place to hide: Facing shame so we can find self-respect.* New York: Simon & Schuster.

Nichols, M. P., & Schwartz, R. C. (1995). *Family therapy: Concepts and methods* (2nd ed.). Boston: Allyn & Bacon.

Novas, H. (1994). *Everything you need to know about Latino history.* New York: Penguin.

Ogbu, J. (1987). Variability in minority school performance: A problem in search of an explanation. *Anthropology and Education Quarterly, 18*(4), 312–334.

Ogbu, J. U., & Matute-Bianchi, M. A. (1986). Understanding sociocultural factors: Knowledge, identity, and social adjustment. In California State Department of Education, Bilingual Education Office, *Beyond language: Social and cultural factors in schooling* (pp. 73–142). Sacramento: California State University, Los Angeles, Evaluation, Dissemination and Assessment Center.

Okagaki, L., & Sternberg, R. J. (1993). Parental beliefs and children's school performance. *Child Development, 64,* 36–56.

Ortiz, V. (1995). The diversity of Latino families. In R. E. Zambrana (Ed.), *Understanding Latino families: Scholarship, policy, and practice.* Thousand Oaks, CA: Sage.

Ortiz, V., & Arce, C. H. (1984). Language orientation and mental health status among persons of Mexican descent. *Hispanic Journal of Behavioral Sciences 6*(2), 127–143.

Ortiz-Colón, R. (1985). *Acculturation, ethnicity and education: A comparison of Anglo teachers' and Puerto Rican mothers' values regarding behaviors and skills.* Unpublished doctoral dissertation, Harvard University.

Padilla, A. M. (1980). The role of cultural awareness and ethnic loyalty in acculturation. In A. M. Padilla (Ed.), *Acculturation: Theory, models and some new findings* (pp. 47–84). Boulder, CO: Westview Press.

Padilla, A. M. (1994). Bicultural development: A theoretical and empirical examination. In R. G. Malgady & O. Rodriguez (Eds.), *Theoretical and conceptual issues in Hispanic mental health.* Malabar, FL: Krieger.

Padilla, A. M., Ruíz, R. A., & Alvarez, R. (1976). Community mental health services for the Spanish speaking/surnamed population. *American Psychologist, 30,* 892–905.

Papajohn, J., & Spiegel, J. (1975). *Transactions in families.* San Francisco: Jossey-Bass.

Paredes, A. (1993). *Folklore and culture on the Texas-Mexican border.* Austin, TX: Center for Mexican American Studies, University of Texas at Austin.

Park, R.E. (1928). Human migration and the marginal man. *American Journal of Sociology, 5,* 881–893.

Parker, P. (1990). For the white person who wants to know how to be my friend. In G. Anzaldúa (Ed.), *Making faces, making soul: Haciendo caras.* San Francisco: An Aunt Lute Foundation Book.

Pathey-Chávez, G. (1993). High school as an arena for cultural conflict and acculturation for Latino Angelinos. *Anthropology and Education Quarterly, 24*(1), 33–60.

Paz, O. (1961). *The labyrinth of solitude: Life and thought in Mexico.* New York: Evergreen Books.

Peñalosa, F. (1968). Mexican family roles. *Journal of Marriage and the Family, 30,* 680–689.

Penn, P. (1985). Feed-forward: Future questions, future maps. *Family Process, 24,* 289–310.

Pérez, M., & Andrés, I. (1977). Spiritualism as an adaptive mechanism among Puerto Ricans in the United States. *Cornell Journal of Social Relations, 12*(2), 125–136.

Phinney, J. S. (1990). Ethnic identity in adolescents and adults: Review of research. *Psychological Bulletin, 108*(3), 499–514.

Phinney, J. S. (1995). Ethnic identity and self-esteem: A review and integration. In A. M. Padilla (Ed.), *Hispanic psychology: Critical issues in theory and research.* Thousand Oaks, CA: Sage.

Phinney, J. S., Lockner, B., & Murphy, R. (1990). Ethnic identity and psychological adjustment. In A. Stiffman & L. Davis (Eds.), *Ethnic issues in adolescent mental health* (pp. 53–72). Newbury Park, CA: Sage.

Pierce, C. (1970). Offensive mechanisms. In F. Barbour (Ed.), *The black seventies.* Boston: Sargent.

Pinderhughes, E. (1989). *Understanding race, ethnicity, and power: The key to efficacy in clinical practice.* New York: Free Press.

Portes, A., & Bach, R. L. (1985). *Latin journey: Cuban and Mexican immigrants in the United States.* Berkeley: University of California Press.

Portes A., & Rumbaut, R. G. (1990a). A foreign world: Immigration, mental health, and acculturation. In *Immigrant America: A portrait* (pp. 143–179). Berkeley: University of California Press.

Portes, A., & Rumbaut, R. G. (1990b). *Immigrant America: A portrait.* Berkeley: University of California Press.

Powell, D. R. (1995a). *Parent education and support programs: The state of the field.* Chicago: Family Resource Coalition.

Powell, D. R. (1995b). Including Latino fathers in parent education and support programs: Development of a program model. In R. E. Zambrana (Ed.), *Understanding Latino families.* Thousand Oaks, CA: Sage.

Powell, D. R., Zambrana, R., & Silva-Palacios, V. (1990). Designing culturally responsive parent programs: A comparison of Mexican and Mexican American mothers' program preferences. *Family Relations, 39,* 298–304.

Prilleltensky, I. (1990). Enhancing the social ethics of psychology: Toward a psychology in the service of social change. *Canadian Psychology 31*(4), 310–319.

Prilleltensky, I. (1994). Psychology and social ethics. *American Psychologist, 49,* 966–967.

Prilleltensky, I. (1997). Community psychology: Reclaiming social justice. In D. Fox & I. Prilleltensky (Eds.), *Critical psychology: An introduction* (pp. 166–184). London: Sage.

Rabkin, J., & Struening, E. L. (1976). *Ethnicity, social class and mental illness* (Paper Series no. 17). New York: Institute of Pluralism and Group Identity.

Ramírez, M. III. (1984). Assessing and understanding biculturalism: Multiculturalism in Mexican-American adults. In J. F. Martínez & R. H. Mendoza (Eds.), *Chicano psychology* (pp. 77–94). San Diego, CA: Academic Press.

Ramírez, O., & Arce, C. H. (1981). The contemporary Chicano family: An empirically based review. In A. Baron Jr. (Ed.), *Explorations in Chicano psychology* (pp. 3–28). New York: Praeger.

Ramírez, R. (1979). A bridge rather than a barrier to family and marital counseling. In P. P. Martin (Ed.), *La frontera perspective* (pp. 61–62). Tucson, AZ: La Frontera Center.

Ramírez, S. (1977). *El Mejicano, psicología de sus motivaciones.* Mexico D. F.: Editorial Grijalbo.

Ramos-McKay, J., Comas-Díaz, L., & Rivera, L. (1988). Puerto Ricans. In L. Comas-Díaz & E. H. Griffith (Eds.), *Clinical guidelines in cross cultural mental health* (pp. 204–232). New York: Wiley.

Rashid, H. M. (1984). Promoting biculturalism in young African-American children. *Young Children, 39,* 13–23.

Riding, A. (1989). *Distant neighbors.* New York: Vintage Books.

Rivera, E. (1982). First communion. In H. Augenbraum & I. Stavans (Eds.), *Growing up Latino: Memoirs and stories.* Boston: Houghton Mifflin.

Rivera, T. (1987). . . . *Y no se lo tragó la tierra: And the earth did not devour him.* Houston: Arte Público Press.

Rodríguez, G. (1994). The AVANCE family support and education program: Strengthening families in the pre-school years. In J. Szapocznik (Ed.), *A Hispanic/Latino family approach to substance abuse prevention* (Center for Substance Abuse Prevention Cultural Competence Series No. 2, pp. 155–170). Rockville, MD: National Clearinghouse for Alcohol and Drug Information.

Rodríguez, L. (1993). *Always running.* New York: Simon & Schuster.

Rodríguez, L. (1996). Forgive me mother for my crazy life. In A. Castillo (Ed.), *Goddess of the Americas, la diosa de las Américas: Writings on the Virgin of Guadalupe.* New York: Riverhead Books.

Rodríguez, O. (1987). *Hispanics and human services: Help-seeking in the inner city* (Monograph No. 14). Bronx: Hispanic Research Center, Fordham University.

Rodríguez, R. (1989). *Hunger of memory: The education of Richard Rodríguez.* New York: Bantam.

Rodríguez, R. (1992). *Days of obligation: An argument with my Mexican father.* New York: Viking.

Rogers, C., & Leichter, H. (1964). Laterality and conflict in kinship ties. In W. Goode (Ed.), *Readings on the family and society.* Englewood Cliffs, NJ: Prentice-Hall.

Rogler, L., Barreras, O., & Cooney, R. (1981). Coping with distrust in a study of intergenerational Puerto Rican families in New York City. *Hispanic Journal of Behavioral Sciences, 3*(1), 1–17.

Rogler, L. H., Cortés D. E., & Malgady, R. G. (1991). Acculturation and mental health status among Hispanics. *American Psychologist, 46*(6), 585–597.

Rogler, L. H., Malgady, R. G., Constantino, G., & Blumenthal, R. (1987). What does culturally sensitive mental health services mean? The case of Hispanics. *American Psychologist, 47,* 565–570.

Roland, A. (1988). *In search of self in India and Japan: Toward a cross-cultural psychology.* Princeton, NJ: Princeton University Press.

Roland, A. (1994). Identity, self, and individualism in a multicultural perspective. In E. P. Salett & D. R. Koslow (Eds.), *Race, ethnicity, and self.* Washington, DC: NMCI Publications.

Rosaldo, R. (1989). *Culture and truth: The remaking of social analysis.* Boston: Beacon Press.

Ross, C. E., Mirowsky, J., and Cockerham, W. C. (1983). Social class, Mexican culture and fatalism: Their effects on psychological distress. *American Journal of Community Psychology, 11,* 383–399.

Rotter, J. B. (1966). Generalized expectancies for internal versus external control of reinforcement. *Psychological Monographs, 80*(1, Whole No. 609).

Rouse, R. (1992). Making sense of settlement: Class transformation, cultural struggle, and transnationalism among Mexican migrants in the United States. In N. G. Schiller, L. Basch, & C. Blanc-Szanton (Eds.), *Towards a transnational perspective on migration.* New York: New York Academy of Sciences.

Rueschenberg, E., & Buriel, R. (1989). Mexican American family functioning and acculturation: A family systems perspective. *Hispanic Journal of Behavioral Sciences, 11*(3), 232–244.

Rumbaut, R. G., Chávez, L. R., Moser, R. J., Pickwell, S. M., & Wishik, S. M. (1988). The politics of migrant health care: A comparative study of Mexican immigrants and Indochinese refugees. *Research in the Sociology of Health Care, 7,* 143–202.

Rumbaut, R. G., & Cornelius, W. A. (Eds.). (1995). *California's immigrant children: Theory, research and implications for educational policy.* San Diego: Center for U.S.-Mexican Studies, University of California.

Saba, G. W., Karrer, B. M., & Hardy, K. V. (1989). *Minorities and family therapy.* New York: Haworth Press.

Sampson, E. E. (1993). Identity politics: Challenges to psychology's understanding. *American Psychologist, 48* (12), 1219–1230.

Sandoval, M. (1977). *Santería:* Afro-Cuban concepts of disease and its treatment in Miami. *Journal of Operational Psychiatry, 8,* 52–63.

Santiago, E. (1993). *When I was Puerto Rican.* New York: Addison-Wesley.

Santiago, M. (1994). *A Puerto Rican view of death and dying.* Presentation at quadrennial meeting of *Family Process Journal,* San Juan, Puerto Rico.

Scheffler, L. (1983). *Magia y brujería en México.* Mexico, D. F.: Panorama Editorial.

Schiller, N. G., Basch, L., & Blanc-Szanton, C. (Eds.). (1992). *Towards a transnational perspective on migration: Race, class, ethnicity, and nationlism reconsidered.* New York: New York Academy of Sciences.

Schwartzman, J. (1983). Family ethnography: A tool for clinicians. In C. J. Falicov (Ed.), *Cultural perpectives in family therapy.* Rockville, MD: Aspen.

Seltzer, W. (1995). *Cultural narratives and child psychotherapy.* Presentation at University of San Diego, Marriage and Family Therapy program.

Seltzer, W. J., & Seltzer, M. R. (1983). Material, myth and magic: A cultural approach to family therapy. *Family Process, 22,* 3–4.

Selvini Palazzoli, M., Boscolo, L., Cecchin, G., & Prata, G. (1978). A ritualized prescription in family therapy: Odd days and even days. *Journal of Marriage and Family Counseling, 4,* 3–9.

Shapiro, E. R. (1994). *Grief as a family process: A developmental apporach to clinical practice.* New York: Guilford Press.

Shapiro, E. R. (1995). Family development in cultural context: Implications for prevention and early intervention with Latino families. New England Journal of *Public Policy, 14*(3), 235–144.

Shorris, E. (1992). *Latinos: A biography of the people.* New York: Norton.

Shuval, J. T. (1982). Migration and stress. In L. Goldberger & S. Breznitz (Eds.), *Handbook of stress: Theoretical and clinical aspects* (2nd ed., pp. 641–657). New York: Free Press.

Simmen, E. (1972). *Pain and promise: The Chicano today.* New York: New American Library.

Simpson, G., & Yinger, J. M. (1958). *Racial and cultural minorities.* New York: Harper & Bros.

Sluzki, C. (1979). Migration and family conflict. *Family Process, 18*(4), 379–390.

Sluzki, C. (1982). The Latin lover revisited. In M. McGoldrick, J. K. Pearce, & J. Giordano (Eds.), *Ethnicity and family therapy* (pp. 492–498). New York: Guilford Press.

Sluzki, C. (1983). The sounds of silence. In C. J. Falicov (Ed.), *Cultural perspectives in family therapy* (pp. 68–77). Rockville, MD: Aspen.

Sluzki, C. E. (1989). Network disruption and network reconstruction in the process of migration/relocation. *The Berkshire Medical Center Department of Psychiatry Bulletin, 2*(3), 2–4.

Solís, J. (1995). The status of Latino children and youth: Challenges and prospects. In R. E. Zambrana (Ed.), *Understanding Latino families: Scholarship, policy, and practice.* Thousand Oaks, CA: Sage.

Soto, E., & Shaver, P. (1982). Sex-role traditionalism, assertiveness, and symptoms of Puerto Rican women living in the United States. *Hispanic Journal of Behavioral Sciences, 4*(1), 1–19.

Spiegel, J. (1971). *Transactions: The interplay between individual, family, and society.* New York: Science House.

Steinberg, L., Dornbusch, S. M., & Brown, B. B. (1992). Ethnic differences in adolescent achievement. *American Psychologist 47*(6), 723–729.

Stonequist, E. V. (1935). The problem of marginal man. *American Journal of Sociology, 7,* 1–12.

Suárez-Orozco, C. (1993). *Generational discontinuities: A cross-cultural comparison of Mexican, Mexican immigrant, Mexican American and white non-Hispanic adolescents.* PhD dissertation, California School of Professional Psychology.

Suárez-Orozco, C., & Suárez-Orozco, M. (1994). The cultural psychology of Hispanic immigrants. In T. Weaver (Ed.), *The handbook of Hispanic cultures in the United States.* Houston: Arte Publico Press.

Suárez-Orozco, M. M., & Suárez-Orozco, C. E. (1995). The cultural patterning of achievement-motivation: A comparison of Mexican, Mexican immigrant, Mexican-American and non-Latino white American students. In R. Rumbaut & W. Cornelius (Eds.), *California's immigrant children*. San Diego: Center for U.S.-Mexican Studies, University of California.

Suárez-Orozco, M., & Dundes, A. (1984). The *piropo* and the dual image of women in the Spanish-speaking world. *Journal of Latin American Lore, 10*(1), 111–133.

Sue, D. W., & Sue, D. (1990). *Counseling the culturally different: Theory and practice*. New York: Wiley.

Szapocznik, J., & Kurtines, W. (1980). Acculturation, biculturalism, and adjustment among Cuban Americans. In A. M. Padilla (Ed.), *Acculturation: Theory, models and some new findings*. Washington, DC: American Association for the Advancement of Science.

Szapocznik, J., Santisteban, D., Kurtines, W., Perez-Vidal, A., & Hervis, O. (1984). Bicultural effectiveness training: A treatment intervention for enhancing intercultural adjustment in Cuban American families. *Hispanic Journal of Behavioral Sciences, 6*(4), 317–344.

Szapocznik, J., Santisteban, D., Rio, A., Perez-Vidal, A., & Kurtines, W. M. (1986). Family effectiveness training (FET) for Hispanic families. In H. P. Lefley and P. B. Pedersen (Eds.), *Cross-cultural training for mental health professionals*. Springfield, IL: Charles C. Thomas.

Takaki, R. (1994). *A different mirror*. San Francisco: University of California.

Tannen, D. (1990). *You just don't understand: Women and men in conversation*. New York: Ballantine Books.

Taylor, C., & Gutmann, A. (Eds.). (1994). *Multiculturalism: Examining the politics of recognition*. Princeton, NJ: Princeton University Press.

Terry, L. L., & Domokos-Cheng Ham, M. (1994). *Cultural awareness-responsiveness-advocacy in marriage and family programs*. Paper presented to the annual conference of the American Association for Marriage and Family Therapy, Chicago, IL.

Thomas, P. (1967). *Down these mean streets*. New York: New American Library.

Tomm, K., Suzuki, K., & Suzuki, K. (1990). The Ka-No-Mushi: An inner externalization that enables compromise? *Australian and New Zealand Journal of Family Therapy, 11*(2), 104–107.

Trueba, H. T. (1989). *Raising silent voices: Educating linguistic minorites for the 21st century*. Cambridge, MA: Newbury House.

Trueba, H. T., Rodríguez, Y. Z., & Cintrón, J. (1993). *Healing multicultural America: Mexican immigrants rise to power in rural California*. London: Falmer.

Tseng, W., & McDermott, J. F. Jr. (1981). *Culture mind and therapy: An introduction to cultural psychiatry*. New York: Brunner/Mazel.

Turner, J. E. (1991). Migrants and their therapists: A trans-context approach. *Family Process, 30*, 407–419.

U.S. Bureau of the Census. (1991). *Statistical abstract*. Washington, DC: U.S. Government Printing Office.

Vásquez, M. J. T., & González, A. M. (1981). Sex roles among Chicanos: Stereotypes, challenges, and changes. In A. Barón Jr. (Ed.), *Explorations in Chicano psychology*. New York: Praeger.

Vega, W. A. (1990). Hispanic families in the 1980s: A decade of research. *Journal of Marriage and the Family, 52*, 1015–1024.

Vega, W. A., Kolody, B., & Valle, R. (1988). Marital strain, coping and depression among Mexican American women. *Journal of Marriage and the Family, 50*, 391–403.

Vega, W. A., Kolody, B., Valle, R., & Weir, J. (1991). Social networks, social support, and their relationship to depression among immigrant Mexican women. *Human Organization, 50,* 154–162.

Vélez, C. N., & Ungemack, J. A. (1989). Drug use among Puerto Rican youth: An exploration of generational status differences. *Social Science and Medicine, 29*(6), 779–789.

Vélez, W. (1989). High school attrition among Hispanic and non-Hispanic white youths. *Sociology of Education, 62,* 119–133.

Vigil, J. D. (1988). *Barrio gangs: Street life and identity in Southern California.* Austin: University of Texas Press.

Villareal, J. A. (1970). *Pocho.* Garden City, NY: Doubleday.

Von Bertalanffy, L. (1968). *General systems theory.* New York: George Braziller.

Wagner, R. M. (1988). Changes in extended family relationships for Mexican Americans and Anglo single mothers. In C. A. Everett (Ed.), *Minority and ethnic issues in the divorce process.* New York: Hawthorn Press.

Waldegrave, C. (1990). Social justice and family therapy. *Dulwich Centre Newsletter, 1,* 15–20.

Walsh, F. (1983). Normal family ideologies: Myths and realities. In C. J. Falicov (Ed.), *Cultural perspectives in family therapy.* Rockville, MD: Aspen.

Walsh, F. (in press). *Strengthening family resilience.* New York: Guilford Press.

Walters, M., Carter, B., Papp, P., & Silverstein, O. (1988). *The invisible web: Gender patterns in family relationships.* New York: Guilford Press.

Warheit, G., Vega, W., Auth, J., & Meinhardt, K. (1985). Mexican-American immigration and mental health: A comparative analysis of psychosocial stresss and dysfunction. In W. Vega & M. Miranda (Eds.), *Stress and Hispanic mental health* (pp. 76–109). Rockville, MD: National Institute of Mental Health.

Weingarten, K. (1995). Radical listening: Challenging cultural beliefs for and about mothers. *Journal of Feminist Family Therapy, 7*(1/2), 7–22.

Wells, K. B., Hough, R. L., Golding, J. M., Burnam, M. A., & Karno, M. (1987). Which Mexican-Americans underutilize health services? *American Journal of Psychiatry, 144*(7), 918–922.

Werner, E. (1990). Protective factors and individual resilience. In S. Meisels & J. Shonkoff (Eds.), *Handbook of early childhood intervention* (pp. 97–115). Cambridge, England: Cambridge University Press.

West, C. (1993). *Race matters.* New York: Routledge.

Westermeyer, J. (1989). *Psychiatric care of migrants: A clinical guide.* Washington, DC: American Psychiatric Press.

White, M. (1989). The externalizing of the problem and the reauthoring of lives and relationships. In M. White (Ed.), *Selected papers* (pp. 5–28). Adelaide, Australia: Dulwich Centre Publications.

White, M. (1993). Deconstruction and therapy. In S. Gilligan & R. Price (Eds.), *Therapeutic conversations.* New York: Norton.

Williams, C. L., & Berry, J. W. (1991). Primary prevention of acculturative stress among refugees: Application of psychological theory and practice. *American Psychologist, 46,* 632–641.

Williamson, D. (1981). Termination of the intergenerational hierarchical boundary between the first and second generations: A new stage in the family. *Journal of Marital and Family Therapy, 7*(4), 441–452.

World Health Organization. (1979). Psychological factors and health. In P. I. Ahmed & G. V. Coelho (Eds.), *Toward a new definition of health* (pp. 87–111). New York: Plenum.

Wrenn, C. G. (1962). The culturally encapsulated counselor. *Harvard Educational Review, 32*, 444–449.

Wright Mills, C. (1959). *The sociological imagination.* London: Oxford University Press.

Wright, L. M., Watson, W. L., & Bell, J. M. (1996). *Beliefs: The heart of healing in families and illness.* New York: Basic Books.

Ybarra, L. (1982). Marital decision making and the role of machismo in the Chicano family. *De Colores, 6*, 32–47.

Young, I. M. (1990). *Justice and the politics of difference.* Princeton, NJ: Princeton University Press.

Zamichow, N. (1992, February 10). No way to escape the fear: Stress disorder grips women immigrants. *Los Angeles Times*, San Diego Edition, pp. B2–B4.

Zavala-Martínez, I. (1988). *En la lucha:* The economic and socioemotional struggles of Puerto Rican women. *Women and Therapy, 6*, 13–24.

Zavala-Martínez, I. (1994). *Quién soy?* Who am I? Identity issues for Puerto Rican adolescents. In E. P. Salett & D. R. Koslow (Eds.), *Race, ethnicity, and self: Identity in multicultural perspective.* Washington, DC: National Multicultural Institute.

Zayas, L. H. (1994). Hispanic family ecology and early childhood socialization: Health care implications. *Family Systems Medicine, 12*(3), 315–325.

Zimmerman, J. (1991). Crossing the desert alone: An etiological model of female adolescent suicidality. In C. Gilligan, A. Rogers, & D. Thomas (Eds.), *Women, girls and psychotherapy: Reframing resistance* (pp. 223–240). Binghamton, NY: Harrington Park Press.

Ziv, T. A., & Lo, B. L. (1995). Denial of care to illegal immigrants: Proposition 187 in California. *New England Journal of Medicine, 332*(16), 1095–1098.

# Index